Contemporary Management of

Myeloproliferative Neoplasms

Contemporary Management of

Myeloproliferative Neoplasms

Editors

Brady L Stein MD MHS
Assistant Professor, Department of Medicine
Northwestern University Feinberg School of Medicine
Chicago, Illinois, USA

Brandon J McMahon MD
Associate Professor, Department of Medicine
Northwestern University Feinberg School of Medicine
Chicago, Illinois, USA

JAYPEE *The Health Sciences Publishers*

New Delhi | London | Philadelphia | Panama

Jaypee Brothers Medical Publishers (P) Ltd

Headquarters

Jaypee Brothers Medical Publishers (P) Ltd
4838/24, Ansari Road, Daryaganj
New Delhi 110 002, India
Phone: +91-11-43574357
Fax: +91-11-43574314
Email: jaypee@jaypeebrothers.com

Overseas Offices

J.P. Medical Ltd
83 Victoria Street, London
SW1H 0HW (UK)
Phone: +44 20 3170 8910
Fax: +44 (0)20 3008 6180
Email: info@jpmedpub.com

Jaypee-Highlights Medical Publishers Inc
City of Knowledge, Bld. 237, Clayton
Panama City, Panama
Phone: +1 507-301-0496
Fax: +1 507-301-0499
Email: cservice@jphmedical.com

Jaypee Medical Inc
The Bourse
111 South Independence Mall East
Suite 835, Philadelphia, PA 19106, USA
Phone: +1 267-519-9789
Email: jpmed.us@gmail.com

Jaypee Brothers Medical Publishers (P) Ltd
17/1-B Babar Road, Block-B, Shaymali
Mohammadpur, Dhaka-1207
Bangladesh
Mobile: +08801912003485
Email: jaypeedhaka@gmail.com

Jaypee Brothers Medical Publishers (P) Ltd
Bhotahity, Kathmandu, Nepal
Phone: +977-9741283608
Email: kathmandu@jaypeebrothers.com

Website: www.jaypeebrothers.com
Website: www.jaypeedigital.com

Inquiries for bulk sales may be solicited at: jaypee@jaypeebrothers.com

Contemporary Management of Myeloproliferative Neoplasms

First Edition: **2015**

ISBN: 978-93-5152-362-8

Printed at: Samrat Offset Pvt. Ltd.

Contents

Contributors

Editor

Brady L Stein MD MHS
Assistant Professor, Department of Medicine
Northwestern University Feinberg School of Medicine
Chicago, Illinois, USA

Brandon J McMahon MD
Associate Professor, Department of Medicine
Northwestern University Feinberg School of Medicine
Chicago, Illinois, USA

Contributing Authors

Sonia L Ali MD
Clinical Fellow
Hematology/Oncology, Scripps Clinic
San Diego, California, USA

John Crispino PhD
Professor
Division of Hematology/Oncology
Northwestern University
Chicago, Illinois, USA

Anne M Ditto MD FAAAI FACAAI FISAAI FACP FRSM
Associate Professor of Medicine
Department of Medicine
Division of Allergy-Immunology
Northwestern University Feinberg School of Medicine
Chicago, Illinois, USA

Jonathan M Gerber MD
Director of the Leukemia Program
Department of Hematologic Oncology and Blood Disorders
Levine Cancer Institute
Clinical Assistant Professor of Medicine
University of North Carolina School of Medicine
Charlotte, North Carolina, USA

Laure Gilles PhD
Post-Doctoral Fellow
Division of Hematology/Oncology
Northwestern University
Chicago, Illinois, USA

Jagoda K Jasielec MD
Fellow, Section of Hematology/Oncology
Department of Medicine
The University of Chicago
Burbank, Illinois, USA

Irum Khan MD
Assistant Professor of Medicine
Division of Hematology/Oncology
University of Illinois College of Medicine
Chicago, Illinois, USA

Mahboobeh Mahdavinia MD PhD
Clinical Fellow
Department of Medicine
Division of Allergy-Immunology
Northwestern University Feinberg School of Medicine
Chicago, Illinois, USA

Laura C Michaelis MD
Associate Professor
Malignant Hematology
Medical College of Wisconsin Froedtert Medical Center
Milwaukee, Wisconsin, USA

Alison R Moliterno MD
Associate Professor of Medicine
Division of Hematology
Johns Hopkins University School of Medicine
Baltimore, Maryland, USA

Casey O'Connell MD
Department of Internal Medicine
Jane Anne Nohl Division of Hematology
Keck School of Medicine
University of Southern California
Los Angeles, California, USA

Olatoyosi Odenike MD
Associate Professor of Medicine
Department of Medicine
The University of Chicago Medicine
Comprehensive Cancer Center
Chicago, Illinois, USA

LoAnn C Peterson MD
Director of Hematopathology and Fellowship Program
Northwestern Memorial Hospital
Professor, Department of Pathology
Northwestern University
Chicago, Illinois, USA

Damiano Rondelli MD
Professor of Medicine
Chief, Division of Hematology/Oncology
University of Illinois College of Medicine
Chicago, Illinois, USA

Jamile M Shammo MD FASCP FACP
Associate Professor
Department of Medicine and Pathology
Rush University Medical Center
Chicago, Illinois, USA

Kristy Wolniak MD PhD
Hematopathology Fellow
Department of Pathology
Northwestern University Feinberg School of Medicine
Chicago, Illinois, USA

Preface

The last decade has witnessed major scientific discoveries within the field of BCR-ABL negative myeloproliferative neoplasms (MPNs). These discoveries have translated into breakthroughs in the understanding of disease pathogenesis, a molecular classification that allows for facilitated diagnosis, and targeted therapies that will establish a foundation for future treatments. There is a new era of enthusiasm in these MPN, along with an understanding that the heterogeneity and disease processes are somewhat distinct from their Philadelphia-positive counterpart, chronic myeloid leukemia. Recognition of multiple contributors to the clinical and clonal burden in MPN has led to novel therapeutic strategies, and in the near future, hopefully an identification of rational combination treatments.

In this book, we provide an overview of the diagnostic classification of the MPN, with relevant examples of the histology; this is still critical in establishing a diagnosis, of course complimenting molecular genetic studies. We next provide an overview of relevant contributors to disease pathogenesis, which will provide a background and rationale for the later chapter on novel MPN therapies (Janus kinase-inhibition and others), especially for myelofibrosis (MF). Because thrombotic and bleeding complications can dominate the clinical course during the first decade of disease in essential thrombocythemia (ET) and polycythemia vera (PV), an entire chapter is devoted toward the epidemiology, pathogenic features, risk factors, and management of this set of complications. An in depth review of epidemiology, clinical features, prognosis, and treatment of ET, PV, and MF is provided in chapters 4–6. Because JAK2 V617F is found in virtually all patients with PV, the impact of this mutation is discussed more extensively in chapter 5. Transplantation remains the only curative procedure for the MPN, particularly MF, but the decision to proceed is challenging for physicians and patients alike, and relevant data on prognosis, conditioning regimens, and outcomes are reviewed. Finally, patients with mast cell diseases and hypereosinophilic disorders present challenges in diagnosis and treatment, and the approach to these issues, as well as an update on management of these BCR-ABL negative MPNs is provided in chapters 9 and 10.

This book compliments practical aspects of diagnosis and treatment with insights into disease pathogenesis in a rapidly changing landscape, gearing towards students, residents, fellows, and attendings with a special interest in MPN. We hope the readers will agree, and find this book to be a useful tool for the care of their own MPN patients.

Brady L Stein MD MHS
Assistant Professor
Department of Medicine
Northwestern University Feinberg School of Medicine
Chicago, Illinois, USA

Brandon J McMahon MD
Associate Professor
Department of Medicine
Northwestern University Feinberg School of Medicine
Chicago, Illinois, USA

Acknowledgments

We would like to acknowledge the team from Jaypee Brothers, who have helped us create a book that we are quite proud of. We would like to especially thank Dr Madhu Choudhary, Ms Madhvi Thakur, and Ms Shweta Tiwari for guiding the project from a concept to a finished product. We are grateful for the time spent and contributions from our colleagues, and importantly, to our patients, who we continue to learn from in immeasurable ways.

CHAPTER

1 Diagnostic Criteria in the Myeloproliferative Neoplasms

LoAnn C Peterson, Kristy Wolniak

INTRODUCTION

The myeloproliferative neoplasms (MPNs) comprise several clonal hematopoietic stem cell diseases that share a number of overlapping features including overproduction of one or more myeloid lineages with relatively unaffected maturation. As a consequence, the bone marrow is hypercellular and red blood cells, granulocytes, and/or platelets may be increased in the peripheral blood. Hematopoiesis eventually extends to other organs, such as the spleen and liver, and there is a variable rate of transformation to acute leukemia or MF. The MPNs recognized in the World Health Organization (WHO) classification of MPNs are listed in box 1-1.[1]

Chronic myelogenous leukemia (CML) has long been the prototype for this group of diseases and was the first MPN in which the molecular pathogenesis was defined. The cytogenetic hallmark of CML is the Philadelphia (Ph) chromosome

Box 1-1 WHO Classification of Myeloproliferative Neoplasms[1]

- Myeloproliferative neoplasms (MPNs):
  - Chronic myelogenous leukemia, BCR-ABL1 positive
  - Chronic neutrophilic leukemia
  - Polycythemia vera
  - Primary myelofibrosis
  - Essential thrombocythemia
  - Chronic eosinophilic leukemia, NOS
  - Mastocytosis
  - MPN, unclassifiable
- Myeloid neoplasms with molecular genetic abnormalities:
  - Myeloid and lymphoid neoplasms with PDGFRA abnormalities
  - Myeloid neoplasms with PDGFRB rearrangement
  - Myeloid and lymphoid neoplasms with FGFR1 abnormalities

WHO, World Health Organization; BCR-ABL1, breakpoint cluster region-Abelson murine leukemia viral oncogene homolog 1; NOS, not otherwise specified; PDGFRA, platelet-derived growth factor receptor-alpha; PDGFRB, platelet-derived growth factor receptor-beta.

that results from a reciprocal t(9;22)(q34;q11.2) translocation or its variants t(V;9;22). The molecular consequence of this translocation is the formation of a *BCR-ABL1* (breakpoint cluster region-Abelson murine leukemia viral oncogene homolog 1) gene fusion that encodes a BCR-ABL fusion tyrosine kinase. Whereas the native ABL (Abelson leukemia virus) protein has tightly regulated tyrosine kinase activity, the chimeric BCR-ABL oncoprotein is constitutively activated. Similar to other kinases, the BCR-ABL protein transfers phosphate from adenosine triphosphate (ATP) to tyrosine residues in specific substrate proteins. This activates multiple transduction pathways and results in deregulated cellular proliferation, reduced apoptosis and decreased adherence to the bone marrow stroma. These properties allow the leukemic cells to gradually displace the normal hematopoietic cells. This knowledge of the pathogenesis of CML led to the development of effective targeted therapy in the form of ABL tyrosine kinase inhibitors, such as imatinib.[2-4]

The success of imatinib as a targeted therapy for the fusion tyrosine kinase BCR-ABL in CML established a conceptual framework for identifying the underlying mutations in other MPNs, and great strides have been made over the last few years toward identifying the genetic abnormalities in *BCR-ABL1* negative MPNs. In these diseases, however, it has become apparent that there is a broad and complex array of genetic abnormalities present rather than one defined abnormality as in CML. The discovery of mutations in the tyrosine kinase Janus kinase 2 (JAK2) in different MPN diseases[5-9] made it clear that the model of one molecular abnormality defining one disease is not applicable in many types of MPNs.

It was a major breakthrough in MPN research in 2005 when the activating point mutation [V617F (a change of valine to phenylalanine at the 617 position)] in JAK2 was identified in approximately 95% of patients with polycythemia vera (PV) and approximately 50% of patients with primary myelofibrosis (PMF) or essential thrombocythemia (ET).[10] JAK2 is a cytoplasmic tyrosine kinase that transduces signaling, especially signals triggered by hematopoietic growth factors such as erythropoietin. The *JAK2 V617F* mutation, as well as more recently identified additional *JAK2* mutations and rearrangements,[11] result in a constitutively activated tyrosine kinase that activates proliferation and survival pathways. The JAK-1/2 inhibitor ruxolitinib is available therapeutically and clinical trials have found beneficial effects, such as reduction of spleen size and constitutional symptoms in myelofibrosis (MF) patients.[12,13] Identification of *JAK2* mutations are helpful in diagnosing MPN and guiding therapy; however, *JAK2* mutations are not disease specific and are also found in patients without MPNs.[6,14] The classification of MPNs in the WHO includes the presence of *JAK2* mutations in the criteria; however, *JAK2* mutations are not disease-specific or required for any MPN diagnosis.

Many *BCR-ABL1* negative MPN genetic alterations identified are in genes involved in cell signaling, cell cycle, and apoptosis. Recently, several mutations have also been identified in genes involved in epigenetic regulation.[15,16] Similar to *JAK2* mutations, most of these mutations are not specific to MPNs. Therapies are rapidly being developed to target many of these mutations. As underlying genetic abnormalities are uncovered in MPN with potential therapeutic implications, the classification of MPNs by the WHO has been adapted to include these abnormalities into the diagnostic classification scheme. In the WHO classification, molecular abnormalities can be disease-defining, such as *BCR-ABL1*, or as in the case of *JAK2* mutations, they have been incorporated into the criteria in support of the diagnosis and to help guide therapy.[1]

A recent study identified that a significant portion of patients with essential thrombocythemia and primary myelofibrosis without JAK2 or myeloproliferative leukemia virus oncogene (MPL) mutations have somatic muations of the gene CALR, encoding calreticulin. Identification of CALR mutations may be helpful in the diagnosis of essential thrombocythemia and primary myelofibrosis and initial studies suggest the presence of CALR mutations may have prognostic implications.[17]

There are currently four chronic myeloid neoplasm entities in the WHO with defined molecular abnormalities: CML with *BCR-ABL1*, myeloid and lymphoid neoplasms with platelet-derived growth factor receptor-alpha (*PDGFRA*) rearrangement, myeloid neoplasms with platelet-derived growth factor receptor-beta (*PDGFRB*) rearrangement, and myeloid and lymphoid neoplasms with *FGFR1* abnormalities. The last three entities have been grouped in the WHO into a category separate from the other MPNs and characteristically have a prominent eosinophilic component. Many of the other MPN genetic abnormalities, like mutations of *JAK2*, are useful in helping to diagnose MPN and potentially guide therapy, but at this time are not considered defining of one specific disease. Presumably, with the development of therapies targeting molecular abnormalities, there will be an ever-increasing number of molecularly-defined diseases.

As with CML, the three other molecularly-defined myeloid neoplasms have a fusion gene with an aberrant tyrosine kinase, with potential therapeutic implications. Abnormalities of both the α and β moieties of the platelet-derived growth factor receptor (*PDGFRA* and *PDGFRB*), a surface tyrosine kinase receptor, have been associated with myeloid neoplasms with eosinophilia. Chromosomal translocations involving the *FGFR1* gene at 8p11 give rise to a myeloproliferative disorder characterized by eosinophilia and lymphoblastic lymphoma that frequently progresses to acute myeloid leukemia (AML).[18] The presence of either the *PDGFRA* or *PDGFRB* rearrangement leads to constitutively activated tyrosine kinase and predicts responsiveness to imatinib.[19] Although *FGFR1* inhibitors have been developed, no effective targeted pharmaceutical therapy is available at this time for patients with myeloid and lymphoid neoplasms with *FGFR1* abnormalities.[20]

This chapter summarizes the diagnosis of *BCR-ABL1* negative MPN based on the established WHO criteria including clinical, morphologic, and genetic features. CML is not within the scope of this book, but a brief morphologic description is included here for comparison to the *BCR-ABL1*-negative MPNs. Subsequent chapters will review the newly defined molecular abnormalities in the *BCR-ABL1*-negative MPNs.

CHRONIC MYELOGENOUS LEUKEMIA

Chronic myelogenous leukemia is a chronic MPN causally related to the *BCR-ABL1* fusion gene.[21] The diagnosis is based on characteristic blood and bone marrow findings, and documentation of the presence of *BCR-ABL1* fusion by cytogenetic and/or molecular analysis. The diagnosis is usually established during an initial, indolent or chronic phase. The major hematological finding at diagnosis is an excessive number of mature and immature granulocytes in both the peripheral blood and bone marrow. As the disease progresses, patients advance to an accelerated or blast phase. The accelerated phase often precedes the blast phase and is characterized by clinical deterioration, and changes in blood counts and morphology but without a sufficient number of blasts for diagnosis of acute leukemia. The blast phase represents overt acute leukemia characterized by the rapid expansion of myeloid or lymphoid lineage blasts.[22]

Microscopic Findings

The diagnosis of CML is usually strongly suggested by characteristic peripheral blood findings (Figure 1-1A) that include a neutrophilic leukocytosis. The neutrophil series in the blood is typically represented by all stages of maturation from the myeloblast to the segmented neutrophil with myelocytes and segmented stages usually the most numerous. In rare cases, mature neutrophils predominate. The neutrophils in the chronic phase of the disease do not typically show dysplastic changes. Basophils are increased in absolute number; this characteristic feature aids in distinguishing CML from a reactive neutrophilia. An eosinophilia is, also, common but lacks the diagnostic specificity of basophilia. Circulating immature basophils or eosinophils may be found. Myeloblasts are usually present but generally do not exceed 2–3%. Monocytes may be mildly increased but are usually less than 4% of the leukocyte differential.

The platelets are usually increased in number and platelet morphology is normal although occasional large platelets with decreased or absent granules may be present. Rarely, thrombocytosis may be the predominant feature of a patient presenting with CML with alterations in leukocytes inconspicuous or absent. A normochromic, normocytic anemia, and a small number of nucleated red blood cells are present in most patients.

The bone marrow is hypercellular and shows a marked increase in granulocytes. The neutrophils show normal maturation although a relative increase in

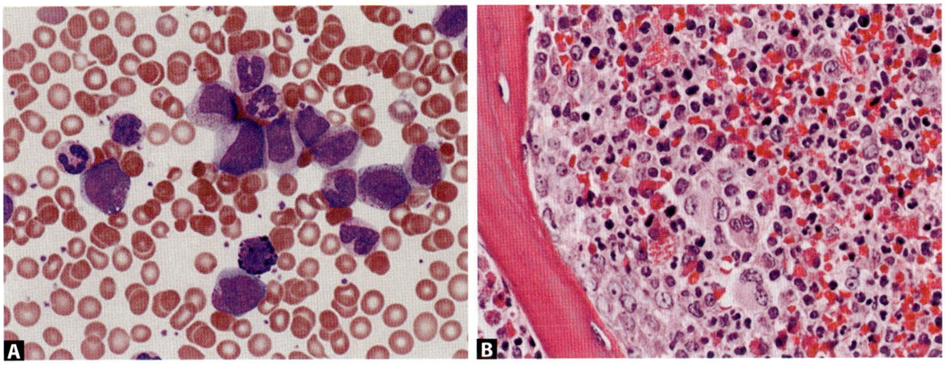

Figure 1-1 Chronic myelogenous leukemia, peripheral blood and bone marrow. **A,** The peripheral blood smear shows a neutrophilia with all stages of maturation represented. A basophil is also present. **B,** The bone marrow is markedly hypercellular with marked granulocytic proliferation. Several megakaryocytes are present in this field. They appear smaller than normal megakaryocytes.

myelocytes or a "myelocyte bulge" is often a prominent feature. The periosteal cuff of promyelocytes and myelocytes is widened, often 5–10 cells thick in comparison to 1-2 cells seen in normal bone marrow biopsies (Figure 1-1B).[23] Basophils and eosinophils are increased and may be abundant. Blasts represent fewer than 10% of the bone marrow cells. Megakaryocytes may be normal in number but they are usually increased; they are scattered throughout the bone marrow biopsy or clustered in small groups. The megakaryocytes tend to be smaller than those found in normal bone marrow biopsies, in contrast to the large megakaryocytes seen in other chronic MPNs, such as ET. Hypolobate megakaryocytes may be observed. Erythroid precursors are often decreased in number. Macrophages containing blue-pigment debris (sea-blue histiocytes) and pseudo-Gaucher cells are found in the bone marrow in about one-third of cases. These macrophages are part of the neoplastic clone and result from increased bone marrow turnover of granulocytes.[24] They are positive with stains for periodic acid-Schiff (PAS) and iron. Lymphoid aggregates are often present and may be prominent, especially following therapy.

Genetic Characteristics

The hallmark genetic abnormality of CML is a reciprocal chromosomal translocation, t(9;22)(q34;q11), that was first discovered as a small chromosome named the Ph chromosome. About 95% of patients with CML exhibit this translocation while another 5% have complex or variant translocations involving additional chromosomes with the same end result—development of the *BCR-ABL* oncogene by fusion of the *BCR* on chromosome 22 to the *ABL* gene on chromosome 9.[25]

BCR-ABL1 NEGATIVE MYELOPROLIFERATIVE NEOPLASMS POLYCYTHEMIA VERA

Polycythemia vera is a chronic MPN characterized by a clonal proliferation of myeloid cells with erythrocytosis being the most prominent manifestation. Virtually all patients with PV carry the *JAK2* V617F or other functionally similar mutation. Such mutations are absent in secondary or reactive causes of erythrocytosis. Elevations in hemoglobin (Hb) and the presence of *JAK2* V617F or other similar *JAK2* mutation serve as major criteria for the diagnosis of PV in the WHO diagnostic criteria for PV shown in box 1-2. Minor criteria for the diagnosis include characteristic bone marrow histopathology for PV, low serum erythropoietin level, and endogenous erythroid colony formation *in vitro*.[26,27]

Clinical Features

The mean age at diagnosis of PV is approximately 60 years with a slight male predominance (1.2: 1). About 7% of patients are diagnosed before the age of 40 years; PV is only rarely diagnosed in children.[28] Most patients at diagnosis are symptomatic with the most common symptoms being headache, dizziness/vertigo, fatigue, and pruritus. Complaints of a prior or current thrombotic event are common. The main physical findings are a ruddy cyanosis, splenomegaly in 70%, hepatomegaly in about 33%, and hypertension in 50%.[29]

Laboratory Findings

The Hb/hematocrit and the red cell mass are elevated.[26] If iron deficiency is present, the Hb/hematocrit may be normal or low. The platelet count is elevated in about

Box 1-2 WHO Criteria for Polycythemia Vera[27]

Diagnosis requires the presence of both major and one minor criterion or the presence of the first major criterion together with two minor criteria

Major criteria:

- Hemoglobin (Hb) more than18.5 g/dL in men, 16.5 g/dL in women, or elevated RBC mass more than 25% above mean normal predicted value, or Hb or hematocrit more than 99th percentile of method-specific reference range for age, sex, altitude of residence or Hb more than 17 g/dL in men, 15 g/dL in women if associated with a documented increase of at least 2 g/dL from an individual's baseline value that cannot be attributed to correction of iron deficiency.
- Presence of Janus kinase 2 (JAK2) V617F or other functionally similar JAK2 mutation

Minor criteria:

- Bone marrow biopsy showing hypercellularity for age and panmyelosis with prominent erythroid, granulocytic, and pleomorphous megakaryocytic proliferation
- Low serum erythropoietin level
- Endogenous erythroid colony formation *in vitro*

WHO, World Health Organization; RBC, red blood cell.

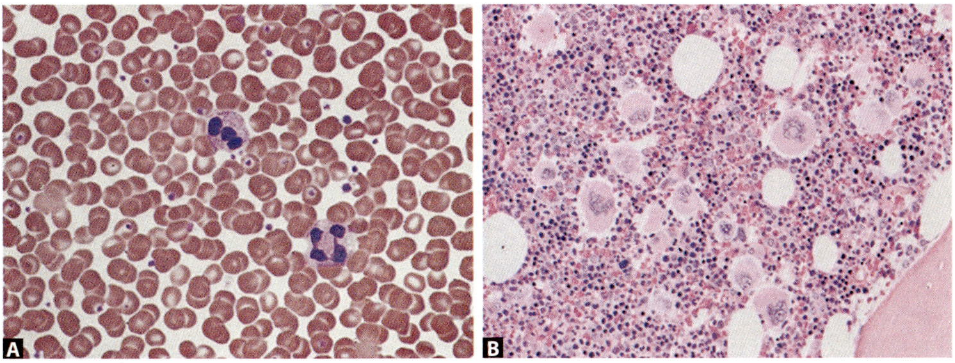

Figure 1-2 Polycythemia vera, peripheral blood, and bone marrow. **A,** The blood smear shows an erythrocytosis with crowding of the red blood cells. **B,** The bone marrow biopsy shows an erythroid hyperplasia with increased numbers of megakaryocytes. The megakaryocytes vary in size and are not dysplastic.

60% of patients and the leukocyte count is elevated in about 60% of patients.[29] A basophilia as well as an eosinophilia may be present. Serum erythropoietin levels are usually low. A common feature of many MPNs, endogenous erythroid colony formation, is characteristic of PV, but testing for this feature is not widely available.[30]

Microscopic Findings

The peripheral blood smear shows an erythrocytosis (Figure 1-2A). The red cells are generally normochromic, normocytic but may be hypochromic, microcytic if the patient is iron deficient. The leukocytes are often increased because of an increased number of neutrophils; occasional immature neutrophils may be apparent. Basophilia and eosinophilia may be present. Platelets are frequently increased and platelet clumps may be observed.

The bone marrow in PV is usually mildly to markedly hypercellular with a panmyelosis that includes erythroid, granulocytic, and megakaryocytic hyperplasia (Figure 1-2B). Erythroid and megakaryocytic proliferation are typically the most prominent. Enlarged islands of erythropoiesis are present. The megakaryocytes vary in size from small to large and lack dysmorphic features. They tend to cluster and may be localized around bone marrow sinusoids or adjacent to bone trabeculae. The granulocyte series shows no shift to immaturity and no increase in blasts is present.[31] Storage iron is almost always absent. Reticulin fibers are usually normal but may be mildly to moderately increased.[32] Lymphoid aggregates may be found in up to 20% of patients.[30]

Genetic Characteristics

Cytogenetic abnormalities are identified at diagnosis in about 25% of patients with PV. The most common recurring aberrations include +8, +9, del(20q), del(13q), and del(1q).[30] Molecular genetic studies including fluorescence *in situ* hybridization (FISH) have identified frequent cryptic abnormalities of chromosome 9p, site of the JAK2 gene.[33] Chromosomal abnormalities are present with increasing frequency as the disease progresses and are found in about 80–90% of patients with post-polycythemic myelofibrosis (post-PVMF) and nearly 100% of patients who develop acute leukemia.[30]

As many as 97% of patients with PV possess the *JAK2 V617F* gene mutation resulting from a point mutation in exon 14.[6,7,34] Loss of heterozygosity through mitotic combination is frequent in PV. In one study the patients homozygous for the mutation had higher Hb levels, higher incidence of pruritus, and a higher rate of fibrotic transformation than patients who were heterozygous.[35] Other *JAK2* mutations with effects similar to those of *JAK2 V617F* have been reported in patients negative for *JAK2 V617F*. These mutations are in-frame deletions or tandem point mutations in exon 12.[36]

Disease Progression

Patients with PV are at risk of transformation to post-PVMF or acute leukemia. The risk of transformation to post-PVMF is about 6% at 15 years; the risk of evolution to acute leukemia is similar at about 7% at 15 years.[37] Duration of disease is a significant risk factor for developing post-PVMF while older age and cytotoxic therapy other than hydroxyurea are risk factors for progression to AML.[38,39]

Transformation of PV to post-PVMF has also been referred to as the "spent phase" of PV. Post-PVMF is characterized be a decrease in Hb, leukoerythroblastosis, and red cell poikilocytosis that often includes tear-drop shaped red cells. The bone marrow exhibits prominent fibrosis and may be hypocellular (Figure 1-3A). The fibrosis can be defined by reticulin staining (Figure 1-3B). Osteosclerosis may be present. Megakaryocytes, often in clusters, may be prominent; unlike those seen at diagnosis, they may be dysmorphic. Erythropoiesis and granulopoiesis are decreased, and

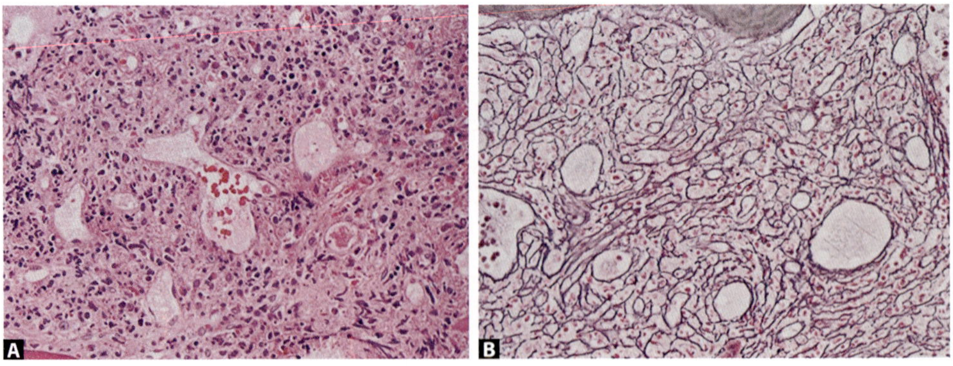

Figure 1-3 Post-polycythemic myelofibrosis, bone marrow. **A,** The bone marrow is fibrotic and hypocellular. **B,** A reticulin stain shows marked reticulin fibrosis.

intrasinusoidal hematopoiesis may be observed. The spleen often enlarges further during this time secondary to extramedullary hematopoiesis. Specific criteria have been proposed by an international consortium for the diagnosis of post-PVMF, requiring the diagnosis of PV and bone marrow fibrosis with at least two of four additional criteria.[40]

The blast phase or acute leukemia that develops in PV is of myeloid origin[41] and is preceded by myelodysplastic features in about 50% of cases.[23]

PRIMARY MYELOFIBROSIS

Primary myelofibrosis is a clonal stem cell disorder characterized by granulocytic and megakaryocytic proliferation, reactive bone marrow fibrosis, and extramedullary hematopoiesis. Other terms that have been used for this disorder include agnogenic myeloid metaplasia, myelosclerosis with myeloid metaplasia, and idiopathic myelofibrosis. This disease evolves from an initial prefibrotic stage characterized by a hypercellular bone marrow with absent or minimal fibrosis to a stage with marked bone marrow fibrosis and, also, frequently osteosclerosis. The fibrotic stage is characterized by a prominent leukoerythroblastic blood picture and the presence of tear drop shaped red blood cells. About 50% of patients with PMF exhibit the *JAK2 V617F* mutation. The WHO criteria for diagnosis of PMF are shown in box 1-3.[26,42]

Although granulocytes and megakaryocytes are the most prominent hematopoietic cells involved in PMF, erythroid precursors, monocytes/macrophages, and, occasionally, B- and T-lymphocytes are derived from the same clonal stem cell.[43] The fibrosis is secondary and nonclonal; its production is stimulated by growth factors secreted by the neoplastic megakaryocytes. Megakaryocyte-derived transforming growth factor-β1 is the major cytokine implicated in the mediation of fibrosis in PMF.[44,45]

Clinical Features

The median age at diagnosis is about 60 years with a male to female ratio of 1.2: 1 to 1.6: 1. Less than 3% of patients present before the age of 30 years; PMF is exceedingly rare in children.[45] The presenting clinical features vary widely and depend on the stage of the disease when the disease is first detected. Compared to ET or PV, most patients are symptomatic at diagnosis, but as many as one-third of patients are asymptomatic at diagnosis. When complaints are present, the most common presenting symptom is fatigue. Other symptoms may include pruritus, bone pain, cough, early saticty, abdominal pain, weight loss, fever, and night sweats.[46]

About 30% of patients are first detected in the prefibrotic or cellular phase. At this time, splenomegaly may be present but is only minimal to modest.[47] Most patients with PMF present when bone marrow fibrosis is present. Splenomegaly secondary to extramedullary hematopoiesis is usually present at that time and may be marked

Box 1-3 WHO Criteria for Primary Myelofibrosis[42]

Diagnosis requires meeting all three major and two minor criteria

Major criteria

- Presence of megakaryocyte proliferation and atypia,* usually accompanied by either reticulin and/or collagen fibrosis, or, in the absence of remarkable reticulin fibrosis, the megakaryocyte changes must be accompanied by marked bone marrow cellularity including granulocytic proliferation and decreased erythroid precursors (i.e., pre-fibrotic cellular-phase disease)
- Not meeting WHO criteria for polycythemia vera, † BCR-ABL1 positive CML, ‡ myelodysplastic syndrome (MDS),§ or other myeloproliferative disorders#

Minor criteria

- Leukoerythroblastosis¶
- Increase in serum lactate dehydrogenase level¶
- Anemia¶
- Splenomegaly¶

WHO, World Health Organisation; BCR-ABL1, breakpoint cluster region-Abelson murine leukemia viral oncogene homolog 1; CML, chronic myelogenous leukemia

*Small to large megakaryocytes with an aberrant nuclear/cytoplasmic ratio and hyperchromatic, bulbous, or irregularly folded nuclei and dense clustering.

†Requires the failure of iron replacement therapy to increase Hb level to the polycythemia vera range in the presence of decreased serum ferritin.

‡Requires the absence of BCR-ABL1.

§Requires absence of dyserythropoiesis and dysgranulopoiesis.

Demonstration of Janus kinase 2 V617F or other clonal marker, or demonstration that bone marrow fibrosis is not secondary to infection, autoimmune disorder or other chronic inflammatory condition, hairy cell leukemia or other lymphoproliferative disorder, metastatic cancer, or toxic (chronic) myelopathies

#It should be noted that patients with conditions associated with reactive myelofibrosis are not immune to PMF and the diagnosis should be considered in such cases if other criteria are met.

Degree of abnormality could be borderline or marked.

with the spleen often extending 10 cm or more below the left costal margin.[48] Symptoms related to splenomegaly, such as early satiety and abdominal discomfort may be prominent. Hepatomegaly is also common.

Laboratory Findings

Thrombocytosis is often the most prominent hematological manifestation in early PMF (prefibrotic or very early fibrotic lesions) with the platelet count reported to exceed 600 × 10^9/L in 86% of patients. Leukocytosis (51%) and anemia (38%) may also be present.[49] Anemia is present in 50–70% of patients who present with fibrotic PMF; 25% manifest a severe anemia (Hb <8 g/dL). The leukocyte count is elevated in approximately 50% of patients and exceeds 30 × 10^9/L in about 10%. Patients can also exhibit a thrombocytopenia at diagnosis, typically with overt PMF.[46]

The absolute number of circulating clusters of differentiation (CD)34+ hematopoietic precursor cells in PMF is reported to be higher than normal controls and also higher than patients with other *BCR-ABL1*-negative chronic MPNs.[50]

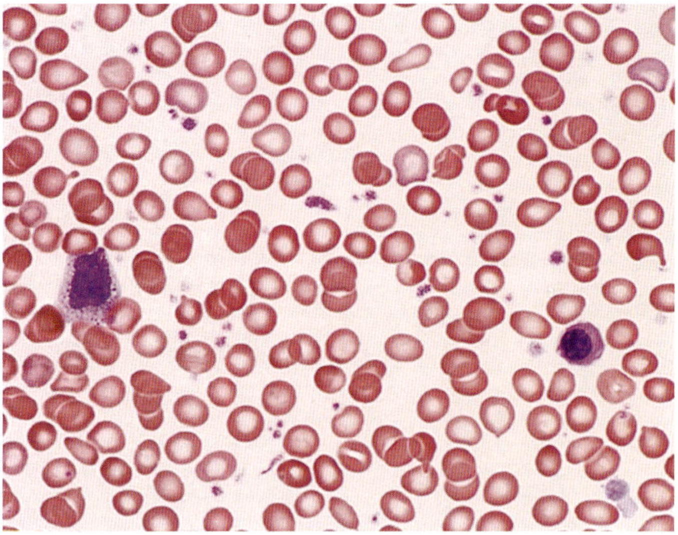

Figure 1-4 Primary myelofibrosis, peripheral blood. This blood smear shows tear drop shaped red cells, a leukoerythroblastic reaction, and increased platelets. The platelets have variable morphology including large, hypogranular platelets.

Other abnormal laboratory results that may be observed include elevations in lactate dehydrogenase (LDH), alkaline phosphatase, uric acid, and vitamin B_{12}.

Microscopic Findings

Blood and Bone Marrow

The characteristic features of the blood smear in PMF are increased poikilocytosis with tear drop shaped red cells (Figure 1-4), a leukoerythroblastic reaction with circulating nucleated red blood cells and granulocyte precursors, and large hypogranular platelets. Micromegakaryocytes and megakaryocyte nuclei are frequently present. These changes are secondary to release from sites of extramedullary hematopoiesis and increase as the disease progresses. These findings may be seen during the prefibrotic stage, but are usually subtle; thrombocytosis often dominates the blood picture at that time. Circulating blasts are often present during the fibrotic stage but should be less than 10% of cells. Blasts more than 10% should raise the possibility of an accelerated phase or acute leukemia.[42]

The bone marrow in the prefibrotic or cellular stage of PMF is hypercellular with minimal or absent reticulin fibrosis (Figures 1-5A to C). Prominent megakaryocytic proliferation is characteristic of this stage of PMF. A granulocytic hyperplasia with a shift to immaturity is typically observed; erythroid precursors are often decreased or exhibit shift to immaturity. The megakaryocytes form clusters and may be located next to bony trabeculae. They vary from small to giant and exhibit prominent

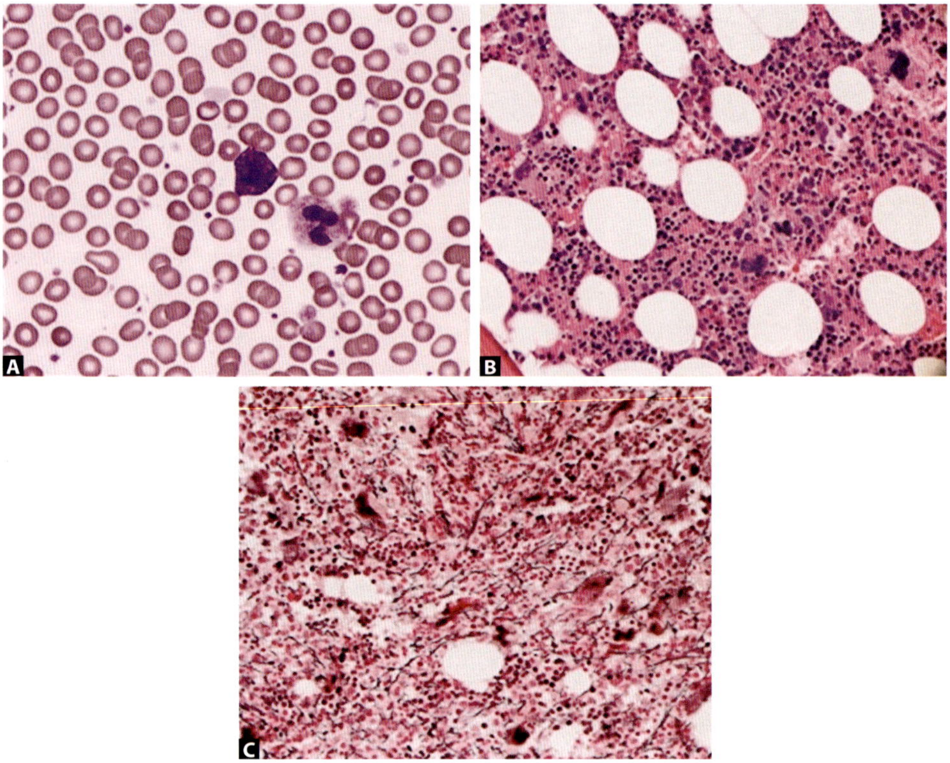

Figure 1-5 Prefibrotic primary myelofibrosis, peripheral blood, and bone marrow. **A,** The blood smear shows increased platelets that vary in size and include large, hypogranular platelets. **B,** The bone marrow is hypercellular; the megakaryocytes are increased and many are morphologically abnormal with increased nuclear/cytoplasmic ratios and hyperchromatic nuclei. **C,** Reticulin stain reveals a focus of slightly increased reticulin fibers.

morphologic abnormalities including hyperchromatic nuclei, hyposegmentation, irregular lobulation, and frequent bare or "naked" megakaryocytic nuclei. Dyserythropoiesis and dysgranulopoiesis are absent. Recognition of the morphologically abnormal megakaryocytes is critical to recognizing the prefibrotic stage and distinguishing it from other myeloproliferative disorders, particularly ET. Reticulin fibrosis, when present, tends to be concentrated around vessels. Vascular proliferation is increased.[31]

As the bone marrow progresses from the prefibrotic to the fibrotic stage, the cellularity decreases, and reticulin and even collagen fibrosis becomes more prominent. The bone marrow is not easily aspirated often resulting in a dry tap. Patches of hematopoietic tissue may be separated by fibrous tissue or fat. The bone marrow sinuses are often dilated and may contain immature hematopoietic cells. Morphologically abnormal megakaryocytes are usually the predominant cells and may occur in clusters or sheets; megakaryocytes may be particularly prominent within dilated sinuses.[31] New bone formation and osteosclerosis often develop. Bone marrow microvessel density is increased.[51] Lymphoid aggregates are also frequent in bone marrow biopsies from patients with PMF.

Extramedullary Findings

Many of the abnormalities observed in the peripheral blood are due to release of cells from sites of extramedullary hematopoiesis into the circulation. Extramedullary hematopoiesis can occur in any organ but is most prominent in spleen and liver. The red pulp of the spleen is expanded by erythroid, granulocytic and megakaryocytic cells located primarily in the sinuses. Megakaryocytes are often the most prominent. Fibrosis of the red pulp cords may be present. The hepatic sinuses may also show extramedullary hematopoiesis; fibrosis and cirrhosis may also occur.[52]

Genetic Characteristics

Conventional cytogenetic analysis reveals clonal abnormalities in about 50% of patients with PMF. The most frequent abnormalities include del(20)(q11;q13), del(13)(q12;q22), trisomy 8, trisomy 9, del(12) (p11;p13), monosomy, or long-arm deletions of chromosome 7 and partial trisomy 1q. None of these abnormalities is specific for PMF. An adverse prognosis has been linked to the following abnormalities: 12p-, +8, and -7/7q-;[45] der(6)t(1;6)(q21-23;p21-23) has been reported to be specific for PMF although it is an uncommon finding.[53] There is no *BCR-ABL1* fusion gene. Comparative genomic hybridization studies have documented gains of chromosome 9p as the most frequent genetic abnormality, occurring in about 50% of patients.[54]

The reported frequency of the *JAK2 V617F* mutation in PMF ranges from 35% to 57%. Homozygosity for this mutation occurs in 9–29% of cases and has been shown to be the result of mitotic recombination. No prognostic significance for the mutation has been found although the presence of the mutation appears to be associated with older age and history of thrombosis or pruritis.[45] Mutations in myeloproliferative leukemia virus oncogene (MPL), receptor for thrombopoietin, have also been described in about 5% of patients with PMF. The clinical significance of this finding is under investigation.[55]

A recent study has also identified mutation of the CALR gene in a significant portion of patients without JAK2 or MPL mutations, and CALR mutations may be associated with a better prognosis.[17]

Disease Progression

The presence of 10–19% blasts in the blood or bone marrow signifies an accelerated phase and 20% or more is diagnostic of acute transformation with the WHO guidelines.[42] An international working group defined acute transformation as 20% or more blasts in the bone marrow, or 20% or more blasts in the peripheral blood that persist for 8 weeks.[56] Acute leukemia occurs in about 8–23% of patients with PMF and does not appear to be related to prior therapy. Most of the leukemic transformations have been myeloid with the most frequent subtypes being acute megakaryoblastic and acute myeloid with varying degrees of maturation. Clonal karyotypic abnormalities are present in most patients with acute leukemia and evidence for clonal evolution is common. Leukemic transformation is associated with a poor prognosis with the median survival of 2.6 months in one series of 91 patients.[57]

Differential Diagnosis

The prefibrotic phase of PMF can be very difficult to distinguish from ET since isolated thrombocytosis is commonly seen in prefibrotic PMF. Careful examination of the peripheral blood and bone marrow biopsy is critical in distinguishing between these two disorders. A leukoerythroblastic reaction or atypical platelet morphology favors a diagnosis of PMF. The megakaryocytes in PMF are often clustered and variably sized with atypical morphology, while the megakaryocytes in ET tend to be scattered or only loosely aggregated, large to giant, and manifest deeply lobulated nuclei and abundant mature cytoplasm. Left-shifted granulocytic hyperplasia is characteristic of prefibrotic PMF but is usually absent in ET. A significant increase in reticulin fibrosis argues against the diagnosis of ET.

The main disorders in the differential diagnosis of the fibrotic stage of PMF are those that cause prominent bone marrow fibrosis. Any of the myeloproliferative disorders can be associated with bone marrow fibrosis. For example, CML with prominent fibrosis and megakaryocyte proliferation can closely resemble PMF. One helpful histological feature that aids in this distinction is that the megakaryocytes in CML are smaller and lack the bizarre morphology characteristic of PMF. Documentation of the *BCR-ABL1* fusion gene will establish the diagnosis of CML. The distinction between the PMF and the fibrotic phase of PV or ET can be very difficult, and requires clinical and hematological history. MF can also occur in myelodysplastic syndrome (MDS), but, in contrast to PMF, MDS with fibrosis typically exhibit prominent dysplasia in one or more cell lines. In addition, the megakaryocytes lack the pleomorphism of those in PMF; they are often small with monolobate nuclei.

Fibrosis can also be associated with acute leukemia. Acute panmyelosis with MF is a rare form of AML in which patients present with prominent constitutional symptoms, little or no splenomegaly and pancytopenia. Unlike PMF, red cell poikilocytosis is minimal and dysplastic changes in the neutrophils are frequent. The bone marrow is variably cellular with a panmyeloid proliferation and predominance of immature cells; blasts often exceed 20% of the cells. Distinction from PMF that has progressed to AML may not be possible.

Fibrosis also occurs in a wide variety of other neoplastic and nonneoplastic disorders that must be considered in the differential diagnosis of PMF including lymphoproliferative disorders, such as hairy cell leukemia, metastatic tumor, inflammatory processes or toxic processes, autoimmune disorders,[58] hyperparathyroidism, and osteopetrosis.

ESSENTIAL THROMBOCYTHEMIA

Essential thrombocythemia is a chronic MPN characterized by persistent thrombocytosis and a proliferation of enlarged, mature megakaryocytes. Reactive causes of thrombocytosis and other myeloproliferative disorders or MDS associated with thrombocytosis must be excluded in order to establish a diagnosis of ET. About 50% of patients with ET exhibit *JAK2 V617F*. The modified WHO diagnostic criteria for ET are shown in box 1-4.[26,59]

Clinical Features

Epidemiologic studies of ET suggest an annual incidence rate of 2.5 cases per 100,000 population per year[60] with a slight female preponderance.[61] The etiology of ET is unknown.

The mean age at diagnosis is about 55 years.[62] ET is extremely rare in children.[63] About one half of patients may be asymptomatic at presentation. However, complications related to microvascular disturbances, such as headaches, lightheadedness, erythromelalgia, and acral paresthesias are relatively common, reported

Box 1-4 WHO Criteria for Essential Thrombocythemia[59]

Diagnosis requires meeting all four criteria.

- Sustained platelet count* more than or equal to $450 \times 10^9/L$
- Bone marrow biopsy specimen showing proliferation mainly of the megakaryocytic lineage with increased numbers of enlarged, mature megakaryocytes. No significant increase, left-shift of neutrophil granulopoiesis or erythropoiesis
- Not meeting WHO criteria for polycythemia vera,† primary myelofibrosis‡ BCR-ABL-positive CML,§ or myelodysplastic syndrome#
- Demonstration of Janus kinase 2 V617F or demonstration that thrombocytosis is not reactive

WHO, world health organisation; BCR-ABL, breakpoint cluster region-Abelson murine leukemia virus; CML, chronic myelogenous leukemia

*Sustained during the work-up process

†Requires the failure of iron replacement therapy to increase Hb level to the polycythemia vera range in the presence of decreased serum ferritin

‡Requires the absence of relevant reticulin fibrosis, collagen fibrosis, peripheral blood leukoerythroblastosis, or markedly hypercellular marrow accompanied by megakaryocyte morphology that is typical for primary myelofibrosis—small to large with an aberrant nuclear/cytoplasmic ratio and hyperchromatic, bulbous or irregularly folded nuclei and dense clustering

§Requires the absence of BCR-ABL

#Requires absence of dyserythropoiesis and dysgranulopoiesis

¶Causes of reactive thrombocytosis include iron deficiency, splenectomy, surgery, infection, inflammation, connective tissue disease, metastatic cancer, and lymphoproliferative disorders. However, the presence of a condition associated with reactive thrombocytosis does not exclude the possibility of ET if other criteria are met.

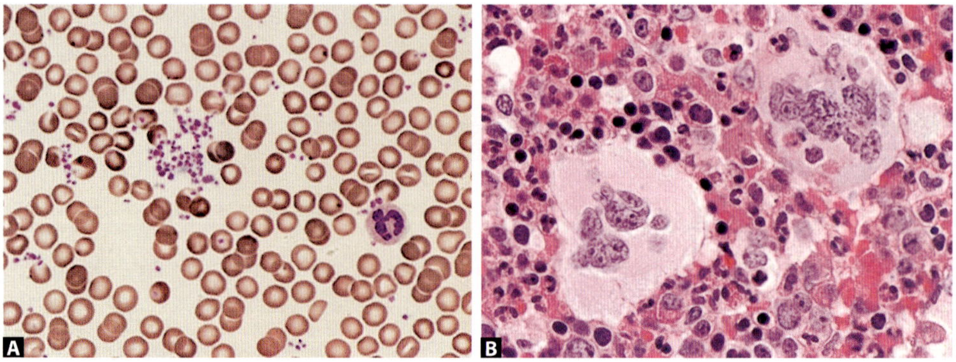

Figure 1-6 Essential thrombocythemia, peripheral blood and bone marrow. **A,** The blood smear exhibits increased platelets with platelet clumping and normal platelet morphology. **B,** The bone marrow has increased megakaryocytes including giant forms with hyperlobulated nuclei

in about 35% of patients.[61,62] Thrombosis and hemorrhage are also common complications of ET. Major thrombosis, primarily arterial, is present in 11–25% of patients at diagnosis and occurs in 11–22% during the course of the disease. Thrombosis accounts for 13–27% of deaths in ET.[64] Bleeding manifestations also occur with major hemorrhage occurring in 2–5% of patients at diagnosis and 1–7% during later follow-up.[64] The risk of hemorrhage is significantly associated with extreme thrombocytosis (platelet count >1 million).[64] First-trimester miscarriages occur in 30–40% of pregnant women with ET.[65] Modest splenomegaly is present in about 35% of patients at diagnosis.[66]

Laboratory Findings

The platelet count is elevated within a wide range but according to the modified WHO criteria must be greater than 450 × 10^9/L.[26] Extremely elevated platelets exceeding 1,000 × 10^9/L may be seen.[67] The Hb and hematocrit are within reference ranges and below the levels defined for the diagnosis of PV.[26] The leukocyte count is usually normal but may be mildly elevated.[68] Serum thrombopoietin levels are normal or elevated, but this measure is not widely available.[69]

Microscopic Findings

The peripheral blood smear shows an increased number of platelets and platelet clumps may be present (Figure 1-6A). Occasional large platelets may be observed but atypical or dysplastic platelets are not present. The erythrocytes are normochromic, normocytic. The leukocytes are morphologically unremarkable with no dysplastic features and leukoerythroblastosis is typically absent.

The cardinal feature of the bone marrow is the presence of increased megakaryocytes in a normocellular to moderately hypercellular bone marrow.

The megakaryocytes are usually dispersed through the bone marrow but may be occasionally found in loose clusters. The megakaryocytes are characteristically large and may be giant (Figure 1-6B), especially in contrast to those seen in CML. They exhibit abundant, mature cytoplasm and deeply lobulated nuclei. Emperipolesis of other bone marrow cells in the megakaryocyte cytoplasm may be present. Grossly atypical or dysplastic megakaryocytes are absent. Granulocytic proliferation is not significantly elevated or left-shifted. Erythroid hyperplasia may be observed if the patient has recently experienced hemorrhage. Reticulin fibrosis is usually absent.[31,70] Storage iron is adequate or, if it is low, a trial of iron therapy fails to increase the Hb levels or red cell mass into the polycythemic range.[68]

Genetic Characteristics

Conventional cytogenetic analysis reveals clonal abnormalities in only about 5% of patients with ET; none are diagnostic. Structural abnormalities include deletions of the long arm of chromosomes 5, 7, 13, 17, and 20. Application of FISH may disclose additional abnormalities of chromosomes 8 and 9 not detected by routine cytogenetic analysis.[62]

About 50% of patients with ET possess the *JAK2 V617F* mutation.[71] The presence of this mutation in ET has been associated with more advanced age at diagnosis, higher leukocyte counts and Hb levels, and higher frequency of thrombotic events than in patients without the mutation.[62,72,73] Mutations of MPL have been reported in less than 5% of patients with ET.[55] As in primary myelofibrosis, mutation of the CALR gene is present in a significant portion of patients without JAK2 or MPL mutations.[17]

The risk of progression of ET to a fibrotic bone marrow picture in one study occurred with a 10-year risk of 0.8%, and at 15 years 9.3%.[74] Progression to AML in patients with ET is unusual in the first 10 years with the risk in one study at 0.7%. The risk at 15 years increased to 2.1%.[74] The progression rates of ET to fibrosis or acute leukemia are significantly lower than those in early/prefibrotic PMF, emphasizing the necessity of accurate diagnosis.[74]

Differential Diagnosis

The first condition that must be ruled out before a diagnosis of ET is established is a reactive thrombocytosis.[62] Numerous conditions can result in a reactive thrombocytosis including iron deficiency anemia, asplenia, trauma, bleeding, hemolysis and a variety of inflammatory processes.[67] However, the presence of such a condition does not rule out ET if other criteria for the diagnosis are met. The identification of an acquired *JAK2* mutation or a clonal cytogenetic abnormality effectively rules out a reactive thrombocytosis. A bone marrow biopsy showing the characteristically increased large, hyperlobulated megakaryocytes also supports a diagnosis of ET.

Identification of the *BCR-ABL*1 translocation establishes the diagnosis of CML and rules out ET. This is of particular importance in those patients who present with isolated thrombocytosis but lack other peripheral blood findings typical for CML. The presence of small megakaryocytes that are characteristic of CML may be a morphologic clue in the bone marrow aspirate and biopsy to the diagnosis of CML.

The main criteria distinguishing PV from ET is the presence of an elevated Hb/hematocrit or red cell mass in PV, and a bone marrow showing panhyperplasia with prominent erythroid and megakaryocytic proliferation. Some patients with PV may present with iron deficiency and decreased or normal Hb levels. In these cases, the blood and bone marrow may closely resemble ET, but the diagnosis of ET should not be made unless iron replacement therapy fails to increase the Hb to a polycythemic range.

The prefibrotic phase of PMF may be very difficult to distinguish from ET. Prefibrotic PMF differs from ET in that the bone marrow is characterized by both a granulocytic and megakaryocytic hyperplasia with morphologically abnormal megakaryocytes. In addition, the blood in prefibrotic PMF may exhibit a leukoerythroblastic reaction or morphologically abnormal platelets.

Therapy with growth factor may produce pronounced megakaryocytic hyperplasia and thrombocytosis that may resemble a myeloproliferative disorder.[75]

Most MDS are associated with thrombocytopenia although occasionally, such as in the 5q-syndrome a thrombocytosis may be observed. The presence of dysplastic morphology in one or more cell lines supports the diagnosis of a MDS rather than ET.

Familial ET is a rare disorder characterized by the excessive production of platelets. It is a heterogeneous disorder with some cases reported to have mutations in the thrombopoietin gene or in the gene for c-Mpl (the thrombopoietin receptor).[76] A careful history is crucial in identifying these patients.

CHRONIC NEUTROPHILIC LEUKEMIA

Chronic neutrophilic leukemia (CNL) is a rare chronic MPN characterized by a persistent mature neutrophilic leukocytosis and a hypercellular bone marrow. Reactive causes of a neutrophilia must be excluded before the diagnosis is made. *BCR-ABL1* positive CML must also be ruled out. CNL achieved formal recognition with the 2001 WHO classification; the WHO diagnostic criteria are listed in box 1-5.[77]

Clinical Features

Chronic neutrophilic leukemia is rare with less than 50 well documented cases published in the literature.[78] The etiology is unknown. The median age at diagnosis is 65.5 years (range 15–86) with approximately equal numbers of females and males. Many patients are asymptomatic at diagnosis. Fatigue is the most common presenting symptom; other symptoms that may be present include weight loss, easy

Box 1-5 WHO Criteria for Chronic Neutrophilic Leukemia[77]

- Peripheral blood leukocytosis more than or equal to $25 \times 10^9/L$
  - Segmented neutrophils and bands more than 80% of white blood cells
  - Immature granulocytes (promyelocytes, myelocytes, metamyelocytes) less than 10% of white blood cells
  - Myeloblasts less than 10% of white blood cells
- Hypercellular bone marrow biopsy
  - Neutrophilic granulocytes increased in percentage and number
  - Myeloblasts less than 5% of nucleated marrow cells
  - Neutrophilic maturation pattern normal
- Hepatosplenomegaly
- No identifiable cause for physiologic neutrophilia
  - No infectious or inflammatory process
  - No underlying tumor, or if present, demonstration of clonality of myeloid cells by genetic or molecular studies
- No Philadelphia chromosome or BCR-ABL1 fusion gene
- No rearrangement of PDGFRA, PDGFRB, or FGFR1
- No evidence of another myeloproliferative disease
  - No evidence of polycythemia vera, i.e., normal red cell mass
  - No evidence of primary myelofibrosis, i.e., no abnormal megakaryocytic proliferation, no reticulin or collagen fibrosis, and no marked red blood cell poikilocytosis
  - No evidence of essential thrombocytosis, i.e., platelets less than $600 \times 10^9/L$, no proliferation of mature, enlarged megakaryocytes
- No evidence of myelodysplastic syndrome or a myelodysplastic/myeloproliferative disorder
  - No granulocytic dysplasia
  - No myelodysplastic changes in other myeloid lineages
  - Monocytes less than $1 \times 10^9/L$

WHO, World Health Organization; BCR-ABL1, breakpoint cluster region-Abelson murine leukemia viral oncogene homolog 1.

bruising, bone pain, and night sweats. Splenomegaly is usually present at diagnosis while lymphadenopathy and hepatomegaly are unusual.[78,79]

Laboratory Findings

The leukocyte count is elevated with a mean leukocyte count of about $50 \times 10^9/L$ (range 10–172 $\times 10^9/L$).[78,80] Mild anemia is often present. The platelet count is frequently normal; it may be deceased but thrombocytopenia, when present, is usually not severe.[78,79]

Serum vitamin B_{12} levels are elevated and neutrophil alkaline phosphatase (NAP) scores are usually elevated.[79]

Microscopic Findings

The blood smear shows a prominent neutrophilic leukocytosis. The majority of the neutrophils are mature; immature neutrophils may be observed but are usually less than 5% of the leukocytes. Blasts are usually absent. The neutrophils frequently exhibit pronounced toxic granulation and Döhle bodies. Dysplasia is absent. Monocytes, basophils, and eosinophils are not increased, and red cell and platelet morphology is normal.[78]

The bone marrow is hypercellular due to marked granulocytic proliferation. Granulocyte maturation appears normal with the majority of neutrophils at the myelocyte to segmented neutrophil stage. Blasts are not increased. Dysplasia is not present. Reticulin fibrosis is absent or only mild.[78-81]

Genetic Characteristics

Cytogenetic abnormalities are present in about 20% of patients at diagnosis and may also develop in a subset of patients during follow-up. The most common aberrations include 20q-, 21+, and 11q-.[78] By definition, no patient has a *BCR-ABL1* fusion. The JAK2 mutation is uncommon in CNL, reported in only one of six patients in one study.[82]

Differential Diagnosis

Reactive causes of neutrophilia must be excluded before a diagnosis of CNL is made. A prominent neutrophilia can also be seen in association with epithelial malignancies and may be secondary to tumor production of cytokines.[78] Therefore, a search for an occult malignancy is warranted before a diagnosis of CNL is made. A disproportionate number of CNL have been reported in association with plasma cell myeloma. The neutrophilia in these cases is likely reactive, and are, also, possibly cytokine driven. Evidence to support this hypothesis includes reports of remissions of the CNL after treatment of the plasma cell disorder and documentation of polyclonal neutrophils in some cases.[78] The WHO recommends that the bone marrow of all cases of CNL be examined for a plasma cell dyscrasia and, if present, clonality of the neutrophil proliferation supported by cytogenetic or molecular studies before a diagnosis of CNL is made.[81] The diagnosis requires the absence of features characteristic of other MPNs. The rare cases of CML that are characterized by a predominance of mature and segmented neutrophils but that exhibit a *BCR-ABL1* fusion gene should be regarded as CML rather than CNL.

Treatment and Prognosis

Optimal therapy for CNL has not been established. Therapy to date has mostly consisted of cytoreductive agents, such a hydroxyurea with about 75% of patients having a decrease in leukocyte count and/or splenomegaly. Successful use of α-interferon has been reported. Allogeneic stem cell transplant has also been reported. Disease progression is marked by refractoriness to therapy, marked splenomegaly, anemia and thrombocytopenia, and the appearance of immature cells in the peripheral blood. Transformation to AML can occur. The median survival of patients with CNL is reported as 23.5 months (range 1–106). The most common causes of death include intracranial hemorrhage and progressive disease.[78,83]

CHRONIC EOSINOPHILIC LEUKEMIA, NOT OTHERWISE SPECIFIED

Hypereosinophilia ($\geq 1.5 \times 10^9$/L) can be divided into three categories: (1) reactive, (2) clonal, and (3) idiopathic. In reactive eosinophilia, the eosinophilia is a response to an underlying disorder, such as an allergic condition or a tissue invasive parasitic infection. The clonal eosinophilias are myeloid malignancies in which eosinophils are part of the neoplastic clone. Examples include AML with inv(16), *BCR-ABL1* positive CML, disorders associated with *JAK2* mutations or other genetic abnormalities, and the separate myeloid neoplasm categories of eosinophilia with *PDGFR* or *FGFR1* rearrangements. In idiopathic eosinophilia, the reason for the eosinophilia is unknown despite a thorough investigation.[84-86]

Chronic eosinophilic leukemia, not otherwise specified (CEL-NOS) is a clonal eosinophilia in which there is an autonomous, neoplastic proliferation of eosinophils leading to a persistent eosinophilia in blood ($\geq 1.5 \times 10^9$/L), bone marrow, and other organs (Box 1-6). This diagnosis requires not only the exclusion of reactive eosinophilias, but also the exclusion of other hematological neoplasms in which the eosinophils are part of the clone (including those with *PDGFR* or *FGFR1* rearrangements). Abnormal T-cell populations with eosinophilia secondary to cytokine production must also be excluded. Evidence documenting clonality in CEL include the identification of a clonal genetic abnormality or an increase in blasts in the blood (>2%) or bone marrow (5–19%).[87] Advances in our understanding of the molecular pathophysiology of these disorders have shifted an increasing proportion of cases from CEL-NOS to other genetically defined eosinophilic disorders.

Box 1-6 WHO Criteria for Chronic Eosinophilic Leukemia, Not Otherwise Specified[86]

- Eosinophilia more than or equal to 1.5×10^9/L
- There is no Ph chromosome or BCR-ABL1 fusion gene or other myeloproliferative neoplasms (MPNs) or MDS/MPN
- There is no t(5;12)(q31-35;p13) or other rearrangement of *PDGFRB*
- There is no *FIP1L1-PDGFRA* fusion gene or other rearrangement of *PDGFRA*
- There is no rearrangement of *FGFR1*
- The blast cell count in the peripheral blood and bone marrow is less than 20%, and there is no inv(16)(p13q22) or t(16;16)(p13;q22) or other feature diagnostic of AML
- Clonal cytogenetic or molecular genetic abnormality, or blast cells are more than 2% in the peripheral blood or more than 5% in the bone marrow

If a patient has eosinophilia but these criteria are not met, the diagnosis may be reactive eosinophilia, idiopathic hypereosinophilia, or idiopathic hypereosinohpilic syndrome.

WHO, World Health Organization; BCR-ABL1, breakpoint cluster region-Abelson murine leukemia viral oncogene homolog 1; MDS, myelodysplastic; AML, acute myeloid leukemia

Clinical Features

Chronic eosinophilic leukemia-NOS can occur at any age but the peak incidence is in the fourth decade.[87] In about 10% of patients, the eosinophilia is discovered incidentally in otherwise asymptomatic individuals. The most common signs and symptoms at presentation include weakness and fatigue, cough, dyspnea, myalgias or angioedema, rash or fever, and rhinitis.[88] The organs most commonly infiltrated by eosinophils are heart, skin, central nervous system, lungs, spleen, liver, eyes, and gastrointestinal tract.[88] Organ damage results from release of cytokines, enzymes, and others proteins into the tissues by the infiltrating eosinophils.

Laboratory Findings

Persistent eosinophilia is the primary feature of CEL ($\geq 1.5 \times 10^9/L$). The leukocyte count is usually modestly elevated in the range of 20–30 $\times 10^9/L$ although higher counts can occur. The percentage of eosinophils is variable but levels of 30–70% are common. Anemia may be present. The platelet count is variable although thrombocytosis is reported to be more common than thrombocytopenia.[88]

Microscopic Findings

The most prominent feature in the peripheral blood is eosinophilia; the majority of the eosinophils are mature although occasional immature eosinophils including myelocytes and promyelocytes may be present. The eosinophils often exhibit some morphologic abnormalities, such as hypogranularity, nuclear hypo- or hypersegmentation, and cytoplasmic vacuolization. These changes can also be seen in reactive eosinophilia and cannot be used to confirm a diagnosis of CEL. A neutrophilia may also be present. Blasts are usually absent.

The bone marrow is hypercellular with an increase in eosinophils and their precursors. Eosinophil maturation is orderly in most cases with no increase in blasts. Charcot-Leyden crystals are often present. Erythroid precursors and megakaryocytes are usually normal appearing. Dysplasia in other cell lineages or increased blasts (<20%) may be present in occasional cases. Reticulin fibrosis is also common.[87]

Genetic Abnormalities

A variety of genetic aberrations have been reported in CEL-NOS although the mechanism for leukemogenesis in these patients is unknown. These abnormalities include those well recognized in other myeloid neoplasms, such as trisomy 8, monosomy 7, iso(17q), and del(20)(q11q12). Loss of the Y chromosome has been reported in several patients. Other abnormalities including trisomy 10, trisomy 15, 17q+, 15q-, trisomy 21, and complex chromosomal rearrangements have also been reported.[89]

Differential Diagnosis

Before making a diagnosis of CEL-NOS, secondary causes of eosinophilia must be ruled out. Worldwide, the most common underlying cause of secondary eosinophilia is helminthic infection; in Europe and North America, it is allergic/atopic disorders. Other reactive causes include medications, vasculitis, collagen vascular diseases, pulmonary disorders, such as Löeffler syndrome, neoplasms including carcinomas, renal allograft rejection, and many other disorders. In these cases, the eosinophils are produced in response to cytokines, such as interleukin-3, interleukin-5, and granulocyte/macrophage colony stimulating factor, usually produced by T-helper lymphocytes.[84]

Reactive eosinophilia can be seen in association with hematological neoplasms, such as Hodgkin lymphoma, non-Hodgkin lymphoma, especially T-cell lymphoma, and acute lymphoblastic leukemia (LBL). Abnormal populations of T-cells, often clinically occult, can also drive an eosinophilia through production of interleukin-5. These T-cells exhibit an aberrant immunophenotype, typically CD3-CD4+ or CD3+CD4-CD8-, and are often clonal by T-cell receptor gene rearrangement. Some of these patients eventually develop an overt T-cell lymphoma.[90]

The diagnosis of CEL should be made only if evidence for clonality is identified. However, some hematopoietic neoplasms are associated with clonal eosinophilia and these should be excluded before the diagnosis of CEL is made. These include acute leukemias associated with eosinophilia, such as AML with inv(16)(p12q22) or t(16;16)(p13;q22), myelodysplastic neoplasms, and other MPNs. The presence of *BCR-ABL1* rules out a diagnosis of CEL. The presence of rearrangements of *PDGFRA, PDGFRB,* and *FGFR1* also rule out the diagnosis of CEL-NOS.

Treatment and Prognosis

Some patients with CEL respond to prednisone alone or in combination with hydroxyurea. Responses to imatinib alone have been reported in some patients 2.5with eosinophilia without known genetic abnormalities; therefore, some advocate a trial of this agent. Allogeneic stem cell transplant can be considered for patients refractory to drug therapy.[84,91]

MASTOCYTOSIS

Mastocytosis is a MPN characterized by a clonal proliferation of mast cells with infiltration of one or more organs.[92,93] Mastocytosis is heterogenous and broadly divided into cutaneous mastocytosis and systemic mastocytosis. In cutaneous mastocytosis, the disease is confined to the skin. Urticaria pigmentosa is the most common form of cutaneous mastocytosis. It occurs most frequently in children and may regress spontaneously. Systemic mastocytosis occurs in adults and is a persistent disease in which there is widespread organ involvement

Box 1-7 WHO Criteria for Systemic Mastocytosis[86]

Diagnosis required major and one minor criteria or at least three minor criteria

Major criterion

Multifocal, dense infiltrates of mast cells (≥15 mast cells in aggregates) detected in sections of bone marrow and/or other extracutaneous organ(s)

Minor criteria

- In biopsy sections of bone marrow or other extracutaneous organs, more than 25% of the mast cells in the infiltrate are spindle-shaped or have atypical morphology or, of all mast cells in bone marrow aspirate smears, more than 25% are immature or atypical
- Detection of an activating point mutation at codon 816 of KIT in bone marrow, blood, or another extracutaneous organ
- Mast cells in bone marrow, blood, or other extracutaneous organs express CD2 and/or CD25 in addition to normal mast cell markers
- Serum total tryptase persistently exceeds 20 ng/mL (unless there is an associated clonal myeloid disorder, in which case this parameter is not valid).

WHO, World Health Organization.

including bone marrow, lymph node, spleen, and liver. Systemic mastocytosis generally occurs in older adults with a similar incidence in males and females. Systemic mastocytosis is divided into indolent systemic mastocytosis, systemic mastocytosis with associated clonal hematological non-mast cell lineage disease, aggressive mastocytosis, mast cell leukemia, mast cell sarcoma, and extracutaneous mastocytoma.[92,94,95] When systemic mastocytosis is preceded by skin lesions, the diagnosis is generally readily established because of the high degree of clinical suspicion. In the absence of cutaneous lesions, the diagnosis may not be recognized because of the rarity of the disorder and the lack of familiarity with the characteristic pathologic findings. The bone marrow is the most common diagnostic biopsy specimen. Diagnosis of systemic mastocytosis as defined by the WHO is the presence of the major criteria and one minor criteria, or at least three minor criteria (Box 1-7).[92]

Clinical Features

A wide variety of symptoms are associated with mastocytosis. They include constitutional symptoms, skin manifestations, mediator-related symptoms, and musculoskeletal symptoms. Constitutional symptoms, such as weakness, fatigue, fever, night sweats, and weight loss are common. Other symptoms frequently present are attributed to chemical mediators released by the mast cells and include generalized pruritis, urticaria, episodic flushing, headache, tachycardia, bronchospasm, nausea, vomiting, and diarrhea. Patients with aggressive disease are less likely to have skin lesions and more likely to have hepatomegaly, splenomegaly, prominent skeletal lesions and/or fractures, malabsorption, anemia, and/or thrombocytopenia.[92]

Laboratory Findings

Peripheral blood findings in systemic mastocytosis are variable. Eosinophilia is present in about one half of patients. Anemia, leukopenia, leukocytosis, and/or thrombocytopenia may be present. Circulating mast cells are rare. Serum tryptase levels may be elevated in systemic mastocytosis. In the absence of any other known clonal myeloid disorders, the presence of a persistently elevated tryptase over 20 ng/mL is a minor criterion for systemic mastocytosis.[92] In addition, recent studies have demonstrated that the coexistent findings of increased serum β_2-microglobulin levels and decreased LDH levels are closely associated with the presence of aggressive systemic mastocytosis.[96,97]

Microscopic Findings

The major criterion for diagnosis of systemic mastocytosis in the bone marrow is the presence of multifocal dense infiltrates of mast cells. The pattern of infiltration is either focal or diffuse. The focal lesions are paratrabecular, perivascular, or randomly distributed. They may be accompanied by a diffuse interstitial infiltrate surrounding the lesions or throughout the bone marrow. The paratrabecular lesions are sometimes associated with fibrosis and widening of the bony trabeculae. The perivascular lesions are usually associated with medial and adventitial hypertrophy of vessel walls. Dense, diffuse infiltration replacing large portions of bone marrow is rare. In most instances, the mast cell lesions in the bone marrow are polymorphous with an admixture of mast cells, lymphocytes, eosinophils, neutrophils, histiocytes, endothelial cells, and fibroblasts in varying proportions. Occasionally, focal lesions are characterized by a central core of lymphocytes surrounded by mast cells giving a “bull’s eye” appearance to the lesions. Some mast cell lesions appear monomorphic, with the cellular population consisting almost entirely of mast cells. Mast cell morphology in bone marrow sections varies considerably from round with abundant cytoplasm to spindle-shaped. Atypical morphology (e.g., spindle shaped) is a minor criterion for diagnosis of systemic mastocytosis.[92]

Because of the fibrosis that is often associated with mast cell lesions, the bone marrow aspiration smears may not reflect the mast cell proliferation. However, mast cells are occasionally present in smears and may be normal appearing, large with abundant cytoplasm and scattered granules, or even spindle shaped.

Mast cells are difficult to identify in hematoxylin and eosin (H&E) stained sections. A particularly useful technique for detection of mast cells in sections is immunohistochemistry for tryptase. This technique is both sensitive and specific for mast cells. Mast cells are, also, positive for chloroacetate esterase but lack myeloperoxidase. Immunophenotyping is also an important aid in diagnosis of systemic mastocytosis. Mast cells express CD45, CD33, and CD117. They lack CD14,

CD15, CD16, as well as B and T-cell markers. Aberrant expression of CD2 and/or CD25 is a minor criterion for diagnosis of systemic mastocytosis.[92]

Genetic Abnormalities

A point mutation in codon 816 of the c-kit proto-oncogene (usually D816V) is detected in most patients with systemic mastocytosis. This mutation results in activation of *KIT* (c-kit receptor tyrosine kinase) tyrosine kinase but patients are resistant to imatinib. Other mutations of exon 17 of *KIT* have also been identified.[92] Clonal cytogenetic abnormalities have been identified in a significant proportion of patients with systemic mastocytosis. Most have been single abnormalities and include those seen in other myeloid malignancies, such as +8, 5q-, del(7), -7, +13, and del(20). In addition, recent studies have identified point mutations in multiple genes including ten-eleven-translocation 2 (TET2), DNA (cytosine-5)-methyltransferase 3 alpha (DNMT3A), additional sex combs-like protein 1 (ASXL1), and casitas B-cell lymphoma (CBL).[95,98] Cytogenetic abnormalities characteristic of other myeloid neoplasias may be identified when the neoplasia is associated with a case of systemic mastocytosis.

Diagnostic Criteria

Studies subsequent to the publication of the 2008 WHO re-evaluated the WHO criteria used for diagnosis and classification of mastocytosis.[96,97] These studies identified subcategories of mastocytosis in addition to those described in the WHO. These additional categories include well-differentiated systemic mastocytosis, indolent systemic mastocytosis with skin lesions, and indolent systemic mastocytosis without skin lesions. The studies also defined clonal mast cell activation disorders which do not fulfill the criteria for systemic mastocytosis.[96,97] Additional diagnostic tests (serum β_2-microglobulin and LDH) were proposed to further refine the diagnosis and classification of mastocytosis.[96,97]

MYELOPROLIFERATIVE NEOPLASM, UNCLASSIFIABLE

Some patients present with features of an MPN but cannot be readily classified into one of the defined diagnostic categories. In these instances, the designation, MPN, unclassifiable, can be used. Some cases may represent early myeloproliferative disorders lacking one or more of the diagnostic criteria. For example, some patients with abdominal vein thrombosis have been found to have a *JAK2 V617F* mutation even though they do not fit the criteria for either ET or PV. While some of these patients subsequently develop erythrocytosis and/or thrombosis, they represent unclassified MPN when first identified.[26,99] Others may represent end stage MPN including those with prominent fibrosis in which the primary MPN cannot be discerned. Still others may represent cases that exhibit features of one or more diagnostic categories.[100]

MYELOID AND LYMPHOID NEOPLASMS WITH EOSINOPHILIA AND ABNORMALITIES OF *PDGFRA, PDGFRB,* OR *FGFR1*

Myeloid and lymphoid neoplasms with eosinophilia and abnormalities of *PDGFRA, PDGFRB,* or *FGFR1* is a newly defined category of myeloid neoplasms in the 2008 WHO classification consisting of three disease categories all resulting from an aberrant tyrosine kinase encoded by a fusion gene.[20] The presentation of all three disease entities may be as MPNs, but not invariably.[20] Due to the pluripotent nature of the mutated cell of origin, the neoplasms may present as AML T-lymphoblastic lymphoma (T-LBL), or precursor B-lymphoblastic leukemia/lymphoma (pre B-ALL). Eosinophilia is a predominant feature in these disease entities, regardless of the nature of the disease presentation. Correctly diagnosing the entities in this category is critical, as the *PDGFRA* and *PDGFRB* neoplasms are responsive to imatinib.[20,101-103]

Myeloid and Lymphoid Neoplasms with *PDGFRA* Rearrangement

Myeloid and lymphoid neoplasms with *PDGFRA* rearrangement is defined as a MPN, AML, or LBL/lymphoma with prominent eosinophilia and presence of a *FIP1L1-PDGFRA* fusion gene or other variants with a *PDGFRA* rearrangement. *BCR-ABL1* fusion gene must not be present for the diagnosis of this neoplasm.

Clinical Features

The presentation of *PDGFRA* neoplasms is heterogenous, but they typically present as CEL with occasional mast cell and neutrophil involvement. *PDGFRA* neoplasms can also present as AML or T-LBL.[19] Patients often have a marked peripheral blood eosinophilia. Organ damage, such as cardiac or pulmonary damage can be present due to infiltration or the tissues by eosinophils and mast cells, and the subsequent cytokine release. Many patients have fatigue and/or pruritus and symptoms of the affected organs. It is far more common in men, and splenomegaly is common.[20,104]

Laboratory Findings

The most prominent laboratory finding in *PDGFRA* neoplasms is a markedly increased peripheral blood eosinophil count (typically $\geq 1.5 \times 10^9$/L). Serum tryptase is usually increased to more than 12 ng/mL and serum vitamin B12 is elevated.[20]

Microscopic Findings

Similar to the morphologic findings in CEL-NOS, the most prominent feature of the majority of myeloid *PDGFRA* neoplasms is a peripheral blood and bone marrow eosinophilia (Figures 1-7A and B). The eosinophils in the peripheral blood are typically mature, though occasional immature eosinophils can be found. Eosinophil abnormalities may be present including altered granulation and nuclear

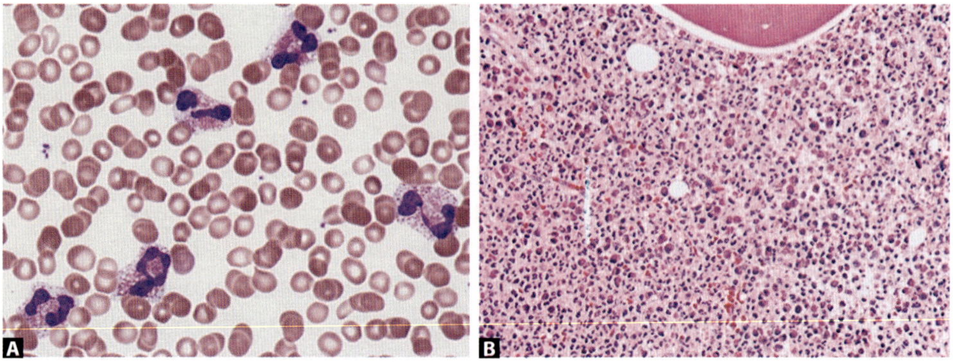

Figure 1-7 Myeloid neoplasm with PDGFRA rearrangement, peripheral blood and bone marrow. **A,** The blood smear exhibited an increase in eosinophils. They appear mature. **B,** The bone marrow biopsy shows a hypercellular bone marrow with a prominent eosinophilia.

hypersegmentation or hyposegmentation.[20] Myeloid *PDGFRA* neoplasms may have mast cell infiltrates which can consist of subtle loose aggregates of mast cells, but most do not meet criteria for systemic mastocytosis.

Genetic Abnormalities

Platelet-derived growth factor receptor-alpha rearrangement usually occurs as a result of a small 800 kb interstitial deletion on chromosome 4q12 that results in fusion of the *PDGFRA* gene to the centromeric *FIP1L1* gene. The protein product of this fusion gene is a constitutively activated tyrosine kinase that is inhibited by imatinib.[10,20] The frequency of the *FIP1L1-PDGFRA* fusion gene in eosinophilic neoplasms is not known as reports have varied widely.[18] The fusion is not apparent on conventional cytogenetic analysis but can be detected by real time-polymerase chain reaction (RT-PCR) or FISH. CHIC2 deletion, detected by FISH, is a surrogate assay for the *FIP1L1-PDGFRA* fusion gene.[105] Analysis suggests that the fusion gene occurs in a pluripotent progenitor cell that may give rise to many cells including eosinophils and mast cells.[106] Other fusion genes associated with similar eosinophilic disorders have also been described including *BCR-PDGFRA, KIF5B-PDGFRA,* and *CDK5RAP2-PDGFRA.*[84]

Myeloid Neoplasms with *PDGFRB* Rearrangement

Myeloid neoplasms with *PDGFRB* rearrangement are defined as myeloid neoplasms occurring with rearrangement of *PDGFRB* at 5q31~33. These neoplasms typically present similar to chronic myelomonocytic leukemia (CMML) with eosinophilia, but can also present similar to other types of myeloid neoplasms including atypical CML, CEL, and AML.

Clinical Features

The myeloid *PDGFRB* neoplasms are more common in men than in women. Though the *PDGFRB* neoplasms can present as various types of myeloid neoplasms, the usual presentation is CMML. Eosinophilia is frequently found, but not always. As with the *PDGFRA* neoplasms, splenomegaly is common, and organ damage occurs from infiltration by eosinophils.[20]

Laboratory Findings

Peripheral blood eosinophilia is frequently found and serum tryptase may be elevated. Giving the heterogeneity of the presentation of the myeloid *PDGFRB* neoplasms, there are few definitive laboratory findings and the diagnosis is based on molecular abnormalities.[20]

Microscopic Findings

The morphology of myeloid *PDGFRB* neoplasms is heterogenous and is dependent on the presentation. In the peripheral blood there is typically a leukocytosis with increased neutrophils, eosinophils, monocytes and immature myeloid cells.[20,107] The bone marrow is hypercellular and there may be an increase of mast cells.[107]

Genetic Abnormalities

The majority of patients with myeloid neoplasms with *PDGFRB* harbor the t(5;12)(q33;p13); this translocation results in fusion of the tyrosine kinase encoding region of *PDGRFB* on chromosome 5q33 to *ETV6* on chromosome 12p13. Other rearrangements involving the *PDGRFB* gene have also been documented.[18,91] These cytogenetic aberrations produce a MPN that is typically associated with prominent eosinophilia and sometimes monocytosis.[20] Patients with *PDGRFB* rearrangements respond to imatinib, making it especially important to recognize patients with this abnormality.[84]

Myeloid and Lymphoid Neoplasms with *FGFR1* Abnormalities

In the myeloid and lymphoid neoplasms with *FGFR1* abnormalities, a mutation in a pluripotent stem cell results in a MPN featuring eosinophilia or lymphoblastic lymphoma, usually precursor T-cell type. The disease morphology is heterogenous, but around 90% of patients with this disease will have eosinophilia. This disorder frequently progresses to AML 1–2 years after diagnosis and is associated with poor prognosis. Also known as 8p11 myeloproliferative syndrome, multiple translocations with a chromosomal 8p11 breakpoint can give rise to the *FGFR1* fusion genes. *FGFR1* can have multiple fusion partners, all giving rise to the aberrantly activated tyrosine kinase.[19] This neoplasm is not responsive to any imatinib or other current therapies, and the outcome is poor. In vitro studies suggest the *FGFR1* inhibitor ponatinib may have efficacy in this neoplasm, but clinical trials have not been completed to test the effects on patients.[108]

Clinical Features

The clinical findings are heterogeneous in neoplasms with *FGFR1* abnormalities. Some patients present with lymphoma and some patients present with splenomegaly as a result of myeloproliferation. Given the systemic nature of the neoplasms, systemic symptoms like fever, and weight loss may be present.[20,104]

Laboratory Findings

Peripheral blood eosinophilia is commonly found in neoplasms with *FGFR1* abnormalities. Other laboratory findings are widely variable and are dependent on the type of presentation of the neoplasm.

Microscopic Findings

There are also widely variable findings in the morphology in the presentation of neoplasms with *FGFR1* abnormalities.[20,109] The most common feature is eosinophilia, occurring in about 90%.[20] Patients presenting in both chronic phase and acute leukemic or lymphoblastic phases can have eosinophilia.[20,104] Patients presenting with a lymphoma may have eosinophilic infiltration in the lymphoma.[20] In the chronic form of the neoplasm, neutrophils and occasionally monocytes are also elevated in the peripheral blood. Lymphoblasts and myeloblasts will be present in the peripheral blood or bone marrow in the acute presentation of the neoplasm.[20]

Genetic Abnormalities

The most common translocation is t(8;13)(p11;q12). In this translocation, the *FGFR1* is fused to the *ZNF198* gene on chromosome 13q12 which results aberrant *FGFR1* tyrosine activity.[18] Other translocations include t(8;9)(p11;q33), t(6;8)(q27;p11), and t(q8;22)(p11;q22).[91]

REFERENCES

1. Vardiman J, Brunning R, Arber D, et al. Introduction and overview of the classification of the myeloid neoplasms. In: Swerdlow SH, Campo E, Harris NL, Jaffe ES, Pileri SA, Stein H, editors. WHO Classification of Tumours of Haematopoietic and Lymphoid Tissues. 4th ed. Lyon, USA: International Agency for Research on Cancer Press; 2008.
2. Deininger M, Buchdunger E, Druker BJ. The development of imatinib as a therapeutic agent for chronic myeloid leukemia. *Blood.* 2005;105(7):2640-53.
3. Druker BJ, Guilhot F, O'Brien SG, et al. Five-year follow-up of patients receiving imatinib for chronic myeloid leukemia. *N Engl J Med.* 2006;355(23):2408-17.
4. Goldman JM, Melo JV. Chronic myeloid leukemia--advances in biology and new approaches to treatment. *N Engl J Med.* 2003;349(15):1451-64.
5. James C, Ugo V, Le Couédic JP, et al. A unique clonal JAK2 mutation leading to constitutive signalling causes polycythaemia vera. *Nature.* 2005;434(7037):1144-48.
6. Jones AV, Kreil S, Zoi K, et al. Widespread occurrence of the JAK2 V617F mutation in chronic myeloproliferative disorders. *Blood.* 2005;106(6):2162-8.
7. Tefferi A, Gilliland DG. The JAK2V617F tyrosine kinase mutation in myeloproliferative disorders: status report and immediate implications for disease classification and diagnosis. *Mayo Clin Proc.* 2005;80(7):947-58.
8. Levine RL, Wadleigh M, Cools J, et al. Activating mutation in the tyrosine kinase JAK2 in polycythemia vera, essential thrombocythemia, and myeloid metaplasia with myelofibrosis. *Cancer Cell.* 2005;7(4):387-97.

9. Kralovics R, Passamonti F, Buser AS, et al. A gain-of-function mutation of JAK2 in myeloproliferative disorders. *N Engl J Med.* 2005;352(17):1779-90.
10. Cools J, DeAngelo DJ, Gotlib J, et al. A tyrosine kinase created by fusion of the PDGFRA and FIP1L1 genes as a therapeutic target of imatinib in idiopathic hypereosinophilic syndrome. *N Engl J Med.* 2003;348(13):1201-14.
11. Pardanani A, Reeder T, Porrata LF, et al. Imatinib therapy for hypereosinophilic syndrome and other eosinophilic disorders. *Blood.* 2003;101(9):3391-7.
12. Mesa RA. Ruxolitinib, a selective JAK1 and JAK2 inhibitor for the treatment of myeloproliferative neoplasms and psoriasis. *IDrugs.* 2010;13(6):394-403.
13. Harrison C, Kiladjian JJ, Al-Ali HK, et al. JAK inhibition with ruxolitinib versus best available therapy for myelofibrosis. *N Engl J Med.* 2012;366(9):787-98.
14. Flach J, Dicker F, Schnittger S, et al. Mutations of JAK2 and TET2, but not CBL are detectable in a high portion of patients with refractory anemia with ring sideroblasts and thrombocytosis. *Haematologica.* 2010;95(3):518-9.
15. Martinez-Avilés L, Besses C, Alvarez-Larran A, et al. TET2, ASXL1, IDH1, IDH2, and c-CBL genes in JAK2- and MPI -negative myeloproliferative neoplasms. *Ann Hematol.* 2012; 91(4):533-41.
16. Brecqueville M, Rey J, Bertucci F, et al. Mutation analysis of ASXL1, CBL, DNMT3A, IDH1, IDH2, JAK2, MPL, NF1, SF3B1, SUZ12, and TET2 in myeloproliferative neoplasms. *Genes Chromosomes Cancer.* 2012;51(8):743-55.
17. Klampfl T, Gisslinger H, Harutyunyan A, et al. Somatic mutations of calreticulin in myeloproliferative neoplasms. *N Engl J Med.* 2013;369:2379-90.
18. Gotlib J, Cross NC, Gilliland DG. Eosinophilic disorders: molecular pathogenesis, new classification, and modern therapy. *Best Pract Res Clin Haematol.* 2006;19(3):535-69.
19. Wadleigh M, DeAngelo DJ, Griffin JD, et al. After chronic myelogenous leukemia: tyrosine kinase inhibitors in other hematologic malignancies. *Blood.* 2005;105(1):22-30.
20. Bain B, Gilliland D, Horny H, Vardiman J. Myeloid and lymphoid neoplasms with eosinophilia and abnormalities of PDGFRA, PDGFRB, or FGFR1. In: Swerdlow SH, Campo E, Harris NL, Jaffe ES, Pileri SA, Stein H, et al., editors. WHO Classification of Tumours of Haematopoietic and Lymphoid Tissues. 4th ed. Lyon, USA: International Agency for Research on Cancer Press; 2008.
21. Deininger MW, Goldman JM, Melo JV. The molecular biology of chronic myeloid leukemia. *Blood.* 2000;96(10):3343-56.
22. Vardiman J, Velo J, Baccarani M, Thiele J. Chronic myelogenous leukemia, BCR-ABL1 positive. In: Swerdlow SH, Campo E, Harris NL, Jaffe ES, Pileri SA, Stein H, et al., editors. WHO Classification of Tumours of Haematopoietic and Lymphoid Tissues, 4th ed. Lyon, USA: International Agency for Research on Cancer Press; 2008.pp.32-7.
23. Dickstein JI, Vardiman JW. Hematopathologic findings in the myeloproliferative disorders. *Semin Oncol.* 1995;22(4):355-73.
24. Anastasi J, Musvee T, Roulston D, et al. Pseudo-Gaucher histiocytes identified up to 1 year after transplantation for CML are BCR/ABL-positive. *Leukemia.* 1998;12(2):233-7.
25. Sawyers CL. Chronic myeloid leukemia. *N Engl J Med.* 1999;340(17):1330-40.
26. Tefferi A, Thiele J, Orazi A, et al. Proposals and rationale for revision of the World Health Organization diagnostic criteria for polycythemia vera, essential thrombocythemia, and primary myelofibrosis: Recommendation from an ad hoc international expert panel. Blood. 2007:110(4):1092-7.
27. Thiele J, Kvasnicka H, Orazi A, Tefferi A, Birgegard G. Polycythaemia vera. In: Swerdlow SH, Campo E, Harris NL, Jaffe ES, Pileri SA, Stein H, et al., editors. WHO Classification of Tumors of Hematopoietic and Lymphoid Tissues. 4th ed. Lyon, USA: International Agency for Research on Cancer Press; 2008.

28. Tefferi A. Polycythemia vera: a comprehensive review and clinical recommendations. Mayo Clin Proc. 2003;78(2):174-94.
29. Berlin N. Polycythemia vera. *Hematol Oncol Clin North Am.* 2003;17(5):1191-210.
30. Pierre R, Imbert M, Thiele J, Vardiman JW, Brunning RD, Flandrin G. Polycythaemia vera. In: Jaffe ES HNL, Stein H, Vardiman JW, editors. World Health Organization Classification of Tumours: Pathology and Genetics of Tumours of Haematopoietic and Lymphoid Tissues. Lyon, USA: International Agency for Research on Cancer Press; 2001.pp.32-4.
31. Thiele J, Kvasnicka HM, Vardiman J. Bone marrow histopathology in the diagnosis of chronic myeloproliferative disorders: A forgotten pearl. *Best Pract Res Clin Haematol.* 2006;19(3):413-37.
32. Peterson P, Ellis J. The bone marrow in polycythemia vera. In: Wasserman L, Berk P, Berlin N, editors. Polycythemia vera and the Myeloproliferative Disorders. Philadelphia: WB Saunders; 1995.p.31.
33. Najfeld V, Montella L, Scalise A, et al. Exploring polycythaemia vera with fluorescence in situ hybridization: additional cryptic 9p is the most frequent abnormality detected. *Br J Haematol.* 2002;119(2):558-66.
34. Baxter EJ, Scott LM, Campbell PJ, et al. Acquired mutation of the tyrosine kinase JAK2 in human myeloproliferative disorders. *Lancet.* 2005;365(9464):1054-61.
35. Tefferi A, Lasho TL, Schwager SM, et al. The clinical phenotype of wild-type, heterozygous, and homozygous JAK2V617F in polycythemia vera. *Cancer.* 2006;106(3):631-5.
36. Scott LM, Tong W, Levine RL, et al. JAK2 exon 12 mutations in polycythemia vera and idiopathic erythrocytosis. *N Engl J Med.* 2007;356(5):459-68.
37. Passamonti F, Rumi E, Pungolino E, et al. Life expectancy and prognostic factors for survival in patients with polycythemia vera and essential thrombocythemia. *Am J Med.* 2004;117(10):755-61.
38. Marchioli R, Finazzi G, Landolfi R, et al. Vascular and neoplastic risk in a large cohort of patients with polycythemia vera. *J Clin Oncol.* 2005;23(10):2224-32.
39. Finazzi G, Caruso V, Marchioli R, et al. Acute leukemia in polycythemia vera: an analysis of 1638 patients enrolled in a prospective observational study. *Blood.* 2005;105(7):2664-70.
40. Barosi G, Mesa RA, Thiele J, et al. Proposed criteria for the diagnosis of post-polycythemia vera and post-essential thrombocythemia myelofibrosis: a consensus statement from the International Working Group for Myelofibrosis Research and Treatment. *Leukemia.* 2008;22(2):437-38.
41. Hernández JM, Orfao A, González M, et al. Immunophenotypic characterisation of acute leukaemia after polycythemia vera. *J Clin Pathol.* 1993;46(7):668-71.
42. Thiele J, Kvasnicka H, Tefferi A, Barosi G, Orazi A, Vardiman J. Primary myelofibrosis. In: Swerdlow SH, Campo E, Harris NL, Jaffe ES, Pileri SA, Stein H, et al., editors. WHO Classification of Tumours of Haematopoietic and Lymphoid Tissues, 4th ed. Lyon, USA: International Agency for Research on Cancer Press; 2008.
43. Reeder TL, Bailey RJ, Dewald GW, et al. Both B and T lymphocytes may be clonally involved in myelofibrosis with myeloid metaplasia. *Blood.* 2003;101(5):1981-3.
44. Chagraoui H, Komura E, Tulliez M, et al. Prominent role of TGF-beta 1 in thrombopoietin-induced myelofibrosis in mice. *Blood.* 2002;100(10):3495-503.
45. Tefferi A. New insights into the pathogenesis and drug treatment of myelofibrosis. *Curr Opin Hematol.* 2006;13(2):87-92.
46. Barosi G. Myelofibrosis with myeloid metaplasia. *Hematol Oncol Clin North Am.* 2003; 17(5):1211-26.
47. Thiele J, Kvasnicka HM, Boeltken B, et al. Initial (prefibrotic) stages of idiopathic (primary) myelofibrosis (IMF) - a clinicopathological study. *Leukemia.* 1999;13(11):1741-8.

48. Dupriez B, Morel P, Demory JL, et al. Prognostic factors in agnogenic myeloid metaplasia: a report on 195 cases with a new scoring system. *Blood.* 1996;88(3):1013-8.
49. Thiele J, Kvasnicka HM, Zankovich R, et al. Early-stage idiopathic (primary) myelofibrosis--current issues of diagnostic features. *Leuk Lymphoma.* 2002;43(5):1035-41.
50. Barosi G, Viarengo G, Pecci A, et al. Diagnostic and clinical relevance of the number of circulating CD34(+) cells in myelofibrosis with myeloid metaplasia. *Blood.* 2001;98(12):3249-55.
51. Mesa RA, Hanson CA, Rajkumar SV, et al. Evaluation and clinical correlations of bone marrow angiogenesis in myelofibrosis with myeloid metaplasia. *Blood.* 2000;96(10):3374-80.
52. Thiele J, Pierre R, Imbert M, Vardiman J, Brunning R, Flandrin G. Chronic idiopathic myelofibrosis. In: Jaffe ES HN, Stein H, Vardiman JW, editors. World Health Organization Classification of Tumours: Pathology and Genetics of Tumours of Haematopoietic and Lymphoid Tissues. Lyon: International Agency for Research on Cancer Press; 2001.pp. 35-8.
53. Dingli D, Grand FH, Mahaffey V, et al. Der(6)t(1;6)(q21-23;p21.3): a specific cytogenetic abnormality in myelofibrosis with myeloid metaplasia. *Br J Haematol.* 2005;130(2):229-32.
54. Al-Assar O, Ul-Hassan A, Brown R, et al. Gains on 9p are common genomic aberrations in idiopathic myelofibrosis: a comparative genomic hybridization study. *Br J Haematol.* 2005;129(1):66-71.
55. Pardanani AD, Levine RL, Lasho T, et al. MPL515 mutations in myeloproliferative and other myeloid disorders: a study of 1182 patients. *Blood.* 2006;108(10):3472-6.
56. Tefferi A, Barosi G, Mesa RA, et al. International Working Group (IWG) consensus criteria for treatment response in myelofibrosis with myeloid metaplasia, for the IWG for Myelofibrosis Research and Treatment (IWG-MRT). *Blood.* 2006;108(5):1497-503.
57. Mesa RA, Li CY, Ketterling RP, et al. Leukemic transformation in myelofibrosis with myeloid metaplasia: a single-institution experience with 91 cases. *Blood.* 2005;105(3):973-7.
58. Pullarkat V, Bass RD, Gong JZ, et al. Primary autoimmune myelofibrosis: definition of a distinct clinicopathologic syndrome. *Am J Hematol.* 2003;72(1):8-12.
59. Thiele J, Kvasnicka H, Orazi A, Tefferi A, Gisslinger H. Essential thrombocythaemia. In: Swerdlow S, Campo E, Harris N, et al.,(Eds). WHO Classification of Tumours of Haematopoietic and Lymphoid Tissues. Lyon: International Agency for Research on Cancer Press; 2008.
60. Mesa RA, Silverstein MN, Jacobsen SJ, et al. Population-based incidence and survival figures in essential thrombocythemia and agnogenic myeloid metaplasia: an Olmsted County Study, 1976-1995. *Am J Hematol.* 1999;61(1):10-15.
61. Fenaux P, Simon M, Caulier MT, et al. Clinical course of essential thrombocythemia in 147 cases. *Cancer.* 1990;66(3):549-56.
62. Tefferi A. Essential thrombocythemia: scientific advances and current practice. *Curr Opin Hematol.* 2006;13(2):93-8.
63. Dame C, Sutor AH. Primary and secondary thrombocytosis in childhood. *Br J Haematol.* 2005;129(2):165-77.
64. Elliott MA, Tefferi A. Thrombosis and haemorrhage in polycythaemia vera and essential thrombocythaemia. *Br J Haematol.* 2005;128(3):275-90.
65. Wright CA, Tefferi A. A single institutional experience with 43 pregnancies in essential thrombocythemia. *Eur J Haematol.* 2001;66(3):152-59.
66. Wolanskyj AP, Lasho TL, Schwager SM, et al. JAK2 mutation in essential thrombocythaemia: clinical associations and long-term prognostic relevance. *Br J Haematol.* 2005;131(2):208-13.
67. Schafer AI. Thrombocytosis. *N Engl J Med.* 2004;350(12):1211-19.
68. Imbert M, Pierre R, Thiele J, Vardiman J, Brunning R, Flandrin G. Essential thrombocythemia. In: ES Jaffe NH, Stein H, JW Vardiman, editors. World Health Organization Classification of Tumours Pathology and Genetics of Tumours of the Haematopoietic and Lymphoid Tissues. Lyon: International Agency for Research on Cancer Press; 2001.pp.39-41.

69. El-Kassar N, Hetet G, Briére J, et al. Clonality analysis of hematopoiesis and thrombopoietin levels in patients with essential thrombocythemia. *Leuk Lymphoma.* 1998;30(1-2):181-8.
70. Thiele J, Kvasnicka HM. A critical reappraisal of the WHO classification of the chronic myeloproliferative disorders. *Leuk Lymphoma.* 2006;47(3):381-96.
71. Campbell PJ, Scott LM, Buck G, et al. Definition of subtypes of essential thrombocythaemia and relation to polycythaemia vera based on JAK2 V617F mutation status: a prospective study. *Lancet.* 2005;366(9501):1945-53.
72. Heller PG, Lev PR, Salim JP, et al. JAK2V617F mutation in platelets from essential thrombocythemia patients: correlation with clinical features and analysis of STAT5 phosphorylation status. *Eur J Haematol.* 2006;77(3):210-6.
73. Cheung B, Radia D, Pantelidis P, et al. The presence of the JAK2 V617F mutation is associated with a higher haemoglobin and increased risk of thrombosis in essential thrombocythaemia. *Br J Haematol.* 2006;132(2):244-5.
74. Barbui T, Thiele J, Passamonti F, et al. Survival and disease progression in essential thrombocythemia are significantly influenced by accurate morphologic diagnosis: an international study. *J Clin Oncol.* 2011;29(23):3179-84.
75. Douglas VK, Tallman MS, Cripe LD, et al. Thrombopoietin administered during induction chemotherapy to patients with acute myeloid leukemia induces transient morphologic changes that may resemble chronic myeloproliferative disorders. *Am J Clin Pathol.* 2002; 117(6):844-50.
76. Ding J, Komatsu H, Wakita A, et al. Familial essential thrombocythemia associated with a dominant-positive activating mutation of the c-MPL gene, which encodes for the receptor for thrombopoietin. *Blood.* 2004;103(11):4198-200.
77. Bain B, Brunning R, Vardiman J, Thiele J. Chronic neutrophilic leukemia. In: Swerdlow SH, Campo E, Harris NL, Jaffe ES, Pileri SA, Stein H, et al., editors. WHO Classification of Tumours of Haematopoietic and Lymphoid Tissues. 4th ed. Lyon: International Agency for Research on Cancer Press; 2008.
78. Elliott MA. Chronic neutrophilic leukemia and chronic myelomonocytic leukemia: WHO defined. *Best Pract Res Clin Haematol.* 2006;19(3):571-93.
79. Elliott MA, Hanson CA, Dewald GW, et al. WHO-defined chronic neutrophilic leukemia: a long-term analysis of 12 cases and a critical review of the literature. *Leukemia.* 2005;19(2): 313-7.
80. Reilly JT. Chronic neutrophilic leukaemia: a distinct clinical entity? *Br J Haematol.* 2002; 116(1):10-8.
81. Imbert M, Bain B, Pierre R, Vardiman J, Brunning R, Flandrin G. Chronic neutrophilic leukemia. In: Jaffee ES HN, Stein H, Vardiman JW, editors. World Health Organization Classification of Tumours: Pathology and Genetics of Tumours of Haematopoietic and Lymphoid Tissues. Lyon: International Agency for Research on Cancer Press; 2001 pp 27-8.
82. Steensma DP, Dewald GW, Lasho TL, et al. The JAK2 V617F activating tyrosine kinase mutation is an infrequent event in both "atypical" myeloproliferative disorders and myelodysplastic syndromes. *Blood.* 2005;106(4):1207-9.
83. Tefferi A, Elliott MA, Pardanani A. Atypical myeloproliferative disorders: diagnosis and management. *Mayo Clin Proc.* 2006;81(4):553-63.
84. Fletcher S, Bain B. Diagnosis and treatment of hypereosinophilic syndromes. *Curr Opin Hematol.* 2007;14(1):37-42.
85. Tefferi A, Patnaik MM, Pardanani A. Eosinophilia: secondary, clonal and idiopathic. *Br J Haematol.* 2006;133(5):468-92.
86. Bain B, Gilliland D, Vardiman J, Horny H. Chronic eosinophilic leukemia, not otherwise specified. In: Swerdlow SH, Campo E, Harris NL, Jaffe ES, Pileri SA, Stein H, et al., editors. WHO Classification of Tumours of Haematopoietic and Lymphoid Tissues. 4th ed. Lyon: International Agency for Research on Cancer Press; 2008.

87. Bain B, Pierre R, Imbert M, JW V, RD B, Flandrin G. Chronic eosinophilic leukemia and the hypereosinophilic syndrome. In: Jaffee ES HN, Stein H, Vardiman JW, editors. World Health Organization Classification of Tumours Pathology and Genetics of Tumours of the Haematopoietic and Lymphoid Tissues. Lyon: International Agency for Research on Cancer Press; 2001. pp. 29-31.
88. Gotlib J, Cools J, Malone JM, et al. The FIP1L1-PDGFRalpha fusion tyrosine kinase in hypereosinophilic syndrome and chronic eosinophilic leukemia: implications for diagnosis, classification, and management. *Blood.* 2004;103(8):2879-91.
89. Bain BJ. Cytogenetic and molecular genetic aspects of eosinophilic leukaemias. *Br J Haematol.* 2003;122(2):173-9.
90. Simon HU, Plotz SG, Dummer R, et al. Abnormal clones of T cells producing interleukin-5 in idiopathic eosinophilia. *N Engl J Med.* 1999;341(15):1112-20.
91. Tefferi A. Blood eosinophilia: a new paradigm in disease classification, diagnosis, and treatment. *Mayo Clin Proc.* 2005;80(1):75-83.
92. Horny H, Metcalfe D, Bennett J, et al. Mastocytosis. In: Swerdlow SH, Campo E, Harris NL, Jaffe ES, Pileri SA, Stein H, et al., editors. WHO Classification of Tumours of Haematopoietic and Lymphoid Tissues, 4th ed. Lyon: International Agency for Research on Cancer Press; 2008 pp 54-63.
93. Pardanani A. Systemic mastocytosis in adults: 2012 Update on diagnosis, risk stratification, and management. *Am J Hematol.* 2012;87(4):401-11.
94. Pardanani A, Lim KH, Lasho TL, et al. WHO subvariants of indolent mastocytosis: clinical details and prognostic evaluation in 159 consecutive adults. *Blood.* 2010;115(1):150-1.
95. Traina F, Visconte V, Jankowska AM, et al. Single nucleotide polymorphism array lesions, TET2, DNMT3A, ASXL1 and CBL mutations are present in systemic mastocytosis. *PLoS One.* 2012;7(8):e43090.
96. Alvarez-Twose I, Morgado JM, Sánchez-Munoz L, et al. Current state of biology and diagnosis of clonal mast cell diseases in adults. *Int J Lab Hematol.* 2012;34(5):445-60.
97. Sánchez-Munoz L, Alvarez-Twose I, Garcia-Montero AC, et al. Evaluation of the WHO criteria for the classification of patients with mastocytosis. *Mod Pathol.* 2011;24(9):1157-68.
98. Tefferi A, Levine RL, Lim KH, et al. Frequent TET2 mutations in systemic mastocytosis: clinical, KITD816V and FIP1L1-PDGFRA correlates. *Leukemia.* 2009;23(5):900-4.
99. Patel RK, Lea NC, Heneghan MA, et al. Prevalence of the activating JAK2 tyrosine kinase mutation V617F in the Budd-Chiari syndrome. *Gastroenterology.* 2006;130(7):2031-8.
100. Kvasnicka H, Bain B, Thiele J, Orazi A, Horny H, Vardiman J. Myeloproliferative neoplasm, unclassifiable. In: Swerdlow SH, Campo E, Harris NL, Jaffe ES, Pileri SA, Stein H, Thiele J, Vardiman JW, et al., editors. WHO Classification of Tumours of Haematopoietic and Lymphoid Tissues, 4th ed. Lyon: International Agency for Research on Cancer Press; 2008.
101. Rathe M, Kristensen TK, Møller MB, et al. Myeloid neoplasm with prominent eosinophilia and PDGFRA rearrangement treated with imatinib mesylate. *Pediatr Blood Cancer.* 2010;55(4):730-2.
102. Curtis CE, Grand FH, Musto P, et al. Two novel imatinib-responsive PDGFRA fusion genes in chronic eosinophilic leukaemia. *Br J Haematol.* 2007;138(1):77-81.
103. David M, Cross NC, Burgstaller S, et al. Durable responses to imatinib in patients with PDGFRB fusion gene-positive and BCR-ABL-negative chronic myeloproliferative disorders. *Blood.* 2007;109(1):61-4.
104. Bain BJ. Myeloid and lymphoid neoplasms with eosinophilia and abnormalities of PDGFRA, PDGFRB or FGFR1. *Haematologica.* 2010;95(5):696-8.
105. Pardanani A, Ketterling RP, Brockman SR, et al. CHIC2 deletion, a surrogate for FIP1L1-PDGFRA fusion, occurs in systemic mastocytosis associated with eosinophilia and predicts response to imatinib mesylate therapy. *Blood.* 2003;102(9):3093-6.

106. Robyn J, Lemery S, McCoy JP, et al. Multilineage involvement of the fusion gene in patients with FIP1L1/PDGFRA-positive hypereosinophilic syndrome. *Br J Haematol.* 2006; 132(3): 286-92.
107. Walz C, Metzgeroth G, Haferlach C, et al. Characterization of three new imatinib-responsive fusion genes in chronic myeloproliferative disorders generated by disruption of the platelet-derived growth factor receptor beta gene. Haematologica. 2007;92(2):163-9.
108. Lierman E, Smits S, Cools J, et al. Ponatinib is active against imatinib-resistant mutants of FIP1L1-PDGFRA and KIT, and against FGFR1-derived fusion kinases. *Leukemia.* 2012;26(7):1693-5.
109. Mayeur-Rousse C, Sorel N, Voldoire M, et al. Unique association of systemic mastocytosis and myeloid/lymphoid neoplasm in blast crisis with abnormality of FGFR1 gene. *Leuk Res.* 2012;36(3):377-81.

CHAPTER

2 Insights into Disease Pathogenesis of the Myeloproliferative Neoplasms

Laure Gilles, John Crispino

INTRODUCTION

The myeloproliferative neoplasms (MPNs) are a heterogeneous group of malignant hematopoietic disorders which include polycythemia vera (PV), essential thrombocythemia (ET), primary myelofibrosis (PMF), and chronic myeloid leukemia (CML). The classification also includes other rare hematopoietic disorders, such as chronic neutrophilic leukemia, chronic eosinophilic leukemia, mastocytosis, and unclassified MPNs. All of these diseases are clonal hematopoietic disorders that result from the transformation of a pluripotent hematopoietic progenitor cell, which in turn causes increased hematopoiesis and an overproduction of normal and differentiated blood cells. In several subtypes, myeloproliferation occurs as a result of genetic changes that lead to cytokine independence. The type of blood cell that is preferentially amplified is specific to the disease: the granulocytic lineage (neutrophils, eosinophils, and basophils) in CML, the erythroid lineage in PV, the megakaryocytic lineage (and its derivative, platelets) in ET, and the granulocytic/megakaryocytic lineages in PMF.

In more than 95% of cases, CML is associated with the chromosomal translocation (9;22)(q34;q11.2), commonly known as the Philadelphia chromosome. The translocation leads to the presence of the oncogenic breakpoint cluster region (BCR)-Abelson leukemia virus (ABL) fusion protein in hematopoietic stem cells (HSCs). As a consequence of this fusion, there is constitutive activation of the ABL kinase and related pathways. The myeloproliferative chronic phase of the disease is followed by an accelerated phase during which normal maturation of hematopoietic cells ceases and transformation to acute myeloid leukemia (AML) occurs. This translocation is not seen in other forms of MPNs: thus, PV, ET, and PMF are commonly known as BCR-ABL negative MPNs.

In contrast to CML, whose genetic basis was described in 1973, the molecular pathogenesis of BCR-ABL negative MPNs remained poorly understood until the discovery of Janus kinase 2 (JAK2) V617F (a change of valine to phenylalanine at the 617 position) mutation in 2005.[1–5] The JAK2V617F alteration is present in PV, ET and PMF at different frequencies. Since this seminal discovery, a plethora of mutations have been identified in MPNs. Early investigations focused on mutations in signaling pathways and led to the identification of defects in myeloproliferative leukemia (*MPL*), *LNK*, casitas B-cell lymphoma (*CBL*), suppressor of cytokine signaling (SOCS) 1, SOCS2, and SOCS3, *NRAS*, and neurofibromatosis 1 gene (*NF1*) (Figure 2-1). Other genes implicated in pathogenesis of MPNs include transcription factors, such as *RUNX1* and *IKZF1* (IKAROS family zinc finger 1) and cell cycle and apoptosis regulators, including *RB1* and *TP53*. More recently, insights into the importance of epigenetic gene regulation have resulted in the discovery of new class of mutations. This latter group includes genes that are responsible for deoxyribonucleic acid (DNA) methylation and histone modifications such as ten-eleven-translocation 2 (*TET2*), additional sex combs-like protein 1 (*ASXL1*), enhancer of zeste homolog 2 (*EZH2*), isocitrate dehydrogenases 1 and 2 (*IDH1*, *IDH2*), and DNA (cytosine-5)-methyltransferase 3 alpha (*DNMT3A*) (Figure 2-2).

This chapter will focus on the molecular events implicated in the initiation, development and transformation of BCR-ABL negative disorders.

MUTATIONS IN GENES REGULATING SIGNAL TRANSDUCTION PATHWAYS

Janus Kinase 2

The JAK2 V617F mutation was identified in 2005 and currently represents the most prevalent mutation in BCR-ABL negative MPN. This mutation is present in 95–99% of PV, 50–70% of ET and 40–50% of PMF patients.[6] The JAK2 V617F mutation affects the non-catalytic pseudo-kinase domain (JH2) and is the result of a somatic G to C mutation, which leads to the substitution of a valine to phenylalaline at the 617 codon. The pseudo-kinase domain is required for inhibiting the basal activity of the JH1 kinase domain of JAK2. When the mutation is present, the protein remains phosphorylated even in the absence of any cytokine, which leads to the constitutive activation of downstream signaling pathways.

Janus kinase 2 interacts with three homodimeric receptors: (1) the erythropoietin receptor (EPO-R); (2) myeloproliferative leukemia (MPL) [the thrombopoietin (TPO) receptor]; and (3) granulocyte colony-stimulating factor (G-CSF) receptor. In normal cells, binding of cytokines to their respective receptors induces JAK2 phosphorylation, which results in recruitment of STAT (signal transducer and activator of transcription) proteins and activation of phosphoinositide-3-kinase (PI3K)-Akt [akt kinase (protein kinase B)] and the mitogen-activated protein kinase (MAPK) signaling pathways. Activation of this signaling cascade drives cell proliferation and survival. In the presence of JAK2 V617F, cells continue to proliferate and escape apoptosis.

Different mouse models have been developed to mimic the human diseases. In the first- generation model, bone marrow cells were retrovirally transduced by JAK2

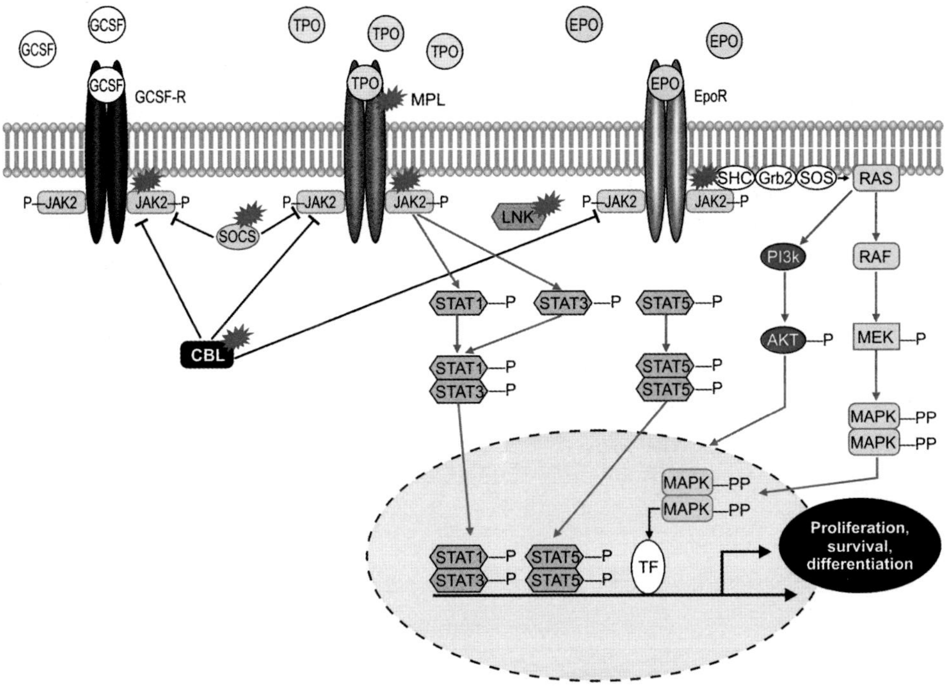

JAK, Janus kinase 2; STAT, signal transducer and activator of transcription; G-CSF, granulocyte colony-stimulating factor; TPO, thrombopoietin; EPO, erythropoietin; PI3K, phosphoinositide-3-kinase; Akt, akt kinase (protein kinase B); MAPK, mitogen-activated protein kinase; CBL, casitas B-cell lymphoma; SOCS, suppressor of cytokine signaling; MPL, myeloproliferative leukemia; MPNs, myeloproliferative neoplasms.

Figure 2-1 Schematic of JAK/STAT cytokine signaling pathways. Signaling downstream of G-CSF, TPO and EPO proceeds through activation of JAK2, which in turn activates STAT family members by phosphorylation. STAT dimers translocate to the nucleus to modulate gene expression, leading to survival, proliferation and differentiation. Binding of these cytokines to their cognate receptors also activates the PI3K/Akt and MAPK pathways. Signaling is negatively regulated by several factors including CBL, SOCS and LNK. Activating mutations in MPL and JAK2, as well as inactivating mutations in CBL, SOCS, and LNK are associated with the MPNs.

V617F and then transplanted to reconstitute lethally irradiated mice. In C57Bl6 mice, these cells principally lead to erythropoiesis and sometimes myelofibrosis (MF) with a long latency, while in BALB/c mice, the phenotype observed was more severe and was characterized by expanded erythropoiesis followed by myelofibrosis.[7,8] Multiple second-generation mouse models with knock-in mutations of JAK2 V617F showed a similar PV phenotype,[9-11] with the exception of one model whose disease more closely resembled ET.[12]

Although most PV patients carry the JAK2 V617F mutation, a minority are JAK2 V617F negative. Moreover, a larger proportion of PMF and ET patients are negative for this mutation, suggesting existence of other mutations in the JAK/STAT pathway.

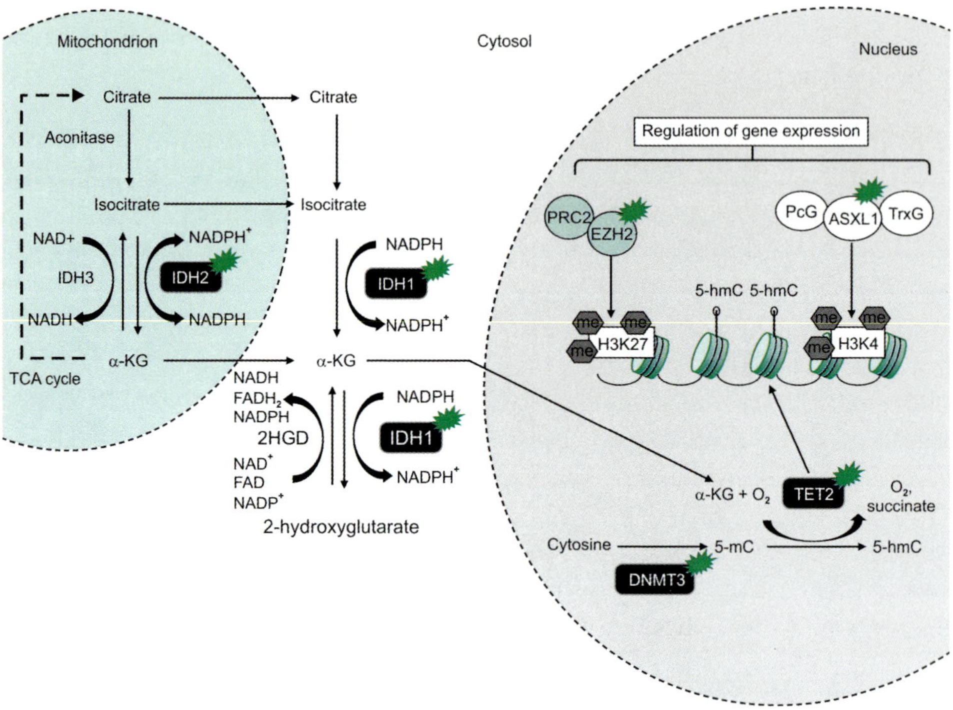

MPNs, myeloproliferative neoplasms; ASXL1, additional sex combs-like protein 1; EZH2, enhancer of zeste homolog 2; DNMT3A, DNA (cytosine-5)-methyltransferase 3 alpha; TET2, ten-eleven-translocation 2; NADPH, reduced form of nicotinamide adenine dinucleotide phosphate; PRC2, polycomb repressive complex 2; PcG, polycomb-group; 5-hmC, 5-hydroxymethylcytosine; 5-mC, 5-methylcytosine; TCA, tricarboxylic acid.

Figure 2-2 Schematic of epigenetic regulators mutated in the MPNs. Genes that regulate gene expression by modification of chromatin that are also mutated in the MPNs include ASXL1, EZH2, DNMT3A and TET2. Other epigenetic factors that can be affected in the MPNs include the isocitrate dehydrogenases 1 and 2 (IDH1, IDH2). These enzymes catalyze the interconversion of isocitrate to α-ketoglutarate (αKG) and α-ketoglutarate (αKG) to 2-hydroxyglutarate (2HG), while simultaneously reducing nicotinamide adenine dinucleotide phosphate (NADP+) to NADPH. It is thought that the production of 2HG negatively regulates the activity of epigenetic regulators such as TET2.

Sequencing of JAK2 in JAK2 V617F negative patients identified other mutations in exon 12.[13,14] As observed with JAK2 V617F, these mutations result in EPO-independent colony growth and interleukin (IL)3-independent proliferation of Baf3 cells carrying these exon 12 mutations.

Because of the importance of JAK2 signaling in cell proliferation and survival, researchers searched for mutations in JAK2 associated receptors, leading to the identification of the activating MPLW515L [a somatic activating mutation in the transmembrane domain of MPL (W515L)] mutation. Interestingly, no mutations in

EPO or G-CSF receptors were found in MPN patients. Other important mutations that have been discovered in MPN patients affect negative regulators of the signaling pathways, such as *CBL* and *LNK*.

Myeloproliferative Leukemia

Soon after the identification of JAK2 V617F, mutations in myeloproliferative leukemia (*MPL)* were found in approximately 5% of ET and 10% of PMF patients, but not in PV patients.[15,16] Of note, *MPL* mutations have also been reported in acute megakaryocytic leukemia and familial thrombocytosis.[17]

Myeloproliferative leukemia encodes the receptor for thrombopoietin, the cytokine that plays a role key in megakaryocyte survival, proliferation, and differentiation. The most frequent mutation affecting MPL is the MPLW515L substitution. Other substitutions in this codon have been described (MPLW515K and MPLW515A) but they represent a lower percentage.[18,19] Amino acid 515 is located in the intracellular region of MPL that lies immediately after the transmembrane domain. This region plays a major role in the cytosolic conformation of the receptor and prevents its autoactivation. Thus, mutations in this domain are sufficient to elicit spontaneous activation of the receptor and as a consequence, downstream signaling pathways.

As was previously observed in the case of JAK2 V617F, *MPL* mutations transform hematopoietic cells to factor-independent growth and induce JAK-STAT pathway activation.[16] However, even though *MPL* and *JAK2* mutations activate the same pathways and result in similar phenotypes *in vitro*, the *in vivo* models show striking differences. Indeed, expression of MPL W515L in mice leads to a lethal myeloproliferative disorder with thrombocytosis and MF.[16] This phenotype, therefore, mimics many of the phenotypes of human ET and PMF.

Casitas B-cell Lymphoma

The CBL protein family includes three homologs (c-CBL, CBL-b, and CBL-c) with ubiquitin ligase activity that targets different tyrosine kinases. The first mutation in *CBL* was described in AML patients.[20,21] Later, *CBL* mutations were identified in chronic myeloid disorders: 17% of chronic myelomonocytic leukemia (CMML) and less than 10% PMF are affected.[22,23] The main function of c-CBL is to participate in the ubiquitination of growth factor receptors, which induces their internalization and degradation.[24] Important targets of CBL are the fetal liver tyrosine kinase-3 receptor (*Flt3-R*), c-kit and MPL.

Mutations found in *CBL* affect two domains of the protein: the "linker" and the "ring". The linker domain is necessary for interaction with the tyrosine kinase binding, while the ring domain, is essential for the negative regulatory function of CBL.[21] Then, the consequence of *CBL* mutations is loss of its inhibitory function.

In vitro over-expression of the CBL mutant results in constitutive activation of the *Flt3* pathway and the phenotype of the cells resembles that of *Flt-3* mutated receptor tyrosine kinase.[25]

LNK

LNK, also known as Src homology (SH2) B3, belongs to a family of adaptor proteins. This family is characterized by the presence of three main domains: (1) proline-rich motifs in N-terminus; (2) a pleckstrin homology domain; and (3) an SH2 domain responsible for the negative activity of the protein. LNK is an intracellular protein, which acts as negative regulator of TPO and EPO pathways. Indeed, LNK negatively inhibits JAK2 through binding its SH2 domain.[26,27]

The murine LNK loss of function model displays an increased HSC pool with enhanced self-renewal capacity and increased quiescence,[28] two characteristics of HSCs controlled by TPO. In addition, *Lnk*$^{-/-}$ mice present abnormal megakaryopoiesis and erythropoiesis due to the absence of negative regulation of JAK/STAT signaling. This loss of control results in the development of thrombocytosis, splenomegaly and fibrosis.[29] In the MPNs, mutations in *LNK* are found in less than 5% of PMF and ET patients, but they are more frequently seen in patients that have undergone leukemic transformation.[30] Mutations almost always target a hot spot (codons 208 to -234) in the PH domain, which is believed to recognize phosphoinositide and control cell membrane localization.[31,32]

Suppressor of Cytokine Signaling

Another family of JAK2 negative regulators is Suppressor of Cytokine Signaling (SOCS). This group includes three members, *SOCS1, SOCS2,* and *SOCS3*.[33] These proteins bind JAK2 and inhibit its catalytic activity.[34] SOCS activity is regulated by methylation of their promoter. Hypermethylation of SOCS1 and SOCS3 promoters have been reported in JAK2 V617F PV and ET and in JAK2 V617F-negative and MPLW515F-negative ET.[35,36] In this condition, SOCS expression level is decreased.

Mutations in *SOCS1*, first described in B-cell lymphoma,[37] lead to their loss of function and, as a consequence, excess JAK/STAT signaling. In the MPNs, *SOCS1* is mutated in 14–25% of ET, 11–13% of PV, and 17% of PMF[35, 36] while *SOCS3* mutations are found in 10% of ET and 22% of PV[18,35,38,39] and *SOCS2* is mutated in 28% of MPNs.[40]

IMPLICATIONS

Currently, tests for *JAK2* and *MPL* mutations, but not other signal transduction genes, are available for clinical use. It should be noted that even though *JAK2* and *MPL* mutations are not found in all cases, JAK inhibitors are equally effective in mutation-positive and mutation-negative patients. This observation can be explained by the finding that patients without JAK2 or MPL mutations frequently show activated JAK/STAT signaling. As discussed above, this pathway can be activated by mutations in other genes, such as LNK. It is likely that screening for mutations in these other regulators will be made available for clinical use.

MUTATIONS IN EPIGENETIC REGULATORS

Epigenetic modifications include DNA methylation and post-translational modification of histone proteins. DNA methylation is involved in key cellular processes including X-chromosome inactivation, imprinting, and transcriptional silencing of specific genes and repetitive elements. DNA methylation patterns are frequently perturbed in human diseases, such as cancer and imprinting disorders including Beckwith–Wiedemann syndrome, Silver–Russell syndrome, Angelman syndrome, and Prader–Willi syndrome. Modifications of histones influence chromatin conformation, which regulates gene expression. As a consequence of these alterations, a wide range of cell metabolism and growth processes are impacted.

Ten-eleven-translocation 2

Ten-eleven-translocation 1, TET2, and TET3 are three homologous proteins, which convert 5-methylcytosine (5-mC) into 5-hydroxymethylcytosine (5-hmC).[41,42] All three have two conserved C-terminal regions responsible for the catalytic activity. Contrary to TET1, TET2 and TET3 do not harbor a DNA- binding domain, suggesting that they interact with partner proteins to associate with DNA.

Ten-eleven-translocation TET1 was identified as the mixed lineage leukemia (MLL) partner AML-associated translocation t(10;11)(q22;q23), and named ten-eleven-translocation.[43] Later, the *TET2* location on chromosome (4q24) was described as a region of rearrangement in few cases of AML.[44] Mutations in *TET2* have been found thanks to whole genome array analysis and molecular cytogenetics. Mutations are present all along the coding sequence of the gene and they can be nonsense, missense and frameshift mutations.[45,46] In MPNs, approximately 16% of PV, 5% of ET and 17% of PMF patients carry a mutation in *TET2*. Mutations are also found in a wide range of myeloid malignancies, including 12% of myelodysplastic syndromes (MDS), 12% of myeloproliferative disorders and 22% of secondary AML.[45]

The main known function of TET2 is to convert 5-mC to 5-hmC. The role of 5-mC in gene regulation has been widely studied and it is associated with multiple effects on gene regulation, genomic imprinting, X-chromosome inactivation, and cancer development. The role of 5-hmC is less well understood, but several studies report that 5-hmC prevents the interaction of 5-mC with protein partners and represents a step toward cytosine demethylation.[47]

To determine the role of TET2 in hematologic malignancies, short-hairpin ribonucleic acid (shRNAs) against the gene were introduced to into murine stem cells harvested from bone marrow. A reduction of TET2 level led to an increase in the proportion of hematopoietic stem/progenitor cells and a reduction of normal differentiation of granulocytes and monocytes.[48] Soon after, hematopoietic conditional knockouts of *TET2* were developed. These animals show an increase in stem cell self-renewal that is eventually accompanied by myeloproliferation with splenomegaly, monocytosis, and extramedullary hematopoiesis. Heterozygous mice also display increased stem cell self-renewal and extramedullary hematopoiesis.[49] A second knockout model of *TET2* has the same phenotype in Hematopoietic Stem Cells and a fatal disorder that mimics the human myeloid disorder. In this latter model, the authors also discovered defects in the lymphoid compartment with impairment in B and T cell differentiation.[50]

A recent study also reports that mutations in *TET2* can be detected in elderly individuals with clonal hematopoiesis, but without a detectable hematological malignancy. As observed in malignant context, in these healthy individuals the alterations in *TET2* are associated with modification of DNA methylation.[51] This study supports the model that *TET2* mutations enhance self-renewal and clonal expansion of HSCs when mutated. Furthermore, the data place mutations in *TET2* as potential early events in the development of hematologic malignancies. These results differ from those that describe *TET2* mutation as a late event in the progression of MPN to leukemic transformation[52-55] and suggest that a conserved order of genetic alterations is not required for MPN development.

Isocitrate Dehydrogenases 1 and 2

Isocitrate dehydrogenases 1 and 2 (IDH1, IDH2) are nicotinamide adenine dinucleotide phosphate ($NADP^+$) dependent enzymes, which catalyze the interconversion of isocitrate to α-ketoglutarate (αKG) and α-ketoglutarate (αKG) to 2-hydroxyglutarate (2HG), while simultaneously reducing nicotinamide adenine dinucleotide phosphate ($NADP^+$) to NADPH.[56,57] This reaction is required for protecting cells from oxidative stress-induced tumorigenesis. Mutations in *IDH1* and *IDH2* were first described in glioma[58] where they are mutually exclusive. Subsequently, they were found in 5–9% of AML and post-MPN AML. More recently, a comprehensive screen of 200 MPNs patients showed that nearly 21% of patients in blast-phase MPN carry a mutation in *IDH* while only 4% of PMF have an *IDH* mutation.[59] Furthermore, no mutations were found in PV and ET. Using a larger cohort of patients, however, another study reported *IDH* mutations in 0.8% of ET and 1.9% in PV.[60]

With respect to function, mutations in *IDH* affect arginine residues that are important for the activity of the protein (mutations R132S or R132G in IDH1 and codons R140 and R172 in IDH2). The presence of these mutated proteins leads to over-production of 2-hydroxyglutarate at the expense of α-ketoglutarate (αKG). As a consequence, αKG-dependent enzymes, including TET2, are affected, resulting in a decrease of 5-hmc among other changes.[48]

Additional Sex Combs-like Protein 1

Additional sex combs-like protein 1 (l *ASXL1* gene encodes the additional sex combs-like protein 1 and is located in chromosomal region 20q11. It belongs to a family of three enhancers of trithorax and polycomb proteins, which regulate the expression of developmental genes by chromatin remodeling.[61,62] ASXL1 has a double function since it is required to maintain both activation and silencing of Hox (homeobox) genes in flies and mice depending on the cell context.[62] The mechanism of action of ASXL1 remains poorly understood, but the protein is involved in chromatin organization through its participation in multiprotein complexes. One such complex is the polycomb repressive deubiquitinase complex, in which BAP1 (a ubiquitin carboxy-terminal hydrolase) removes monoubiquitin from histone 2A in nucleosomes.[63] In another complex, ASXL1 heterochromatin protein-1 (HP-1) associates with the histone demethylase LSD, which promotes repression of RAR (retinoic acid receptor)-mediated transcription.[62]

ASXL1$^{-/-}$ mice present a mild phenotype, although they do show defects in the frequency of differentiated lymphoid and myeloid progenitors. The absence of ASXL1 seems to have no effect on HSC, multipotent progenitors and peripheral blood. Notably, the mice do not appear to spontaneously develop myelodysplastic phenotypes or leukemia.[64]

Mutations in *ASXL1* include frameshift mutations, nonsense mutations, and large 20q11 deletions. These are found in 10–15% of MPNs (less than 7% of ET and PV, but 20–40% of PMF) and MDS, 40% of CMML and 15–20% of acute leukemia.[65,66] In most of the cases, mutations occur in exon 12 and result in synthesis of a truncated protein that lacks the PHD domain (C-terminal plant homeodomain), which is involved in protein-protein interactions.

Enhancer of Zeste Homolog 2

Enhancer of zeste homolog 2 is located on 7q36.1 and encodes for the PcG (poly-comb-group) EZH 2 protein, which belongs to the polycomb repressive complex 2 (PRC2). This complex regulates cell proliferation, differentiation, cell-identity maintenance, aging, and plasticity by modification of chromatin structure.[67,68] Through the SET domain of EZH2, the PRC2 complex methylates histone H3 at lysine 27,[69] which is a marker of transcriptionally active status. EZH2 can also be associated with DNA-methyltransferases (DNMT) to contribute to DNA methylation regulation.

Mutations in *EZH2* were first described in solid tumors, where they appear to induce dedifferentiation.[70] In myeloid disorders, missense, nonsense mutations, and premature codon stops are found all along the *EZH2* sequence. The mutations can be monoallelic or biallelic and, in contrast to solid tumors, they result in loss of function of the protein.[71,72] In the MPNs, *EZH2* mutations have been reported in 13% of patients with PMF, and 3% of PV. They are also described in MDS, demonstrating that *EZH2* mutations are not specific to a disease. In MDS, these mutations are usually associated with a poor prognosis.[73]

DNA (Cytosine-5)-Methyltransferase 3 Alpha

DNA (cytosine-5)-methyltransferase 3 alpha is a DNMT that catalyzes methylation of cytosines in genomic DNA. This methylation process plays an important role in gene repression and maintenance of active chromatin states, which in turn controls genomic imprinting, X-chromosome inactivation, and proper gene expression.[74,75] *DNMT3A* is located on chromosome 2p23.3 and is mutated in 4–22% of *de novo* AML[76] and approximately 8% of MDS patients.[77] A recent study showed that *DNMT3A* is mutated in 7% of PMF patients, but never found in CMML, blast-phase MPN's or post-PV/ET MF.[78] Nevertheless, larger cohort of patients is necessary to definitely rule out presence of *DNMT3A* mutation in these diseases. Functional studies to determine the effect of the mutations on DNMT3A function and hematopoiesis are underway.

Clinical Relevance

Currently, testing for mutations in these epigenetic regulators is not available for clinical use, but it is likely that future knowledge of the complete mutational profile will inform management of these patients. For example, recent studies have suggested that ASXL1 and IDH1/2 mutations may independently contribute to an adverse prognosis.[79,80] A more complete knowledge of the complete repertoire of mutations in patients may help identify those who would benefit from "epigenetic therapies" including hypomethylating agents and histone deacetylases (HDACs) (discussed in Chapter 8).

DISCUSSION

The discovery of JAK2 V617F mutation marked a huge advance in the understanding of the molecular biology of BCR-ABL negative MPNs, but it also presented new questions. The most important is how a single mutation can be responsible for the development of three different diseases. Even though many studies have provided novel insights, the question remains unanswered. Because the cell lineages impaired in PV, ET, and PMF are different from one another, it was first proposed that progenitor cells of the lineage uniquely harbored the mutation, which then led to the different phenotypes. However, evidence that ET, PV, and PMF are derived from stem cell clone able to give rise to granulocytic, erythroid, and megakaryocytic lineages rules out this model.[81]

Another model proposed that the mutation occurs in HSC, while the level and the duration of JAK2V617F expression determines the disease type.[82] In this model, low level of expression of the mutated kinase would lead an ET phenotype while high level of expression (consequence of a second event) would lead to PV. This model is supported by the examination of patient zygosity, which reveals that 93–100% of ET patients are heterozygous for JAK2 V617F, whereas 21–35% of PV and 0–21% of PMF are homozygous.[83] Animal models also support this dosage model.[84] Nevertheless, the presence of a *JAK2* mutation and its expression level alone are unable to explain the differential development of PV, PMF, and ET. Indeed, *JAK2* is not mutated in every patient. It is likely that the combination of additional mutations contributes to the specific phenotype.

A recent model of MPN development suggests that an initial inherited or acquired mutation, such as *TET2*, is present in the HSC leading to a premalignant state.[51] *ASXL1*, *TET2*, deletion of the chromosome 20q, which frequently precede *JAK2* mutation, may cause this pre-malignant condition. A second event, including mutagenesis of *JAK2*, *MPL*, *KIT*, or *CBL* may promote the MPN phenotype. More recently this model has been contested as several studies described *TET2* mutation as a late event in the progression of MPN to leukemic transformation.[52-55] Indeed, as in CML, BCR-ABL negative MPNs have the propensity to evolve to AML. Thus, MPN can be considered as a transition state that, with the addition of other events, leads to leukemic transformation.

Finally, a recent study argues that the order in mutational events can vary among patients.[85] Additionally, the effects of *TET2* or *ASXL1* mutations are different depending on when they occur, during the MPN pathogenesis or leukemic transformation.[54] Thus, a better understanding of the pathogenesis of MPN and molecular events involved in leukemic transformation are necessary to give a new direction in drug discovery research. Although ruxolitinib is approved for use as a therapy for Primary Myelofibrosis,[86] it is unable to cure the disease.[87] Thus, the best hope for patients lies in the development of rational combinations of other agents, such as immunotherapy (lenalidomide, thalidomide, and pomalidomide), interferons, and epigenetic therapies (azacitidine, decitabine, and HDAC inhibitors) with a JAK inhibitor. The best therapies could then be tailor-made to target the specific set of mutations in an individual patient.

REFERENCES

1. Levine RL, Wadleigh M, Cools J, et al. Activating mutation in the tyrosine kinase JAK2 in polycythemia vera, essential thrombocythemia, and myeloid metaplasia with myelofibrosis. *Cancer Cell.* 2005;7(4):387-97.

2. Baxter EJ, Scott LM, Campbell PJ, et al. Acquired mutation of the tyrosine kinase JAK2 in human myeloproliferative disorders. *Lancet.* 2005;365(9464):1054-61.
3. Kralovics R, Passamonti F, Buser AS, et al. A gain-of-function mutation of JAK2 in myeloproliferative disorders. *N Engl J Med.* 2005;352(17):1779-90.
4. James C, Ugo V, Le Couédic JP, et al. A unique clonal JAK2 mutation leading to constitutive signalling causes polycythaemia vera. *Nature.* 2005;434(7037):1144-8.
5. Zhao R, Xing S, Li Z, et al. Identification of an acquired JAK2 mutation in polycythemia vera. *J Biol Chem.* 2005;280(24):22788-92.
6. Tefferi A, Vainchenker W. Myeloproliferative neoplasms: molecular pathophysiology, essential clinical understanding, and treatment strategies. *J Clin Oncol.* 2011;29(5):573-82.
7. Lacout C, Pisani DF, Tulliez M, et al. JAK2V617F expression in murine hematopoietic cells leads to MPD mimicking human PV with secondary myelofibrosis. *Blood.* 2006;108(5):1652-60.
8. Wernig G, Mercher T, Okabe R, et al. Expression of Jak2V617F causes a polycythemia vera-like disease with associated myelofibrosis in a murine bone marrow transplant model. *Blood.* 2006;107(11):4274-81.
9. Mullally A, Lane SW, Ball B, et al. Physiological Jak2V617F expression causes a lethal myeloproliferative neoplasm with differential effects on hematopoietic stem and progenitor cells. *Cancer Cell.* 2010;17(6):584-96.
10. Marty C, Lacout C, Martin A, et al. Myeloproliferative neoplasm induced by constitutive expression of JAK2V617F in knock-in mice. *Blood.* 2010;116(5):783-7.
11. Akada H, Yan D, Zou H, et al. Conditional expression of heterozygous or homozygous Jak2V617F from its endogenous promoter induces a polycythemia vera-like disease. *Blood.* 2010;115(17):3589-97.
12. Li J, Spensberger D, Ahn JS, et al. JAK2 V617F impairs hematopoietic stem cell function in a conditional knock-in mouse model of JAK2 V617F-positive essential thrombocythemia. *Blood.* 2010;116(9):1528-38.
13. Scott LM, Tong W, Levine RL, et al. JAK2 exon 12 mutations in polycythemia vera and idiopathic erythrocytosis. *N Engl J Med.* 2007;356(5):459-68.
14. Butcher CM, Hahn U, To LB, et al. Two novel JAK2 exon 12 mutations in JAK2V617F-negative polycythaemia vera patients. *Leukemia.* 2008;22(4):870-3.
15. Pardanani AD, Levine RL, Lasho T, et al. MPL515 mutations in myeloproliferative and other myeloid disorders: a study of 1182 patients. *Blood.* 2006;108(10):3472-6.
16. Pikman Y, Lee BH, Mercher T, et al. MPLW515L is a novel somatic activating mutation in myelofibrosis with myeloid metaplasia. *PLoS Med.* 2006;3(7):e270.
17. Hussein K, Bock O, Theophile K, et al. MPLW515L mutation in acute megakaryoblastic leukaemia. *Leukemia.* 2009;23(5):852-5.
18. Chaligne R, James C, Tonetti C, et al. Evidence for MPL W515L/K mutations in hematopoietic stem cells in primitive myelofibrosis. *Blood.* 2007;110(10):3735-43.
19. Beer PA, Campbell PJ, Scott LM, et al. MPL mutations in myeloproliferative disorders: analysis of the PT-1 cohort. *Blood.* 2008;112(1):141-9.
20. Sargin B, Choudhary C, Crosetto N, et al. Flt3-dependent transformation by inactivating c-Cbl mutations in AML. *Blood.* 2007;110(3):1004-12.
21. Caligiuri MA, Briesewitz R, Yu J, et al. Novel c-CBL and CBL-b ubiquitin ligase mutations in human acute myeloid leukemia. *Blood.* 2007;110(3):1022-4.
22. Grand FH, Hidalgo-Curtis CE, Ernst T, et al. Frequent CBL mutations associated with 11q acquired uniparental disomy in myeloproliferative neoplasms. *Blood.* 2009;113(24):6182-92.
23. Sanada M, Suzuki T, Shih LY, et al. Gain-of-function of mutated C-CBL tumour suppressor in myeloid neoplasms. *Nature.* 2009;460(7257):904-8.
24. Dikic I, Szymkiewicz I, Soubeyran P. Cbl signaling networks in the regulation of cell function. *Cell Mol Life Sci.* 2003;60(9):1805-27.

25. Reindl C, Quentmeier H, Petropoulos K, et al. CBL exon 8/9 mutants activate the FLT3 pathway and cluster in core binding factor/11q deletion acute myeloid leukemia/ myelodysplastic syndrome subtypes. *Clin Cancer Res.* 2009;15(7):2238-47.
26. Tong W, Lodish HF. Lnk inhibits Tpo-mpl signaling and Tpo-mediated megakaryocytopoiesis. *J Exp Med.* 2004;200(5):569-80.
27. Tong W, Zhang J, Lodish HF. Lnk inhibits erythropoiesis and Epo-dependent JAK2 activation and downstream signaling pathways. *Blood.* 2005;105(12):4604-12.
28. Takaki S, Morita H, Tezuka Y, et al. Enhanced hematopoiesis by hematopoietic progenitor cells lacking intracellular adaptor protein, Lnk. *J Exp Med.* 2002;195(2):151-60.
29. Velazquez L, Cheng AM, Fleming HE, et al. Cytokine signaling and hematopoietic homeostasis are disrupted in Lnk-deficient mice. *J Exp Med.* 2002;195(12):1599-611.
30. Pardanani A, Lasho T, Finke C, et al. LNK mutation studies in blast-phase myeloproliferative neoplasms, and in chronic-phase disease with TET2, IDH, JAK2 or MPL mutations. *Leukemia.* 2010;24(10):1713-8.
31. Gery S, Gueller S, Chumakova K, et al. Adaptor protein Lnk negatively regulates the mutant MPL, MPLW515L associated with myeloproliferative disorders. *Blood.* 2007;110(9):3360-4.
32. Bersenev A, Wu C, Balcerek J, et al. Lnk controls mouse hematopoietic stem cell self-renewal and quiescence through direct interactions with JAK2. *J Clin Invest.* 2008;118(8):2832-44.
33. Fujimoto M, Naka T. Regulation of cytokine signaling by SOCS family molecules. *Trends Immunol.* 2003;24(12):659-66.
34. Krebs DL, Hilton DJ. SOCS: physiological suppressors of cytokine signaling. *J Cell Sci.* 2000;113(Pt 16):2813-9.
35. Jost E, do O N, Dahl E, et al. Epigenetic alterations complement mutation of JAK2 tyrosine kinase in patients with BCR/ABL-negative myeloproliferative disorders. *Leukemia.* 2007;21(3):505-10.
36. Teofili L, Martini M, Cenci T, et al. Epigenetic alteration of SOCS family members is a possible pathogenetic mechanism in JAK2 wild type myeloproliferative diseases. *Int J Cancer.* 2008;123(7):1586-92.
37. Melzner I, Bucur AJ, Brüderlein S, et al. Biallelic mutation of SOCS-1 impairs JAK2 degradation and sustains phospho-JAK2 action in the MedB-1 mediastinal lymphoma line. *Blood.* 2005;105(6):2535-42.
38. Fourouclas N, Li J, Gilby DC, et al. Methylation of the suppressor of cytokine signaling 3 gene (SOCS3) in myeloproliferative disorders. *Haematologica.* 2008;93(11):1635-44.
39. Suessmuth Y, Elliott J, Percy MJ, et al. A new polycythaemia vera-associated SOCS3 SH2 mutant (SOCS3F136L) cannot regulate erythropoietin responses. *Br J Haematol.* 2009;147(4):450-8.
40. Quentmeier H, Geffers R, Jost E, et al. SOCS2: inhibitor of JAK2V617F-mediated signal transduction. *Leukemia.* 2008;22(12):2169-75.
41. Tahiliani M, Koh KP, Shen Y, et al. Conversion of 5-methylcytosine to 5-hydroxymethylcytosine in mammalian DNA by MLL partner TET1. *Science.* 2009;324(5929):930-5.
42. Ito S, D'Alessio AC, Taranova OV, et al. Role of Tet proteins in 5mC to 5hmC conversion, ES-cell self-renewal and inner cell mass specification. *Nature.* 2010;466(7310):1129-33.
43. Lorsbach RB, Moore J, Mathew S, et al. TET1, a member of a novel protein family, is fused to MLL in acute myeloid leukemia containing the t(10;11)(q22;q23). *Leukemia.* 2003;17(3):637-41.
44. Viguie F, Aboura A, Bouscary D, et al. Common 4q24 deletion in four cases of hematopoietic malignancy: early stem cell involvement? *Leukemia.* 2005;19(8):1411-5.
45. Delhommeau F, Dupont S, Della Valle V, et al. Mutation in TET2 in myeloid cancers. *N Engl J Med.* 2009;360(22):2289-301.
46. Langemeijer SM, Kuiper RP, Berends M, et al. Acquired mutations in TET2 are common in myelodysplastic syndromes. *Nat Genet.* 2009;41(7):838-42.
47. Dahl C, Gronbaek K, Guldberg P. Advances in DNA methylation: 5-hydroxymethylcytosine revisited. *Clin Chim Acta.* 2011;412(11-12):831-6.

48. Figueroa ME, Abdel-Wahab O, Lu C, et al. Leukemic IDH1 and IDH2 mutations result in a hypermethylation phenotype, disrupt TET2 function, and impair hematopoietic differentiation. *Cancer Cell.* 2010;18(6):553-67.
49. Moran-Crusio K, Reavie L, Shih A, et al. Tet2 loss leads to increased hematopoietic stem cell self-renewal and myeloid transformation. *Cancer Cell.* 2011;20(1):11-24.
50. Quivoron C, Couronne L, Della Valle V, et al. TET2 inactivation results in pleiotropic hematopoietic abnormalities in mouse and is a recurrent event during human lymphomagenesis. *Cancer Cell.* 2011;20(1):25-38.
51. Busque L, Patel JP, Figueroa ME, et al. Recurrent somatic TET2 mutations in normal elderly individuals with clonal hematopoiesis. *Nat Genet.* 2012;44(11):1179-81.
52. Schaub FX, Looser R, Li S, et al. Clonal analysis of TET2 and JAK2 mutations suggests that TET2 can be a late event in the progression of myeloproliferative neoplasms. *Blood.* 2010;115(10):2003-7.
53. Beer PA, Delhommeau F, LeCouedic JP, et al. Two routes to leukemic transformation after a JAK2 mutation-positive myeloproliferative neoplasm. *Blood.* 2010;115(14):2891-900.
54. Abdel-Wahab O, Manshouri T, Patel J, et al. Genetic analysis of transforming events that convert chronic myeloproliferative neoplasms to leukemias. *Cancer Res.* 2010;70(2):447-52.
55. Kosmider O, Delabesse E, de Mas VM, et al. TET2 mutations in secondary acute myeloid leukemias: a French retrospective study. *Haematologica.* 2011;96(7):1059-63.
56. Yen KE, Bittinger MA, Su SM, et al. Cancer-associated IDH mutations: biomarker and therapeutic opportunities. *Oncogene.* 2010;29(49):6409-17.
57. Dang L, Jin S, Su SM. IDH mutations in glioma and acute myeloid leukemia. *Trends Mol Med.* 2010;16(9):387-97.
58. Parsons DW, Jones S, Zhang X, et al. An integrated genomic analysis of human glioblastoma multiforme. *Science.* 2008;321(5897):1807-12.
59. Pardanani A, Patnaik MM, Lasho TL, et al. Recurrent IDH mutations in high-risk myelodysplastic syndrome or acute myeloid leukemia with isolated del(5q). *Leukemia.* 2010;24(7):1370-2.
60. Tefferi A, Lasho TL, Abdel-Wahab O, et al. IDH1 and IDH2 mutation studies in 1473 patients with chronic-, fibrotic- or blast-phase essential thrombocythemia, polycythemia vera or myelofibrosis. *Leukemia.* 2010;24(7):1302-9.
61. Cho YS, Kim EJ, Park UH, et al. Additional sex comb-like 1 (ASXL1), in cooperation with SRC-1, acts as a ligand-dependent coactivator for retinoic acid receptor. *J Biol Chem.* 2006; 281(26):17588-98.
62. Lee SW, Cho YS, Na JM, et al. ASXL1 represses retinoic acid receptor-mediated transcription through associating with HP1 and LSD1. *J Biol Chem.* 2010;285(1):18-29.
63. Scheuermann JC, de Ayala Alonso AG, Oktaba K, et al. Histone H2A deubiquitinase activity of the polycomb repressive complex PR-DUB. *Nature.* 2010;465(7295):243-7.
64. Fisher CL, Pineault N, Brookes C, et al. Loss-of-function additional sex combs like 1 mutations disrupt hematopoiesis but do not cause severe myelodysplasia or leukemia. *Blood.* 2010;115(1):38-46.
65. Carbuccia N, Murati A, Trouplin V, et al. Mutations of ASXL1 gene in myeloproliferative neoplasms. *Leukemia.* 2009;23(11):2183-6.
66. Tefferi A. Novel mutations and their functional and clinical relevance in myeloproliferative neoplasms: JAK2, MPL, TET2, ASXL1, CBL, IDH and IKZF1. *Leukemia.* 2010;24(6):1128-38.
67. Sauvageau M, Sauvageau G. Polycomb group proteins: multi-faceted regulators of somatic stem cells and cancer. *Cell Stem Cell.* 2010;7(3):299-313.
68. De Haan G, Gerrits A. Epigenetic control of hematopoietic stem cell aging the case of Ezh2. *Ann N Y Acad Sci.* 2007;1106:233-9.
69. Cao R, Zhang Y. The functions of E(Z)/EZH2-mediated methylation of lysine 27 in histone H3. *Curr Opin Genet Dev.* 2004;14(2):155-64.
70. Simon JA, Lange CA. Roles of the EZH2 histone methyltransferase in cancer epigenetics. *Mutat Res.* 2008;647(1-2):21-9.

71. Ernst T, Chase AJ, Score J, et al. Inactivating mutations of the histone methyltransferase gene EZH2 in myeloid disorders. *Nat Genet.* 2010;42(8):722-6.
72. Nikoloski G, Langemeijer SM, Kuiper RP, et al. Somatic mutations of the histone methyltransferase gene EZH2 in myelodysplastic syndromes. *Nat Genet.* 2010;42(8):665-7.
73. Bejar R, Stevenson K, Abdel-Wahab O, et al. Clinical effect of point mutations in myelodysplastic syndromes. *N Engl J Med.* 2011;364(26):2496-506.
74. Tadokoro Y, Ema H, Okano M, et al. De novo DNA methyltransferase is essential for self-renewal, but not for differentiation, in hematopoietic stem cells. *J Exp Med.* 2007;204(4): 715-22.
75. Jurkowska RZ, Jurkowski TP, Jeltsch A. Structure and function of mammalian DNA methyltransferases. *Chembiochem.* 2011;12(2):206-22.
76. Yamashita Y, Yuan J, Suetake I, et al. Array-based genomic resequencing of human leukemia. *Oncogene.* 2010;29(25):3723-31.
77. Walter MJ, Ding L, Shen D, et al. Recurrent DNMT3A mutations in patients with myelodysplastic syndromes. *Leukemia.* 2011;25(7):1153-8.
78. Abdel-Wahab O, Pardanani A, Rampal R, et al. DNMT3A mutational analysis in primary myelofibrosis, chronic myelomonocytic leukemia and advanced phases of myeloproliferative neoplasms. *Leukemia.* 2011;25(7):1219-20.
79. Guglielmelli P, Biamonte F, Pereira A, et al. (2012). Prognostic impact of mutations in a large series of patients with myelofibrosis. *Blood.* 2012;120:Abstract 431.
80. Lasho T, Gangat N, Finke C, et al. (2012). Prognostic interactions between SRSF2, ASXL1, and IDH mutations in primary myelofibrosis and determination of added value to cytogenetic risk stratification and DIPSS-Plus. *Blood.* 2012;120:Abstract 430.
81. Fialkow PJ, Faguet GB, Jacobson RJ, et al. Evidence that essential thrombocythemia is a clonal disorder with origin in a multipotent stem cell. *Blood.* 1981;58(5):916-9.
82. Villeval JL, James C, Pisani DF, et al. New insights into the pathogenesis of JAK2 V617F-positive myeloproliferative disorders and consequences for the management of patients. *Semin Thromb Hemost.* 2006;32(4 Pt 2):341-51.
83. Tefferi A, Vainchenker W. Myeloproliferative neoplasms: molecular pathophysiology, essential clinical understanding, and treatment strategies. *J Clin Oncol.* 2011;29(5):573-82.
84. Tiedt R, Hao-Shen H, Sobas MA, et al. Ratio of mutant JAK2-V617F to wild-type Jak2 determines the MPD phenotypes in transgenic mice. *Blood.* 2008;111(8):3931-40.
85. Swierczek SI, Yoon D, Bellanne-Chantelot C, et al. Extent of hematopoietic involvement by TET2 mutations in JAK2V(6)(1)(7)F polycythemia vera. *Haematologica.* 2011;96(5):775-8.
86. Verstovsek S, Kantarjian H, Mesa RA, et al. Safety and efficacy of INCB018424, a JAK1 and JAK2 inhibitor, in myelofibrosis. *N Engl J Med.* 2010;363(12):1117-27.
87. Tefferi A. JAK inhibitors for myeloproliferative neoplasms: clarifying facts from myths. *Blood.* 2012;119(12):2721-30.

CHAPTER 3 Thrombotic and Bleeding Complications in BCR-ABL Negative MPN

Brandon J McMahon

INTRODUCTION

The breakpoint cluster region (BCR)-Abelson leukemia virus (ABL) negative, classical myeloproliferative neoplasms (MPNs) include polycythemia vera (PV), essential thrombocythemia (ET), and primary myelofibrosis (PMF). These are a heterogeneous group of clonal stem cell disorders characterized by overproduction of mature myeloid cells. Despite some overlap of their pathophysiology, the diseases follow different clinical courses. PV and ET are more common, and tend to follow a more benign clinical course, than myelofibrosis (MF). That stated, patients with PV and ET still have a lower life expectancy than age- and sex-matched controls, with a median survival on the order of approximately 15–20 years.[1-3] The MPNs share a potential for transformation to myelodysplastic syndrome, acute leukemia, and in the cases of PV and ET, a myelofibrotic stage. Considerable emphasis is placed on the possible evolution to these less favorable diseases, which carry poorer overall prognoses. Transformation to these more aggressive states occur at low rates, however, with myelofibrotic transformation at 10 years estimated at 0.7% and 0.8%, respectively, for ET and PV. The risk for leukemic transformation is estimated at less than 5% and less than 10% for these two diseases in the same time frame.[4-9]

Thrombotic and bleeding complications are much more common, resulting in a significant degree of morbidity, and have also been reported to contribute in up to 45% of MPN deaths.[10] Thromboses can be arterial or venous, involve unusual vascular sites, and have been reported to be present in up to a third of patients at time of MPN diagnosis.

Despite the high rate of thromboses, and to a lesser degree bleeding events, little is known about the mechanisms as to why they occur. More information is emerging with the discovery of the acquired somatic mutations identified with Philadelphia-negative MPN, particularly the Janus kinase 2 (JAK2) V617F (a change of valine to phenylalanine at the 617 position) mutation. This is estimated to be present in greater than 90% of patients with PV, and approximately half of those with ET or MF.[11] This chapter focuses on thrombotic and bleeding tendencies in the classical MPNs, reviewing proposed mechanisms, risk factors for occurrence, and clinical data to support primary and secondary prevention of these complications.

THROMBOTIC EVENTS

Incidence

It is not uncommon for thromboembolic events to be the presenting issue that leads to the initial MPN diagnosis. It has been estimated that thrombosis is present in approximately one-third of patients with PV, 10–29% with ET, and 13% of those with MF at the time of diagnosis.[12-14] These estimates are even higher when considering specific populations. In one study, 70% of patients presented with a portal vein thrombosis as the first manifestation of an MPN.[15] Following an established diagnosis of an MPN, the cumulative rate of thrombosis has been reported to be 2.5–5.0% per patient year in those with PV, with similar rates of 1.9–3.0% in ET and 1.75–2.2% in MF.[10,13,16,17]

Recurrence following incident thrombosis in MPN remains high, and involvement of the same vascular bed as the initial event is common. Indeed, recurrence rates of 8–19% in PV, 8–31% in ET, and 9–10.7% in MF have been reported.[12-14,16] Approximately one-third of a large cohort of almost 500 patients with either PV or ET and associated thrombosis suffered a recurrent event, corresponding to an incidence of 7.6% patient-years.[18] In this study, age greater than 60 years, and leukocytosis at time of initial thrombosis in those less than 60 years, were predictive for recurrence.

Thromboses occur at both the macro- and microvascular level in MPNs. Clinical manifestations of the latter include erythromelalgia, headache, transient visual loss, digital ischemia/discoloration, numbness, paresthesias, or dizziness. In the larger vascular territories, arterial involvement (cerebrovascular accident, acute coronary syndrome, and peripheral arterial thrombosis) is more common than venous, comprising over three quarters of events reported in several publications.[12] Site of involvement may differ by age and gender, as it has been demonstrated that abdominal venous thrombosis is often a presenting feature of young women.[12,15]

Thrombosis in Unusual Sites

Patients with MPN often present with thrombosis at unusual sites, including cerebral sinus vessels, the inferior vena cava, and splanchnic vessels. As previously stated, these unusual thrombotic events can often be their presenting feature.[19,20] Up to half of patients with the otherwise rare Budd-Chiari syndrome have been reported to have an underlying MPN.[21] In another study of patients presenting with cerebral, portal, or mesenteric vein thrombosis, approximately 14% filled criteria for having PV or ET at time of presentation, almost all of which were *JAK2 V617F* positive.[22] Interestingly, some were *JAK2* positive despite having no other overt findings of an MPN present. For those specifically having a portal vein thrombosis with no other findings of a MPN, the incidence of a JAK2 mutation was fairly high at 43%. These results are similar to another study, where 17% of patients with a portal or mesenteric venous thrombosis were found to harbor the JAK2 mutation.[23] While the majority did not otherwise have evidence for an underlying MPN at presentation, almost a third of these patients were eventually diagnosed with either MF or PV at a median follow-up of 41 months. The prevalence of the JAK2 mutation in patients presenting with splanchnic thrombosis has ranged from 7% to 70%, with a rate of 39% in one of the largest series of 241 patients.[13,15,20] Even if peripheral counts are seemingly normal, consideration for an underlying MPN should, therefore, be given to those patients presenting with these otherwise uncommon thromboses in the absence of another cause, including portal hypertension or intra-abdominal malignancy.

MECHANISMS

Platelet Activation

The pathophysiology corresponding to the thrombotic complications in MPN is incompletely understood. Microvascular disturbances may explain a number of the vasomotor symptoms experienced, including headache, dizziness, visual disturbances, and lightheadedness/dizziness. Platelet and endothelial pathology has been demonstrated to in part to mediate erythromelalgia, manifesting symptomatically as erythema and pain affecting the hands and feet.[24] Patients with ET suffering from erythromelalgia were found to have higher levels of the platelet-specific protein beta-2 thromboglobulin compared to controls and those ET patients without the phenomenon. Skin biopsies demonstrated microthrombi that were positive for von Willebrand's factor, but weak thrombin staining, indicating platelet aggregation is more of a problem in this microvascular process. Symptomatic improvement with aspirin further supports this.

Other abnormalities in platelet function have also been demonstrated in MPN, including a tendency toward spontaneous activation and aggregation, in part due to aberrant glycoprotein expression.[25] Increased thromboxane synthesis and urinary metabolites of platelet activation were shown in ET and PV patients, and P-selectin, another marker, correlated with *JAK2 V617F* positivity.[26,27] These activated platelets have been found to have a predilection toward the endothelium, adding to the potential for pathologic vascular events.[28] The enhanced platelet function seen in MPN may help explain the fact that arterial events are more common than venous thrombosis in these diseases.

Leukocytosis and Erythrocytosis

Leukocytes may also play a significant role in the pathogenesis of MPN-related thrombosis. Activation of platelets and their endothelial displacement is enhanced by leukocytosis.[29,30] Markers of neutrophil activation, including the neutrophil membrane clusters of differentiation (CD)11b, leukocyte alkaline phosphatase expression, elastase, and myeloperoxidase have been shown to parallel markers of coagulation.[31] These included higher levels of thrombin-antithrombin complexes, prothrombin 1+2, and d-dimer levels with increased levels of neutrophil activation. Corresponding markers of endothelial activation were also demonstrated in this study. As will be discussed later in this chapter, leukocytosis may indicate a higher risk for thrombosis in the MPNs.

Much focus has been placed on erythrocytosis and thrombotic tendency in PV. Theoretically, the increased viscosity associated with higher hematocrit (HCT) levels could predispose to thrombosis. The thrombotic risk may be further enhanced by an increased tendency of erythrocytes to adhere to the endothelium.[32] Further evidence for a mechanistic role of erythrocytosis in MPN-associated thrombosis comes indirectly from studies demonstrating decreased risk in patients with HCT levels less than 45%, including a recent prospective randomized control trial.[33,34] This will be discussed further under *Management* section later in this chapter.

Microparticles

Microparticles are subcellular plasma membrane fragments released from apoptotic or stimulated cells that have been demonstrated to contribute to hemostatic and inflammatory responses. These are often not detectable in healthy subjects, but can be significantly increased in certain disease states, adding to thrombotic tendency.[35] There is growing evidence that these procoagulant-bearing microparticles play an important role in a number of hypercoagulable states, including heparin-induced thrombocytopenia (HIT) and malignancy.[36] The increased cellular turnover as well as treatments with cytoreductive or cytotoxic agents can lead to the release of cellular debris in the form of microparticles. These cellular fragments express phosphatidylserine and tissue factor, which lead to the blood clotting enzyme complex and initiation of the coagulation cascade.[37] Higher levels of platelet-derived microparticles were found in patients with ET compared to controls, and this was further associated with an increase in thrombin generation.[38,39] Increased circulating procoagulant activity associated with microparticles was found in another study of PV and ET patients, again compared to healthy control subjects. Thrombin generation assays additionally suggested a role for thrombomodulin resistance in the hypercoagulability of MPN, with a lack of inhibition of thrombin production in the presence of activated protein C.[40] Interestingly, the extent of thrombomodulin resistance and *JAK2* allele burden were proportional. These results implicate abnormalities in the protein C pathway in MPN that can add to the overall hypercoagulability in these diseases. Future prospective studies may clarify the role of tissue factor bearing MPs in the thrombotic tendency seen in MPN.

JAK2 V617F Mutation

The *JAK2* mutation itself may not only represent a risk for development of thrombosis in patients with MPN, particularly at unusual sites, but also directly play an important role in the pathogenesis of thromboses. There has been considerable clinical data demonstrating presence of the mutation being associated with increased risk for thrombosis. Venous thromboembolic events are higher in those patients with ET who are *JAK2* positive compared to those who are *JAK2* negative.[41,42] In a large study of over 800 patients with ET, rates of major thrombosis were 1.4% patients per year versus 2.4% patients per year, in those who were *JAK2* negative and positive, respectively.[41] Interestingly, although *JAK2* status correlated with rates of venous thrombosis in this study, rates of arterial thrombosis were not statistically significant. Another systematic review reported *JAK2* positivity being associated with both arterial and venous thrombosis in ET, but not in MF.[43] This latter finding differs from a more recent study of 707 patients with MF, which reported the overall rate of cardiovascular death and nonfatal thrombotic complications to be 7.2%, corresponding to 1.75 events per 100 patient years.[16] Presence of *JAK2 V617F* was significantly associated with this endpoint on multivariate analysis, and patients with the mutation along with leukocytosis ($>15.0 \times 10^9$/L) were at particular risk, with an event rate of 3.92 events per 100 patient years.

JAK2 V617F allele burden has also been demonstrated to correlate with thrombotic risk.[44,45] In one study, ET patients homozygous for the mutation had higher adverse cardiovascular events compared to those heterozygous, as well as wild type.[46]

The mechanism for the *JAK2* mutation's role in thrombosis may be primarily through its interaction with the endothelium. Liver endothelial cells were found to be homozygous positive for the *JAK2 V617F* mutation in two patients with PV and Budd-Chiari syndrome, whereas the wild-type *JAK2* was found in the endothelium of two patients with hepatoportal sclerosis without PV.[47] Similar findings were reported in another small study of patients with MPN evaluated for the level of endothelial colony-forming units.[48] The *JAK2 V617F* mutation was exhibited in the endothelial colonies of five of 42 patients, all of which had experienced a thrombotic complication. The *JAK2* positive endothelial cells demonstrated a high proficiency to adhere mononuclear cells, which may add to the thrombotic tendency. While small in number, these findings warrant further investigation, and again indicate that the endothelium may play an important role in the pathophysiology of thrombosis in this patient population.

RISK FACTORS

General

With the high rates and associated morbidity and mortality, prevention of thrombotic complications in MPN is one of the main goals of treatment. Much

Table 3-1 Thrombotic Risk Factors in Myeloproliferative Neoplasms

Major	*Disease specific*	*Others*
Prior thrombotic episode	JAK2 mutation (ET)	Smoking
Age >60 years	JAK2 allele burden	Hyperlipidemia
	Leukocytosis	Diabetes mellitus
		Hereditary thrombophilia

focus has been given to identifying specific risk factors in attempts to better clarify those patients who may benefit from more intensive therapy. There are several risk factors that may be associated with higher rates of thrombosis in MPN; these risk factors are summarized in table 3-1. Many of these are well-established cardiovascular risk factors in general, and include hypertension, diabetes mellitus, hypercholesterolemia, and smoking. Presence of these in MPN may enhance thrombotic tendency and primary prevention strategies aimed at cardiovascular disease should also be employed in MPN. It is interesting to note, for example, that 3-hydroxy-3-methylglutaryl coenzyme A (HMG-coA) reductase agents (statins) have been independently shown to reduce the risk of venous thromboembolism (VTE), in addition to their arterial benefits.[49] However, these general cardiovascular risk factors have not been consistently shown to add considerably to thrombotic rates in MPN, and in fact, some studies have failed to show any additional risk.[50,51] Nevertheless, few would argue the overall health benefits associated with optimizing these factors, including in those with an underlying MPN. The two most widely recognized risks for thrombosis in general, including those with MPN, are age over 60 years and prior thrombotic event.[52,53] These are often used to stratify patients into low- or high-risk categories.[54,55]

Erythrocytosis, Leukocytosis, and Thrombocytosis

There has been considerable emphasis placed on peripheral blood counts and thrombotic risk. Historically, the main interventions recommended in the management of MPN have focused on decreasing HCT and platelet counts with the goal of reducing thrombotic complications.[17,56] There has been conflicting clinical data to support this practice; however, with a number of studies demonstrating that erythrocytosis and thrombocytosis do not parallel thrombotic risk.[3,57,58] In fact, elevated platelet counts may pose more of a concern for hemorrhagic events.[59] Controversy surrounding degree of erythrocytosis and potential for thrombosis lead to the Cytoreductive Therapy in Polycythemia Vera (CYTO-PV) study, randomizing patients with PV to a target HCT of either 45–50%, or to a traditional level of less than 45%.[34] Patients randomized to a lower goal HCT had significantly lower rates of thrombosis and death due to cardiovascular events. This study continues to support the traditional approach of considering PV patients with HCT levels greater than 45% at higher risk for thrombosis.

Leukocytosis has been demonstrated to be an independent risk factor for thrombosis in some studies.[30] For example, a total white blood count greater than 15×10^9/L was associated with a hazard ratio for venous and arterial thrombosis of 1.71 when compared to those with a total white blood count less than 10×10^9/L in one study.[58] This was mainly due to higher rates of myocardial infarction seen in those with leukocytosis. Similarly, increased risk for arterial thrombosis has been seen in those patients with prefibrotic MF and leukocytosis.[60] Elevated white blood counts additionally appear to increase the risk for recurrent thrombotic event; in those less than age 60 years, leukocytosis was associated with a hazard ratio of 3.35 for repeated arterial thrombosis.[61] Despite this evidence, not all studies have confirmed leukocytosis as an independent risk factor for thrombosis in MPN.[30,62] Rationale for high white blood count being linked to thrombosis could be related to *JAK2* allele burden, which as previously stated parallels thrombotic risk. Neutrophil activation may lead to upregulation of coagulation as well, discussed in detail in the Mechanisms section of this chapter.

JAK2 Mutation

The *JAK2V617F* mutation not only appears to be involved in the pathogenesis of thrombosis in MPN, but also is a risk factor. Patients with ET who are JAK2 positive have been shown to have significantly more venous thromboembolic events than those are JAK2 negative.[41,42] In one study of over 800 patients with ET, rates of major thrombosis were 1.4% patients per year in those who were JAK2 negative, versus 2.4% patients per year harboring the JAK2 mutation. Also, as previously discussed, patients with ET who were homozygous for the mutation suffered more cardiovascular events than those who were either heterozygous or wild-type.[46] Thrombotic recurrence has similarly been linked to the mutation, being higher in those ET patients *JAK2*V16F homozygous.[63] While genotype did not result in increased thrombosis among patients with PV, there was a correlation with higher *JAK2* allele burden.[42,44,45,64]

Despite relatively high rates of thrombosis in MPN, and incidence of the *JAK2* mutation with these disorders, screening for the mutation among all those presenting with idiopathic VTE is currently not recommended due to the low prevalence. Excluding those patients presenting with splanchnic thrombosis, less than 3% of those evaluated in a recent meta-analysis of 24 studies involving over 3,000 patients presenting with an idiopathic VTE were found to have the mutation.[65] Evaluating those with a splanchnic vein thrombosis, however, the mean prevalence was 32.7%, corresponding to an odds ratio of 53.98 for its development in those who are *JAK2* positive. As many of these patients will subsequently manifest overt MPN, *JAK2* screening in this specific population is reasonable.

Hereditary Thrombophilia

Hereditary thrombophilia may be a risk factor for venous thrombosis in patients with MPN as well. The prevalence of Factor V Leiden (FVL) heterozygosity in PV and ET patients has been reported to be similar to the general population at 4.6%.[66] Presence of the FVL gene mutation was associated with both incident and recurrent VTE in patients with ET and PV. It was not, however, associated with a higher rate of arterial thrombosis, consistent with other clinical settings outside of MPN. Heterozygosity for the prothrombin gene mutation has a similar impact on VTE rates in PV and ET, being 14.7 per 100 patient-years in those with the mutation versus only 0.8 per 100 patient-years in those without in one cohort of over 200 patients.[67] Despite seemingly raising thrombotic potential, utility of routinely checking for FVL and/or PT gene mutations in MPN, either in the presence or absence of VTE, is questioned given lack of impact on treatment approach. It is likely that other inherited thrombophilias have a similar effect on increasing thrombotic risk in those with MPN; however, their rarity limits adequate evaluation and clinical studies to support this are lacking. Presence of antiphospholipid antibodies, however, was not found to increase laboratory markers associated with higher propensity to clot in patients with MPN, and incidence for antibody presence was similar to controls.[27]

MANAGEMENT (TABLE 3-2)

Primary Prophylaxis

As previously mentioned, there is some debate as to how much standard cardiovascular risk factors, including obesity, hypertension, hyperlipidemia, diabetes mellitus, and tobacco use, affect thrombotic rates in MPN.[50,51] However, few would argue that optimizing risk factors associated with cardiovascular disease in general is in the patient's best interest. As these are common problems in the population at large and have far-reaching implications on overall health, it would be difficult to quantify how much of an impact targeting these factors would have on cardiovascular events, specifically in patients with MPN. Nonetheless, current recommendations are to aggressively manage these risk factors.[54]

Aspirin

The impact of aspirin on MPN disease course has been the subject of several clinical investigations, with disparate results. An early study showed no benefit of high-dose aspirin in PV, and there was actually an increase in gastrointestinal bleeding associated with treatment.[69] Subsequent studies demonstrated that using much lower doses resulted in a desired anti-platelet effect, without increasing hemorrhagic tendency.[70] This laid the foundation for the European Collaboration on Low-dose Aspirin in Polycythemia Vera (ECLAP) study, in which over 500 patients were randomized to 100 mg of acetylsalicylic acid (ASA) daily or supportive

Table 3-2 Therapeutic Strategies for MPN-related Thromboses

Intervention	*Comment*
Optimizing cardiovascular risk factors	• Recommended, however, specific impact on MPN-related thrombosis unclear
Aspirin	• Recommended for PV, JAK2-positive ET, ET with vasomotor symptoms, and for secondary prophylaxis in those with arterial thromboses[54,56] • Cautious use in those at high bleeding risk and with extreme thrombocytosis. Consider von Willebrand testing prior to starting with platelets ≥1,000 × 109/L • Unclear efficacy/safety in myelofibrosis
Phlebotomy	• Target HCT <45% recommended in PV with recent randomized trial demonstrating lower thrombotic potential compared to those >45%[34]
Anticoagulation	• Recommended for secondary prophylaxis in venous thrombosis • Duration of therapy unclear; consideration for long-term use given that MPN is a permanent risk factor, particularly in those with splanchnic thromboses
Cytoreduction:	• Consider for primary prophylaxis in those at high risk, and for secondary prophylaxis in those who have had a thrombotic event • Generally accepted target endpoints include normal leukocyte count, HCT <45%, platelets <400 × 109/L[54]
– HU	• Preferred first-line agent at present[54]
– IFN	• Low thrombotic rates with use may be related to lower white blood count and impact on JAK2 allele burden • Only agent known to result in JAK2 V617F molecular remission
– Anagrelide	• Currently considered second-line to HU given data demonstrating less efficacy in preventing arterial thromboses and increased myelofibrotic potential, noting more recent studies did not duplicate these prior findings[54,68]
JAK-inhibitors	• Role in reducing thrombotic potential has not yet been evaluated

MPN, myeloproliferative neoplasms; PV, polycythemia vera; JAK2, Janus kinase 2; ET, essential thrombocythemia; HCT, hematocrit; HU, hydroxyurea; IFN, interferon; V617F, a change of valine to phenylalanine at the 617 position.

care. Patients enrolled otherwise had no indication for anti-platelet therapy.[56] Those receiving aspirin had a reduced risk of combined end-point of nonfatal myocardial infarction, nonfatal stroke, major venous thrombosis, or death from cardiovascular causes. Interestingly, aspirin resulted in a reduction of both venous as well as arterial thrombosis. Although the relative risk of 0.49 was not statistically significant, this may be related to the small number of patients who fit criteria. Additionally, there was no increase in major bleeding.

Similar benefit has been seen with aspirin use in ET. *JAK2* positive ET patients with concomitant cardiovascular risk factors had reduced rates of both venous and arterial thrombosis when low-dose aspirin was used in one study.[71] However, those patients without other cardiovascular risk factors and those negative for *JAK2* failed to derive significant benefit from aspirin.

With these results, low-dose ASA is currently recommended for all PV patients, as well as ET patients with "microvascular disturbance".[54] There are important considerations to this recommendation. One study suggested that once daily, low-dose aspirin does not completely inhibit thromboxane A2 in ET, an issue that could be overcome by increasing the dosing frequency to twice daily.[72] Whether this results in significant clinical benefit remains to be seen. Additionally, the potential for acquired von Willebrand's disease or other intrinsic platelet aggregation abnormalities at platelet counts greater than $1{,}000 \times 10^9$/L have lead some experts to recommend caution with using aspirin at these levels due to potential hemorrhagic complications (see *Bleeding Complications* section). Data are limited with regards to the safety and efficacy of other antiplatelet agents, including clopidogrel.[73] Additionally, the efficacy of aspirin in preventing thrombosis in MF has yet to be demonstrated in clinical trials.

Phlebotomy

As previously mentioned, erythrocytosis/elevated HCT levels seen in PV result in higher viscosity, and therefore, increase the risk for thrombosis. Indeed, an early observational study published in 1978 reported higher thrombotic risk in those with a HCT greater than 44%.[28] Shortly after the publication of this retrospective study, the potential benefits of phlebotomy were again demonstrated in comparison to other treatments, which included chlorambucil and radioactive phosphorous. However, the improved survival seen in the PV patients treated with phlebotomy compared to other treatment arms was mainly due to a lower rate of leukemic transformation.[74] Additionally, the phlebotomized patients experienced a higher rate of thrombosis in the initial 3 years of treatment. The efficacy of phlebotomy in PV management was further called into question when both the Polycythemia Vera Study Group-01 and ECLAP trials failed to show a clear association between HCT less than 50–52% and thrombotic risk.[53,75,76]

The lack of clear data demonstrating benefit of phlebotomy targeting a HCT less than 45% led to a prospective study carried out by the CYTO-PV collaborative group. Patients were randomized to intensive (goal HCT <45%) or less intensive (goal HCT 45–50%) treatments, and followed for a median of 31 months. Targeting a lower HCT resulted in reduced risk of cardiovascular death or major thrombotic event, being 2.7% versus 9.8% in those in the higher HCT group. There were no significant differences in progression to MF, myelodysplasia, or leukemic transformation between the groups.[34] These findings more definitively support prior recommendations to offer phlebotomy to all PV patients, with a target HCT less than 45%.[54]

Cytoreductive Therapy

Efficacy of cytoreduction in decreasing the thrombotic risk in MPN mainly comes from studies evaluating its use for secondary prevention. Cytoreductive therapy has been shown to reduce the risk for both recurrent arterial and venous thrombosis in patients with PV or ET. In one study of almost 500 patients, use of cytoreduction was associated with a hazard ratio of 0.53 for recurrent thrombosis and particular benefit was seen in those with prior acute coronary syndrome.[18] The majority of the patients in this study were treated with hydroxyurea (HU), the remainder with pipobroman, busulfan, interferon (IFN), or anagrelide. Use of alkylating agents, such as busulfan have since fallen out of favor due to data linking treatment with these to a higher rate of leukemic transformation.

Data demonstrating benefit with cytoreduction in primary prevention of thrombosis in MPN is lacking. However, since it has been shown to be useful in secondary prevention, treatment with cytoreductive agents is currently recommended for those patients considered to be high-risk, classified as those over 60 years, in addition to those with a prior history of arterial or venous thrombosis.[54] Other cardiovascular factors are not universally considered in the risk stratification of MPN.

Hydroxyurea: Despite limited clinical studies providing clear evidence for its use, HU is widely considered to be the first-line cytoreductive agent in patients with classical MPN, especially PV and ET. Being an antimetabolite, HU nonspecifically inhibits deoxyribonucleic acid (DNA) synthesis, resulting in a propensity to lower the white blood count in addition to HCT and platelet levels. This may correlate with a reduced thrombotic potential, given data supporting leukocytosis as a risk factor for thrombosis in PV. Prospective studies are needed to support this claim, however. HU has a favorable side-effect profile, is inexpensive, and initial concerns about leukemogenic potential have been unfounded in clinical studies.[1,77]

The majority of the data demonstrating safety and efficacy of HU for thrombosis prevention in MPN comes from trials in patients with ET. Use of HU to target a platelet count less than 600×10^9/L demonstrated an improved thrombosis-free survival compared to no therapy in 114 patients with high-risk ET, with an absolute risk reduction of over 20% in HU compared to controls.[78] Benefit was seen with regards to both arterial and venous events. HU has also been shown to reduce thrombotic potential in patients with ET in a head-to-head comparison with anagrelide, as discussed below.

Anagrelide: Anagrelide specifically leads to a reduction in platelet production, interfering with megakaryocyte maturation. The exact mechanism is not clear, but appears to be through inhibition of phosphodiesterase. There was initial enthusiasm for anagrelide given a more targeted platelet-lowering effect, and potentially lower risk for leukemic transformation compared to HU. However, this enthusiasm waned after a head-to-head randomized control trial demonstrated HU was superior in lowering risk for arterial thrombosis as well as bleeding rates.[17] Furthermore, there was a higher risk for myelofibrotic transformation in the anagrelide arm. Therefore, HU is currently the preferred treatment in patients with PV or ET who require cytoreductive therapy.[54]

There are additional considerations for choice of agent; however, in the previously mentioned study, anagrelide treatment was associated with a lower VTE risk. In addition, a more recent noninferiority study was completed comparing anagrelide to HU in newly diagnosed or treatment naive ET patients considered to be at high risk for thrombotic or hemorrhagic complications based on clinical criteria.[68] Anagrelide demonstrated similar efficacy and safety to HU, with no significant differences in major thrombotic or bleeding events, or tolerability. Rates of fibrotic or leukemic conversion were also comparable between the two groups. Anagrelide could, therefore, be considered in patients with ET or PV felt to be at higher risk for VTE, and/or are intolerant to HU therapy.

Interferon: The ability of IFN to suppress hematologic progenitors has made it an appealing agent for use in MPN. IFN is an agent with a number of potential biologic effects, including being pro-apoptotic and having immunomodulatory properties. Indeed, 80% of patients with PV and ET treated with IFN demonstrated hematologic responses, and it has also been shown to lower thrombotic risk.[79,80] To date, this is also the only agent that has resulted in a complete molecular remission in *JAK2* positive MPN as well. After a 13-year median follow-up, none of the 55 PV patients treated with IFN had a major or minor thrombotic event.[80] Other studies using pegylated IFN in ET and PV have also reported low thrombotic potental.[81-83] The ability of IFN to lower risk for arterial and venous thrombosis may be due to its corresponding reduction of the white blood count, and/or *JAK2* allele burden.[81,84] Unfortunately, the side-effect profile has limited its use, as symptoms, such as fever, myalgias, and depressed mood can prevent treatment initiation or lead to premature discontinuation. Pegylated forms have been shown to be better tolerated. Lack of approval by the Food and Drug Administration (FDA) for use in MPN at present further limits access to IFN in the United States safety and efficacy of IFN in MPN is the subject of ongoing clinical investigations, and results may alter patterns of future use.

Janus Kinase 2 Inhibitors

Small molecule inhibitors of *JAK2* are in development, with ruxolitinib having completed clinical trials and being FDA approved for use in MF. Ruxolitinib is a not specific in its mechanism of action, with both JAK1 and JAK2 inhibition. Phase III studies demonstrated a reduction in spleen size as well as constitutional symptoms in patients with MF who received ruxolitinib.[85] The favorable results have led to investigation for its use in PV, with phase III studies currently underway. The impact of ruxolitinib on thrombotic or bleeding complications in patients with these disorders has not been specifically evaluated to date, and therefore currently unknown.[85-87] Other JAK inhibitors are in development. Through nonspecific JAK tyrosine-kinase inhibition, and resultant decrease in white blood count, they could theoretically result in a lower risk for thrombosis. However, preliminary data of JAK2 inhibitor lestaurtinib indicated that the drug may not only fail to prevent venous and arterial thromboses, but actually increase their risk with PV and ET.[88] The impact on thrombosis will, therefore, need to be monitored carefully in the clinical development of these agents.

Secondary Prophylaxis

It was previously mentioned that the two biggest risk factors for thrombosis in MPN are age over 60 years, and a prior thrombotic episode. Once a patient with an MPN experiences a thrombotic complication, risk for recurrence ranges from 8% to 31% in PV, ET, and MF.[10,13,16,17] Standard of care to date has been to treat venous thrombosis with anticoagulation, typically with unfractionated or low-molecular-weight heparin as a bridge to a vitamin K antagonist, with a target international normalized ratio of 2.0 and 3.0. Anti-platelet agents are typically used for treatment of arterial events. This approach has been demonstrated to be extremely effective in reducing rates of subsequent thrombotic episodes. For example, the hazard ratio for recurrent VTE was 0.32 with use of anticoagulation in one study.[18] Use of anti-platelet agents resulted in significant reductions in cardiac and cerebral infarction rates, with hazard ratios of 0.30 and 0.33, respectively. While the overall major bleeding rate was only 0.9% per patient year, it was considerably higher (2.8% per patient year) when anticoagulation was used in conjunction with anti-platelet agents. Combination therapy may be required in certain circumstances, but particular attention should be paid to possible bleeding complications, as patients with MPN can have an inherent hemorrhagic tendency as well (*See* Bleeding Complications section).

Unfortunately, data on choice of agent and duration of treatment are currently lacking. Low-molecular-weight heparin has shown superiority over vitamin K antagonists for use of secondary thrombotic prevention in other malignancies, but it is not clear whether this translates into a clear benefit in MPN, specifically.[89] Longer term use of low-molecular-weight heparin could be considered, but use of parenteral anticoagulation as a bridge to a vitamin K antagonist is reasonable. Special attention may be needed for development of HIT, as the rates may be higher in MPN than the general population.[90,91] Safety and efficacy of the newer class of oral anticoagulants such as rivaroxaban, dabigatran and apixaban, in MPN have also yet to be clearly established. Similarly, there is also no clear advantage of one anti-platelet over another in this patient population. Optimal duration of treatment is also unclear. Recent guidelines recommend a minimum of 3–6 months of anticoagulation for VTE in patients with PV or ET.[54] An exception to this is in those who suffer splanchnic thrombosis, in which case lifelong anticoagulation is recommended. Despite these recommendations, if presence of an MPN is considered an ongoing thrombotic risk factor, an argument could be made for long-term anticoagulation.[13] An individualized approach to treatment duration is, therefore necessary, particularly considering possible bleeding risk in this patient population.

Aggressive control of peripheral blood counts should reduce the risk of thrombotic recurrence as well. In the previously mentioned study, cytoreduction halved the risk for subsequent thrombosis.[18] Phlebotomy with a goal HCT less than 45% would also be recommended in those with PV.

Pregnancy

Given the lower prevalence of MPN in women of child-bearing age, clinical data on how to best manage women with an MPN in pregnancy is lacking. As pregnancy is a known independent risk factor for VTE, the concomitant presence of PV, ET, or MF likely further increases the thrombotic potential. A small study of women with PV further demonstrated an increased risk for adverse pregnancy outcome, with higher risk for fetal loss in all trimesters as well as premature delivery.[92] This may or may not be associated with the thrombotic risk associated with the disease and further studies are clearly warranted. Women requiring cytoreductive therapy should be treated with IFN, as HU is contraindicated given the teratogenic potential. Low-dose aspirin is recommended for both ET and PV patients, and a target HCT of less than 45% is recommended with PV to lower the thrombotic potential.[54] Prophylactic anticoagulation is recommended for VTE prevention in the 6 weeks postpartum for all women, and throughout pregnancy in those with a prior history of VTE.[54]

BLEEDING COMPLICATIONS

While less common than thrombotic complications, there is still an association of bleeding diathesis in MPN. Bleeding at diagnosis has been reported to complicate 3–18% of ET cases, and 3–8.1% of those with PV.[93] In this same study, bleeding occurred in 9.3% and 8.1% of ET and PV patients, respectively, at follow-up. Despite these relatively high rates, mechanism, risk factors and best approach to prevent hemorrhagic complications are incompletely understood, but some are shown in figure 3-1.

The mechanism for bleeding tendency appears to be multifactorial, with a particular emphasis on platelet defects. There are reports involving abnormalities in adrenergic receptor expression, decreased aggregation in response to epinephrine, and acquired storage pool deficiencies.[94,95] Primary hemostatic defects may also arise

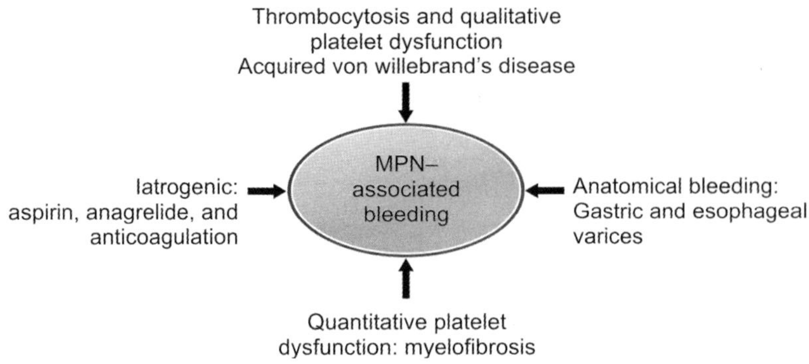

Figures 3-1 Bleeding in classical myeloproliferative neoplasms. The mechanisms resulting in bleeding in MPNs are poorly understood. Qualitative platelet defects, including acquired von Willebrand syndrome, can occur in cases of extreme thrombocytosis. Acquired storage pool disorders and abnormal platelet glycoprotein expression have also been described. Bleeding may occur due to anatomic abnormalities that develop specific to MPNs, including gastric and esophageal varices. Quantitative platelet defects, specifically the thrombocytopenia that can accompany myelofibrosis, may also add to bleeding in some cases. Lastly, bleeding may complicate anticoagulant and/or antiplatelet therapies used in treatment for these diseases.

from aberrancies in platelet glycoprotein expression. There are reports of decreased platelet expression of glycoprotein Ib and IIb/IIa. Subsequent investigations further showed qualitative defects, with impaired fibrinogen binding to the IIb/IIIa receptor.[96,97]

Perhaps the best described defect that could lead to hemorrhagic tendency in MPN is acquired von Willebrand's disease. There can be an inverse relationship between platelet count and the larger, more hemostatically active von Willebrand's multimers.[98] There has also been demonstration of a reduction in the half-life of von Willebrand protein binding to collagen in MPN compared to control subjects.[99] Increased proteolysis of the larger, more hemostatically active von Willebrand's multimers by ADAMTS13 (a disintegrin and metalloproteinase with a thrombospondin type 1 motif, member 13) may lead to these findings. Interestingly, these qualitative abnormalities were able to be corrected through use of cytoreductive therapy in normalization of the platelet counts.

Anatomic issues may also result in increased risk for bleeding. Splenomegaly often accompanies each of the MPN subtypes, particularly MF. This, in turn, can be associated with development of gastric and esophageal varices (via portal hypertension), a potential complication of splanchnic thrombosis as well. Premature platelet clearance from hypersplenism may also result in quantitative platelet dysfunction, which often complicates MF.

Historically, there has been concern for thrombosis associated with elevated platelet counts. However, there is growing evidence that thrombocytosis is more closely associated with hemorrhagic outcomes. In one cohort of 776 patients with ET, a platelet count greater than 450 × 10^9/L was associated with a risk of hemorrhage. The hazard ratio was 3.7 versus those with a normal platelet count. The bleeding risk increased at higher platelet counts.[59] Interestingly, thrombotic events were not found to be higher in those with abnormally high platelet counts in this cohort. Also notable in this study was that leukocytosis was associated with both bleeding and thrombosis.

Rates of bleeding have been reported to be higher in prefibrotic MF compared to ET.[100] In a large study of over 1,000 patients, bleeding rates were 12% in prefibrotic MF versus 6% in those with ET. Prior bleeding episode, use of aspirin and leukocytosis were all independently associated with bleeding risk.

With the growing data demonstrating concern for bleeding events with higher platelet counts in MPN, the standard practice of placing all patients on aspirin has been reexamined. Some experts recommend using caution with use of an anti-platelet agent when the count is greater than 1,000 × 10^9/L, with consideration of checking von Willebrand levels when this occurs.[7] As the acquired von Willebrand's disease pattern is one of loss of the larger multimers (i.e., a type IIa pattern), laboratory evaluation for both the antigen and activity is important, as the quantitative amount of the protein may not be significantly affected, in favor of qualitative defects. Correction of the hemostatic defects with normalization of the platelet counts also raises the question as to the ideal time to begin cytoreductive therapy. There are currently no substantial clinical studies to guide ideal target platelet counts. Further (ideally prospective) clinical studies are needed to help guide recommendations to this end.

CONCLUSION

Thrombotic and bleeding episodes are well recognized complications associated with the classical MPNs. Mechanism, risk factors (beyond age over 60 years and prior event), and optimal treatment are still incompletely understood. Identification of the JAK2 V617F somatic mutation has significantly advanced understanding of these diseases, but its role in thrombosis and bleeding diathesis, and its potential to serve as a therapeutic target specifically to reduce the risk for these complications, has yet to be established. Further clinical studies toward this end, and the identification of other novel biomarkers, may help clinicians provide more individualized therapy in the future.

REFERENCES

1. Passamonti F, Rumi E, Pungolino E, et al. Life expectancy and prognostic factors for survival in patients with polycythemia vera and essential thrombocythemia. *Am J Med.* 2004;117(10):755-61.

2. Rozman C, Giralt M, Feliu E, et al. Life expectancy of patients with chronic nonleukemic myeloproliferative disorders. *Cancer.* 1991;67(10):2658-63.
3. Wolanskyj AP, Schwager SM, McClure RF, et al. Essential thrombocythemia beyond the first decade: life expectancy, long-term complication rates, and prognostic factors. *Mayo Clin Proc.* 2006;81(2):159-66.
4. Noor SJ, Tan W, Wilding GE, et al. Myeloid blastic transformation of myeloproliferative neoplasms--a review of 112 cases. *Leuk Res.* 2011;35(5):608-13.
5. Najean Y, Rain JD. The very long-term evolution of polycythemia vera: an analysis of 318 patients initially treated by phlebotomy or 32P between 1969 and 1981. *Semin Hematol.* 1997;34(1):6-16.
6. Barbui T, Thiele J, Passamonti F, et al. Survival and disease progression in essential thrombocythemia are significantly influenced by accurate morphologic diagnosis: an international study. *J Clin Oncol.* 2011;29(23):3179-84.
7. Tefferi A. Polycythemia vera and essential thrombocythemia: 2012 update on diagnosis, risk stratification, and management. *Am J Hematol.* 2012;87(3):285-93.
8. Crisa E, Venturino E, Passera R, et al. A retrospective study on 226 polycythemia vera patients: impact of median hematocrit value on clinical outcomes and survival improvement with anti-thrombotic prophylaxis and non-alkylating drugs. *Ann Hematol.* 2010;89(7):691-9.
9. Passamonti F, Rumi E, Caramella M, et al. A dynamic prognostic model to predict survival in post-polycythemia vera myelofibrosis. *Blood.* 2008;111(7):3383-7.
10. Marchioli R, Finazzi G, Landolfi R, et al. Vascular and neoplastic risk in a large cohort of patients with polycythemia vera. *J Clin Oncol.* 2005;23(10):2224-32.
11. Tefferi A. Novel mutations and their functional and clinical relevance in myeloproliferative neoplasms: JAK2, MPL, TET2, ASXL1, CBL, IDH and IKZF1. *Leukemia.* 2010;24(6):1128-38.
12. Tefferi A, Elliott M. Thrombosis in myeloproliferative disorders: prevalence, prognostic factors, and the role of leukocytes and JAK2V617F. *Semin Thromb Hemost.* 2007;33(4):313-20.
13. Reikvam H, Tiu RV. Venous thromboembolism in patients with essential thrombocythemia and polycythemia vera. *Leukemia.* 2012;26(4):563-71.
14. Elliott MA, Pardanani A, Lasho TL, et al. Thrombosis in myelofibrosis: prior thrombosis is the only predictive factor and most venous events are provoked. *Haematologica.* 2010; 95(10):1788-91.
15. Hoekstra J, Bresser EL, Smalberg JH, et al. Long-term follow-up of patients with portal vein thrombosis and myeloproliferative neoplasms. *J Thromb Haemost.* 2011;9(11):2208-14.
16. Barbui T, Carobbio A, Cervantes F, et al. Thrombosis in primary myelofibrosis: incidence and risk factors. *Blood.* 2010;115(4):778-82.
17. Harrison CN, Campbell PJ, Buck G, et al. Hydroxyurea compared with anagrelide in high-risk essential thrombocythemia. *N Engl J Med.* 2005;353(1):33-45.
18. De Stefano V, Za T, Rossi E, et al. Recurrent thrombosis in patients with polycythemia vera and essential thrombocythemia: incidence, risk factors, and effect of treatments. *Haematologica.* 2008;93(3):372-80.
19. Richard S, Perrin J, Lavandier K, et al. Cerebral venous thrombosis due to essential thrombocythemia and worsened by heparin-induced thrombocytopenia and thrombosis. *Platelets.* 2011;22(2):157-9.
20. Kiladjian JJ, Cervantes F, Leebeek FW, et al. The impact of JAK2 and MPL mutations on diagnosis and prognosis of splanchnic vein thrombosis: a report on 241 cases. *Blood.* 2008;111(10):4922-9.
21. Darwish Murad S, Plessier A, Hernandez-Guerra M, et al. Etiology, management, and outcome of the Budd-Chiari syndrome. *Ann Intern Med.* 2009;151(3):167-75.
22. De Stefano V, Fiorini A, Rossi E, et al. Incidence of the JAK2 V617F mutation among patients with splanchnic or cerebral venous thrombosis and without overt chronic myeloproliferative disorders. *J Thromb Haemost.* 2007;5(4):708-14.

23. Colaizzo D, Amitrano L, Tiscia GL, et al. The JAK2 V617F mutation frequently occurs in patients with portal and mesenteric venous thrombosis. *J Thromb Haemost.* 2007;5(1):55-61.
24. van Genderen PJ, Lucas IS, van Strik R, et al. Erythromelalgia in essential thrombocythemia is characterized by platelet activation and endothelial cell damage but not by thrombin generation. *Thromb Haemost.* 1996;76(3):333-8.
25. Ginsburg AD. Platelet function in patients with high platelet counts. *Ann Intern Med.* 1975;82(4):506-11.
26. Jensen MK, de Nully Brown P, Lund BV, et al. Increased platelet activation and abnormal membrane glycoprotein content and redistribution in myeloproliferative disorders. *Br J Haematol.* 2000;110(1):116-24.
27. Robertson B, Urquhart C, Ford I, et al. Platelet and coagulation activation markers in myeloproliferative diseases: relationships with JAK2 V6I7 F status, clonality, and antiphospholipid antibodies. *J Thromb Haemost.* 2007;5(8):1679-85.
28. Pearson TC, Wetherley-Mein G. Vascular occlusive episodes and venous haematocrit in primary proliferative polycythaemia. *Lancet.* 1978;2(8102):1219-22.
29. Falanga A, Marchetti M, Vignoli A, et al. Leukocyte-platelet interaction in patients with essential thrombocythemia and polycythemia vera. *Exp Hematol.* 2005;33(5):523-30.
30. Barbui T, Carobbio A, Rambaldi A, et al. Perspectives on thrombosis in essential thrombocythemia and polycythemia vera: is leukocytosis a causative factor? *Blood.* 2009;114(4):759-63.
31. Falanga A, Marchetti M, Evangelista V, et al. Polymorphonuclear leukocyte activation and hemostasis in patients with essential thrombocythemia and polycythemia vera. *Blood.* 2000;96(13):4261-6.
32. Wautier MP, El Nemer W, Gane P, et al. Increased adhesion to endothelial cells of erythrocytes from patients with polycythemia vera is mediated by laminin alpha5 chain and Lu/BCAM. *Blood.* 2007;110(3):894-901.
33. Spivak JL. Polycythemia vera: myths, mechanisms, and management. *Blood.* 2002;100(13):4272-90.
34. Marchioli R, Finazzi G, Specchia G, et al. Cardiovascular events and intensity of treatment in polycythemia vera. *N Engl J Med.* 2013;368(1):22-33.
35. Hugel B, Socie G, Vu T, et al. Elevated levels of circulating procoagulant microparticles in patients with paroxysmal nocturnal hemoglobinuria and aplastic anemia. *Blood.* 1999;93(10):3451-6.
36. Tesselaar ME, Romijn FP, Van Der Linden IK, et al. Microparticle-associated tissue factor activity: a link between cancer and thrombosis? *J Thromb Haemost.* 2007;5(3):520-7.
37. George FD. Microparticles in vascular diseases. *Thromb Res.* 2008;122(Suppl 1):S55-9.
38. Trappenburg MC, van Schilfgaarde M, Marchetti M, et al. Elevated procoagulant microparticles expressing endothelial and platelet markers in essential thrombocythemia. *Haematologica.* 2009;94(7):911-8.
39. Moles-Moreau MP, Ternisien C, Tanguy-Schmidt A, et al. Flow cytometry-evaluated platelet CD36 expression, reticulated platelets and platelet microparticles in essential thrombocythaemia and secondary thrombocytosis. *Thromb Res.* 2010;126(5):e394-6.
40. Duchemin J, Ugo V, Ianotto JC, et al. Increased circulating procoagulant activity and thrombin generation in patients with myeloproliferative neoplasms. *Thromb Res.* 2010;126(3):238-42.
41. Campbell PJ, Scott LM, Buck G, et al. Definition of subtypes of essential thrombocythaemia and relation to polycythaemia vera based on JAK2 V617F mutation status: a prospective study. *Lancet.* 2005;366(9501):1945-53.
42. Carobbio A, Finazzi G, Antonioli E, et al. JAK2V617F allele burden and thrombosis: a direct comparison in essential thrombocythemia and polycythemia vera. *Exp Hematol.* 2009;37(9):1016-21.
43. Lussana F, Caberlon S, Pagani C, et al. Association of V617F Jak2 mutation with the risk of thrombosis among patients with essential thrombocythaemia or idiopathic myelofibrosis: a systematic review. *Thromb Res.* 2009;124(4):409-17.

44. Vannucchi AM, Antonioli E, Guglielmelli P, et al. Prospective identification of high-risk polycythemia vera patients based on JAK2(V617F) allele burden. *Leukemia.* 2007;21(9):1952-9.
45. Antonioli E, Guglielmelli P, Poli G, et al. Influence of JAK2V617F allele burden on phenotype in essential thrombocythemia. *Haematologica.* 2008;93(1):41-8.
46. Vannucchi AM, Antonioli E, Guglielmelli P, et al. Clinical profile of homozygous JAK2 617V>F mutation in patients with polycythemia vera or essential thrombocythemia. *Blood.* 2007;110(3):840-6.
47. Sozer S, Fiel MI, Schiano T, et al. The presence of JAK2V617F mutation in the liver endothelial cells of patients with Budd-Chiari syndrome. *Blood.* 2009;113(21):5246-9.
48. Teofili L, Martini M, Iachininoto MG, et al. Endothelial progenitor cells are clonal and exhibit the JAK2(V617F) mutation in a subset of thrombotic patients with Ph-negative myeloproliferative neoplasms. *Blood.* 2011;117(9):2700-7.
49. Glynn RJ, Danielson E, Fonseca FA, et al. A randomized trial of rosuvastatin in the prevention of venous thromboembolism. *N Engl J Med.* 2009;360(18):1851-61.
50. Cortelazzo S, Viero P, Finazzi G, et al. Incidence and risk factors for thrombotic complications in a historical cohort of 100 patients with essential thrombocythemia. *J Clin Oncol.* 1990;8(3):556-62.
51. Besses C, Cervantes F, Pereira A, et al. Major vascular complications in essential thrombocythemia: a study of the predictive factors in a series of 148 patients. *Leukemia.* 1999;13(2):150-4.
52. Policitemia GI. Polycythemia vera: the natural history of 1213 patients followed for 20 years. Gruppo Italiano Studio Policitemia. *Ann Intern Med.* 1995;123(9):656-64.
53. Radaelli F, Colombi M, Calori R, et al. Analysis of risk factors predicting thrombotic and/or haemorrhagic complications in 306 patients with essential thrombocythemia. *Hematol Oncol.* 2007;25(3):115-20.
54. Barbui T, Barosi G, Birgegard G, et al. Philadelphia-negative classical myeloproliferative neoplasms: critical concepts and management recommendations from European LeukemiaNet. *J Clin Oncol.* 2011;29(6):761-70.
55. Tefferi A, Vainchenker W. Myeloproliferative neoplasms: molecular pathophysiology, essential clinical understanding, and treatment strategies. *J Clin Oncol.* 2011;29(5):573-82.
56. Landolfi R, Marchioli R, Kutti J, et al. Efficacy and safety of low-dose aspirin in polycythemia vera. *N Engl J Med.* 2004;350(2):114-24.
57. Tefferi A, Gangat N, Wolanskyj AP. Management of extreme thrombocytosis in otherwise low-risk essential thrombocythemia; does number matter? *Blood.* 2006;108(7):2493-4.
58. Landolfi R, Di Gennaro L, Barbui T, et al. Leukocytosis as a major thrombotic risk factor in patients with polycythemia vera. *Blood.* 2007;109(6):2446-52.
59. Campbell PJ, MacLean C, Beer PA, et al. Correlation of blood counts with vascular complications in essential thrombocythemia: analysis of the prospective PT1 cohort. *Blood.* 2012; 120(7):1409-11.
60. Buxhofer-Ausch V, Gisslinger H, Thiele J, et al. Leukocytosis as an important risk factor for arterial thrombosis in WHO-defined early/prefibrotic myelofibrosis: an international study of 264 patients. *Am J Hematol.* 2012;87(7):669-72.
61. De Stefano V, Za T, Rossi E, et al. Leukocytosis is a risk factor for recurrent arterial thrombosis in young patients with polycythemia vera and essential thrombocythemia. *Am J Hematol.* 2010;85(2):97-100.
62. Gangat N, Wolanskyj AP, Schwager SM, et al. Leukocytosis at diagnosis and the risk of subsequent thrombosis in patients with low-risk essential thrombocythemia and polycythemia vera. *Cancer.* 2009;115(24):5740-5.
63. De Stefano V, Za T, Rossi E, et al. Increased risk of recurrent thrombosis in patients with essential thrombocythemia carrying the homozygous JAK2 V617F mutation. *Annals Hematol.* 2010;89(2):141-6.
64. Vannucchi AM, Pieri L, Guglielmelli P. JAK2 Allele Burden in the Myeloproliferative Neoplasms: Effects on Phenotype, Prognosis and Change with Treatment. *Ther Adv Hematol.* 2011;2(1):21-32.

65. Dentali F, Squizzato A, Brivio L, et al. JAK2V617F mutation for the early diagnosis of Ph-myeloproliferative neoplasms in patients with venous thromboembolism: a meta-analysis. *Blood.* 2009;113(22):5617-23.
66. Ruggeri M, Gisslinger H, Tosetto A, et al. Factor V Leiden mutation carriership and venous thromboembolism in polycythemia vera and essential thrombocythemia. *Am J Hematol.* 2002;71(1):1-6.
67. Gisslinger H, Mullner M, Pabinger I, et al. Mutation of the prothrombin gene and thrombotic events in patients with polycythemia vera or essential thrombocythemia: a cohort study. *Haematologica.* 2005;90(3):408-10.
68. Gisslinger H, Gotic M, Holowiecki J, et al. Anagrelide compared with hydroxyurea in WHO-classified essential thrombocythemia: the ANAHYDRET Study, a randomized controlled trial. *Blood.* 2013;121(10):1720-8.
69. Tartaglia AP, Goldberg JD, Berk PD, et al. Adverse effects of antiaggregating platelet therapy in the treatment of polycythemia vera. *Semin Hematol.* 1986;23(3):172-6.
70. Low-dose aspirin in polycythaemia vera: a pilot study. Gruppo Italiano Studio Policitemia (GISP). *Br J Haematol.* 1997;97(2):453-6.
71. Alvarez-Larran A, Cervantes F, Pereira A, et al. Observation versus antiplatelet therapy as primary prophylaxis for thrombosis in low-risk essential thrombocythemia. *Blood.* 2010;116(8):1205-10.
72. Pascale S, Petrucci G, Dragani A, et al. Aspirin-insensitive thromboxane biosynthesis in essential thrombocythemia is explained by accelerated renewal of the drug target. Blood. 2012;119(15):3595-603.
73. Squizzato A, Romualdi E, Middeldorp S. Antiplatelet drugs for polycythaemia vera and essential thrombocythaemia. *Cochrane Database Syst Rev.* 2008(2):CD006503.
74. Berk PD, Goldberg JD, Silverstein MN, et al. Increased incidence of acute leukemia in polycythemia vera associated with chlorambucil therapy. *N Engl J Med.* 1981;304(8):441-7.
75. Berk PD, Goldberg JD, Donovan PB, et al. Therapeutic recommendations in polycythemia vera based on Polycythemia Vera Study Group protocols. *Semin Hematol.* 1986;23(2):132-43.
76. Di Nisio M, Barbui T, Di Gennaro L, et al. The haematocrit and platelet target in polycythemia vera. *Br J Haematol.* 2007;136(2):249-59.
77. Bjorkholm M, Derolf AR, Hultcrantz M, et al. Treatment-related risk factors for transformation to acute myeloid leukemia and myelodysplastic syndromes in myeloproliferative neoplasms. *J Clin Oncol.* 2011;29(17):2410-5.
78. Cortelazzo S, Finazzi G, Ruggeri M, et al. Hydroxyurea for patients with essential thrombocythemia and a high risk of thrombosis. *N Engl J Med.* 1995;332(17):1132-6.
79. Kiladjian JJ, Chomienne C, Fenaux P. Interferon-alpha therapy in bcr-abl-negative myeloproliferative neoplasms. *Leukemia.* 2008;22(11):1990-8.
80. Silver RT. Long-term effects of the treatment of polycythemia vera with recombinant interferon-alpha. *Cancer.* 2006;107(3):451-8.
81. Kiladjian JJ, Cassinat B, Chevret S, et al. Pegylated interferon-alfa-2a induces complete hematologic and molecular responses with low toxicity in polycythemia vera. *Blood.* 2008; 112(8):3065-72.
82. Alvarado Y, Cortes J, Verstovsek S, et al. Pilot study of pegylated interferon-alpha 2b in patients with essential thrombocythemia. *Cancer Chemother Pharmacol.* 2003;51(1):81-6.
83. Langer C, Lengfelder E, Thiele J, et al. Pegylated interferon for the treatment of high risk essential thrombocythemia: results of a phase II study. *Haematologica.* 2005;90(10):1333-8.
84. Quintas-Cardama A, Kantarjian H, Manshouri T, et al. Pegylated interferon alfa-2a yields high rates of hematologic and molecular response in patients with advanced essential thrombocythemia and polycythemia vera. *J Clin Oncol.* 2009;27(32):5418-24.
85. Verstovsek S, Kantarjian H, Mesa RA, et al. Safety and efficacy of INCB018424, a JAK1 and JAK2 inhibitor, in myelofibrosis. *N Engl J Med.* 2010;363(12):1117-27.
86. Verstovsek S, Mesa RA, Gotlib J, et al. A double-blind, placebo-controlled trial of ruxolitinib for myelofibrosis. *N Engl J Med.* 2012;366(9):799-807.

87. Harrison C, Kiladjian JJ, Al-Ali HK, et al. JAK inhibition with ruxolitinib versus best available therapy for myelofibrosis. *N Engl J Med.* 2012;366(9):787-98.
88. Moliterno AR RG, Carroll M, Luger S, et al. An open-label study of CEP-701 in patients with JAK2 V617F-positive polycythemia vera and essential thrombocytosis. *ASH Annual Meeting Abstracts.* 2008;112(11):99.
89. Lee AY, Levine MN, Baker RI, et al. Low-molecular-weight heparin versus a coumarin for the prevention of recurrent venous thromboembolism in patients with cancer. *N Engl J Med.* 2003;349(2):146-53.
90. Spectre G, Kalish Y, Schliamser L, et al. Heparin-induced thrombocytopenia in myeloproliferative disorders: a rare or under-diagnosed complication? *Am J Hematol.* 2008;83(5):420-3.
91. Randi ML, Tezza F, Scapin M, et al. Heparin-induced thrombocytopenia in patients with Philadelphia-negative myeloproliferative disorders and unusual splanchnic or cerebral vein thrombosis. *Acta Haematologica.* 2010;123(3):140-5.
92. Robinson S, Bewley S, Hunt BJ, et al. The management and outcome of 18 pregnancies in women with polycythemia vera. *Haematologica.* 2005;90(11):1477-83.
93. Papadakis E, Hoffman R, Brenner B. Thrombohemorrhagic complications of myeloproliferative disorders. *Blood Rev.* 2010;24(6):227-32.
94. Wehmeier A, Fricke S, Scharf RE, et al. A prospective study of haemostatic parameters in relation to the clinical course of myeloproliferative disorders. *Eur J Haematol.* 1990;45(4): 191-7.
95. Kaywin P, McDonough M, Insel PA, et al. Platelet function in essential thrombocythemia. Decreased epinephrine responsiveness associated with a deficiency of platelet alpha-adrenergic receptors. *N Engl J Med.* 1978;299(10):505-9.
96. Mazzucato M, De Marco L, De Angelis V, et al. Platelet membrane abnormalities in myeloproliferative disorders: decrease in glycoproteins Ib and IIb/IIIa complex is associated with deficient receptor function. *Br J Haematol.* 1989;73(3):369-74.
97. Le Blanc K, Lindahl T, Rosendahl K, et al. Impaired platelet binding of fibrinogen due to a lower number of GPIIB/IIIA receptors in polycythemia vera. *Thromb Res.* 1998;91(6):287-95.
98. van Genderen PJ, Budde U, Michiels JJ, et al. The reduction of large von Willebrand factor multimers in plasma in essential thrombocythaemia is related to the platelet count. *Br J Haematol.* 1996;93(4):962-5.
99. van Genderen PJ, Prins FJ, Lucas IS, et al. Decreased half-life time of plasma von Willebrand factor collagen binding activity in essential thrombocythaemia: normalization after cytoreduction of the increased platelet count. *Br J Haematol.* 1997;99(4):832-6.
100. Finazzi G, Carobbio A, Thiele J, et al. Incidence and risk factors for bleeding in 1104 patients with essential thrombocythemia or prefibrotic myelofibrosis diagnosed according to the 2008 WHO criteria. *Leukemia.* 2012;26(4):716-9.

CHAPTER

4 Essential Thrombocythemia

Jamile M Shammo, Laura C Michaelis

INTRODUCTION

Essential thrombocythemia (ET) is a clonal stem cell disorder characterized by dysregulated proliferation of megakaryocytes with a clinical trajectory that is often marked by thrombotic or hemorrhagic complications. Like polycythemia vera (PV), ET can progress to myelofibrosis (MF) and, in rare circumstances, to acute myeloid leukemia (AML). The initial description of the disease entity is often attributed to Emil Epstein and Alfred Goedel who, in 1934 published a case report of a patient with "extreme thrombocytosis, erythrocytosis and mucocutaneous bleeding, and no panmyelosis".[1,2] Dameshek recognized the overlapping clinical features between ET, PV, MF, and chronic myelogenous leukemia (CML) and postulated a shared pathogenesis for these diseases. He speculated that "is it possible that these various conditions—"myeloproliferative disorders"—are all somewhat variable manifestations of proliferative activity of the bone marrow cells, perhaps due to a hitherto undetected stimulus?"[3] The 2005 discovery of the Janus kinase 2 (JAK2) V617F mutation substantiated such a hypothesis.[4-7] Subsequent work has uncovered a cascade of molecular abnormalities in the myeloproliferative neoplasms (MPNs) that may contribute to disease pathogenesis or transformation.[8-10]

Treatment of ET has largely been supportive and has focused on prevention of thrombohemorrhagic complications and amelioration of vasomotor symptoms. To date, our understanding of the inciting molecular events that cause ET or contribute to its transformation is lacking. Currently available therapies for ET do not prevent progression to AML or MF, though this is of fundamental clinical importance. It is hoped that novel therapies targeting the molecular aberrations recently discovered in MPN find their way into the treatment of ET in the years to come.

In this chapter, we will briefly introduce the reader to the epidemiology and pathogenesis of ET, discuss the spectrum of clinical presentations, status of risk stratification, and finally, present an approach to therapy and ongoing research.

EPIDEMIOLOGY

Currently, the annual incidence of ET is estimated at about 1.5–2.5/100,000,[11] with large differences in rates according to geography or ethnicity.[12,13] Understanding the true incidence of this disease has been limited due to disparities in diagnostic criteria and the scarcity of population-based studies. Interestingly, the incidence of this disease has increased—likely secondary to the introduction of automated blood cell counters and the availability of molecular markers, such as JAK2 V617F or myeloproliferative leukemia (MPL) mutations, which have allowed for a rapid and occasionally definitive method for distinguishing clonal from reactive thrombocytosis.[14]

One of the largest epidemiologic studies on ET incidence was published by Mayo Clinic researchers and analyzed a database of individuals in Olmsted County, Minnesota between 1976 and 1995.[11] In the 19 years analyzed, prior to the current World Health Organization (WHO) definition of ET, a total of 39 cases of ET were identified, for an age- and sex-adjusted incidence rate of 2.53/100,000 annually. A Swedish study conducted from 1983 through 1999 found an ET incidence of 1.30 per 100,000 in men and 2.76 per 100,000 in women.[15] Other studies have not confirmed this gender difference in incidence.[11,13]

The introduction of laboratory testing for the JAK2 V617F mutation had practice-changing consequences for the identification and diagnosis of all MPNs including ET. As a result, the diagnostic paradigm changed significantly. Several studies have examined the impact of diagnostic methods on the incidence of the disease. For example, a study, comparing the incidence of ET in the Côte d'Or area of France, before and after the discovery of the JAK-2 mutation in 2005, reported a notable increase in the incidence from 1.2/100,000 in the period of 1980-2004 to 3/100,000 after 2005, underscoring the importance of the availability of accurate diagnostic testing for the appropriate identification of a given disease.[16]

ESSENTIAL THROMBOCYTHEMIA AND JANUS KINASE 2 V617F

In 2004, several groups of scientists detected a critical mutation in the regulatory component of JAK2—a member of the Janus family of cytoplasmic nonreceptor tyrosine kinases (TYK), which also includes JAK1, JAK3, and TYK2. Their collective work, published in 2005, showed that a somatic mutation results in the substitution of valine for phenylalanine at codon 617 of JAK2 (JAK2 V617F).[4-7] About 55% of patients with ET have this mutation, which results in constitutive activation of JAK-STAT (signal transducer and activator of transcription) signaling and consequent enhanced cell survival, proliferation, and differentiation of committed myeloid progenitors. In addition, there is likely recruitment of other signaling molecules that leads to stabilization of this neoplastic cascade.[9] Initially, it was thought that the JAK2 V617F mutation represented a primordial event, similar to the breakpoint cluster region (BCR)-Abelson leukemia virus (ABL) translocation in CML. Since then, however, it has become clear that the MPNs have a more heterogeneous pathogenesis than CML, and that there are likely a multitude of cooperating abnormalities contributing to the final phenotype. Some of these abnormalities involve mutations of the thrombopoietin (TPO) receptor, MPL, and rarely, LNK, ten-eleven-translocation 2 (TET2), additional sex combs-like protein 1 (ASXL1), and others that are described in chapter 2. The frequency of these mutations in ET is low, and their contribution to disease pathogenesis is not well established.[10] There are numerous reports of JAK2 positive mutations in disease entities other than MPNs,[17] supporting the notion that these mutations are cooperative with phenotype, rather than dictating it. Debate continues around models to outline the molecular events that lead to ET, and eventually to fibrotic or leukemic transformation.[18]

Since the discovery of JAK2 V617F, research has also focused on the role of the mutation on the prognosis of ET. So far, the presence of the mutation has not been consistently associated with survival or leukemic transformation in ET.[10] One study, which looked that clinical laboratory and disease characteristics in 275 patients with ET over seven years, found that patients who were JAK2 V617F-positive tended to be older, with higher hemoglobin (Hb) levels and lower platelet counts.[19] The incidence of thrombosis and disease evolution in JAK2 positive and negative patients was comparable. In this study, JAK2 V617F-positive patients had a better response to cytotoxic therapies. A similar study of 118 ET patients concurred, as the rate of thrombotic events and progression to MF and AML did not differ between patients with and without the JAK2 mutation.[20] However, another study suggested that the presence of the JAK2 V617F mutation in ET patients may result in a higher risk of arterial thrombosis,[21] and a lower risk of progression to post-ET MF but was not shown to negatively impact survival.[22] A larger meta-analysis suggests that there is likely an increased rate of thrombosis in patients with ET and JAK2 positivity.[23]

Recently, two groups reported the presence of somatic insertions or deletions in exon 9 of calreticulin (CALR) gene in the majority of patients with MPN's who were lacking an identifiable mutation in JAK2 or MPI.[24,25] This discovery is likely to result in enhancing the diagnostic accuracy of workup conducted in patients suspected of having an MPN.

DIAGNOSTIC WORKUP

The hallmark of ET is a sustained and unexplained thrombocytosis greater than or equal to 450×10^9/L. Therefore, the diagnostic workup should aim to rule out conditions that result in reactive thrombocytosis, and other myeloid disorders that may manifest with thrombocytosis, such as CML, myelodysplastic syndrome (MDS)

Box 4-1 Causes of Thrombocytosis

- Reactive causes:
  - Iron deficiency
  - Acute hemorrhage/blood loss
  - Infections
  - Inflammatory states
  - Hemolysis
  - Asplenia
- Myeloid neoplasms:
  - Essential thrombocytosis
  - Polycythemia vera
  - Myelofibrosis
  - Chronic myelogenous leukemia
  - Myelodysplastic syndrome (RARS-T, deletion 5q)
- Familial causes:
  - MPL, TPO or other unidentified mutations

RARS-T, refractory anemia with ring sideroblasts associated with marked thrombocytosis; MPL, myeloproliferative leukemia; TPO, thrombopoietin.

Box 4-2 World Health Organization (WHO) 2008 Criteria for the Diagnosis of Essential Thrombocythemia

- Platelet count $\geq 450 \times 10^9$/L
- Bone marrow biopsy showing proliferation of mainly the megakaryocytic lineage with increased numbers of the enlarged mature megakaryocytes. No significant increase or left shift of neutrophils granulopoiesis or erythropoiesis
- Not meeting WHO criteria for PV, PMF, CML, MDS, or other myeloid neoplasms
- Demonstration of JAK-2 V617F or other clonal marker, or in the absence of JAK-2 V617F, no evidence for reactive thrombocytosis

PV, polycythemia vera; PMF, primary myelofibrosis; CML, chronic myelogenous leukemia; MDS, myelodysplastic syndrome; JAk-2, Janus kinase 2; V617F, a change of valine to phenylalanine at the 617 position.

[refractory anemia with ring sideroblasts and thrombocytosis (RARS-T), deletion 5q subtype], primary myelofibrosis (PMF), and PV (Box 4-1). In 2008, The WHO set forth four diagnostic criteria for the diagnosis of ET. All four criteria have to be met in order to make such a diagnosis (Box 4-2).[14]

A detailed history and physical examination should be performed to assist in identifying a potential cause for thrombocytosis, and for the detection of splenomegaly, which can be present in 25–50% of patients with ET. Laboratory testing should include a JAK2 V617F mutational analysis, iron studies including ferritin to rule out iron deficiency anemia, inflammatory markers, such as erythrocyte sedimentation rate (ESR) or C-reactive protein (CRP), and an autoimmune profile to rule out connective tissue disorders. A review of peripheral blood smear should be performed to evaluate for dysplasia, or other myeloid neoplasms which can manifest with thrombocytosis.[26] The peripheral smear in ET shows thrombocytosis, platelet anisocytosis, normal red cell morphology, normal white blood cell (WBC) count, a full manual and differential count of the peripheral blood. Although mild leukocytosis may be noted, leukoerythroblastosis and tear drop red cells are not typically seen in ET.

Diagnostic criteria require a bone marrow biopsy to make a diagnosis of ET.[14,26] As described in chapter 1, the bone marrow in ET is normocellular or moderately hypercellular, and exhibits clusters of large megakaryocytes, with lobulated nuclei. However, the presence of bizarre, highly dysplastic megakaryocytes is atypical for ET, and should raise suspicion for other entities, such as PMF or MDS. Mild reticulin fibrosis may be present. Stainable iron is usually identified, unless the patient has experienced hemorrhage and is iron deficient, or has PV. An abnormal karyotype is found in 5–10% cases, but there is no consistent cytogenetic abnormality specific to ET. It is essential to distinguish ET from prefibrotic PMF, because patients with "true" ET have been shown to have a lower risk of evolution to MF and acute leukemia (AL) and they tend to have a better survival than patients with prefibrotic MF.[27] Patients with prefibrotic PMF, rather than ET, tend to have lower Hb levels and higher levels of leukocytes, serum lactate dehydrogenase, circulating clusters of differentiation (CD)34-positive cells, and incidence of palpable splenomegaly.

COMPLICATIONS

Multiple studies have compared the overall survival (OS) of individuals with ET and the general population.[13,28-31] In general, for ET patients is similar to that of the general population,[32] at least in the first decade following diagnosis.[33] A report of survival patterns of over 9,000 patients with MPN in a Swedish Cancer Registry, who were followed for over three decades, demonstrated a decreased life expectancy for all MPN patients including those with ET.[34] Recently, an International Prognostic Score for patients with ET (IPSET) has been proposed to predict survival at diagnosis. The score is calculated by assigning scores to three variables: (1) age greater than 60 years; (2) WBC greater than 11×10^9/L, and (3) history of thrombosis, which defined five categories—with a median survival not reached for the lowest risk category and median OS of 8.8 years for the highest risk category. In that report, an association between leukocytosis and worse survival was further confirmed.[22]

A small number of patients do progress after many years of living with ET to MF (post-ETMF), such patients develop anemia, elevated lactate dehydrogenase (LDH), massive splenomegaly, constitutional symptoms, a leukoerythroblastic picture noted upon examination of the peripheral smear, and significant bone marrow fibrosis. The 2008 WHO classification for myeloid neoplasms has defined a set of diagnostic criteria to facilitate an accurate diagnosis of this entity.[35] This long-term risk for the development of MF or AML, in true ET, is estimated at 9% and 2% at 15 years.[27]

In most cases, the most common concern is the development of thrombosis and less likely, hemorrhagic complications. Thrombotic complications are the major cause for morbidity in affected ET patients and represent a primary trigger for treatment. In fact, one study suggested that thrombosis accounts for half of the causes of death in ET.[22] A concern unique to younger women with ET is a significantly increased risk of fetal loss.[36-38]

Thrombosis

Thrombotic complications more commonly involve the arterial system, and can result in transient ischemic attack, ischemic stroke, acute myocardial infarction, and peripheral arterial occlusion. This complication is discussed in chapter 3 of this textbook as well. Insults to the venous system can manifest with deep venous thrombosis of the lower extremities, splanchnic thrombosis, and cerebral venous thrombosis. One of the more challenging presentations is when patients are initially discovered with Budd-Chiari syndrome (BCS) or portal vein thrombosis (PVT). Patients that present in this manner are more likely to be young and may have normal blood counts—which can render the diagnosis of MPN difficult. A 2008 review of patients with splanchnic vein thrombosis found that a high percentage of these individuals are JAK2 V617F-positive (>30%),[39] and a 2012 meta-analysis demonstrated that in primary BCS, the prevalence of MPN is 40%.[40] In non-cirrhotic, non-malignant PVT, the prevalence of an MPN was 31.5%. Of particular concern in BCS is progression to hepatic failure. These studies suggest that all cases of otherwise unprovoked mesenteric, splanchnic vein thrombosis, and likely cerebral sinus and vein thrombosis should be tested for JAK2 V617F to identify patients with an occult MPN even in the face of a seemingly "normal" complete blood count (CBC).

Various series differ on the incidence of thrombosis at diagnosis—depending on definition of "major" thrombotic event. A large Italian study rigorously vetted patients for a WHO-defined diagnosis of ET and reported thrombosis rates of 12% with a higher incidence of arterial compared to venous events.[21] Thrombotic complications are more common in patients over 60 years in age, those with a prior history of a thrombotic event;[41] and some suggest increased risk in individuals with cardiovascular risk factors, including tobacco use, hypertension, or diabetes mellitus.[42-44] While an elevated platelet count may be associated with an increased risk of hemorrhage, no study has shown an association between platelet count and risk of thrombosis in ET; however, there is some evidence in the literature suggesting that leukocytosis is a much more powerful prognostic factor for thrombotic complications in ET.[21] It should be noted that such data were derived from retrospective analyses. A recently published report described an attempt to prospectively investigate the tendency for developing vascular complications in ET relative to blood counts in 776 such patients (PT-1 cohort). Interestingly, no association between blood counts at diagnosis and future risk of thrombosis was found; however, an elevated platelet count during follow-up was associated with an immediate risk of major hemorrhage, and elevated white cell count during follow-up correlated with thrombosis and major hemorrhage.[45] Very high platelet counts, likely through the presence of an acquired von Willebrand's syndrome, may be protective against thrombosis, but may represent a risk factor for major hemorrhage.[46]

Vasomotor Disturbances

Patients may also present with vasomotor symptoms, such as erythromelalgia, headaches, dizziness, acrocyanosis, and paresthesias. In one series of 74 young women with essential thrombocytosis, 40% reported vasomotor symptoms.[47] Constitutional symptoms, such as night sweats, weight loss, and fever are uncommon in ET, but neurologic vasomotor symptoms can be dramatic. Headache has been cited as the most common neurologic manifestation, and there is a high incidence of transient ischemic attacks involving both the anterior and posterior cerebral circulation.[48] Additional transient neurologic symptoms have been noted, including unsteadiness, dysarthria, dysphoria, motor hemiparesis, scintillating scotomas, amaurosis fugax, vertigo, dizziness, migraine-like symptoms, syncope, and seizures and are thought to be manifestations of microvascular disturbances.

Bleeding

Bleeding events can also complicate ET and tend to associate with extreme thrombocytosis (platelets above 1,000 × 10^9/L). Bleeding complications tend to affect mucosal membranes of the gastrointestinal or upper respiratory tracts, and may be associated with acquired von Willebrand's disease or aspirin use. Studies estimate that between 3% and 14% of patients will experience a hemorrhagic event, some of which are the reasons for diagnosis and some of which occur after initiation of antiplatelet therapy or cytotoxic interventions.[41] Risk factors for bleeding include splenomegaly, leukocyte count greater than 11,000/mL, and platelets higher than 1,000 × 10^9/L.[19] The subsequent platelet dysfunction is characterized by deficits in platelet aggregation.[49] Acquired von Willebrand's disease is a well-described phenomenon.[30,50-54] In the setting of extreme thrombocytosis—(typically above 1,000 × 10^9/L), patients can develop acquired type 2 von Willebrand syndrome due to the proteolysis of large von Willebrand factor (vWF) multimers. The syndrome is reversible with reduction in the platelet count.

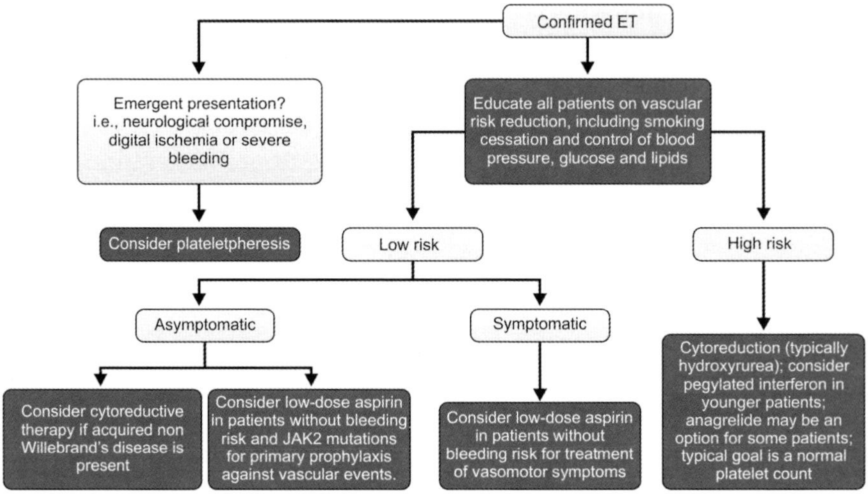

ET, essential thrombocythemia; JAK2, Janus kinase 2.

Figure 4-1 Treatment of essential thrombocythemia.

TREATMENT (FIGURE 4-1)

Emergencies

Occasionally, patients will present with hematologic emergencies in the context of extreme thrombocytosis. In the absence of a medical history, it can be difficult to determine if the patient's platelet count is causative for the vascular event or reactive to it. Typically, patients with secondary (reactive) thrombocytosis do not require platelet-lowering or antiplatelet treatment because the abnormal platelet count itself does not place them at risk for hemostatic or vascular events.[55] An exception to that may be in patients with extreme reactive thrombocytosis and the subsequent development of acquired von Willebrand's disease.[56]

However, in ET, there is anecdotal support for emergent plateletpheresis.[55,57-59] While there have been no prospective trials on the use of plateletpheresis, expert consensus is that those with life-threatening neurological compromise, digital ischemia or bleeding due to acquired von Willebrand's disease may benefit. Because plateletpheresis lowers the platelet count only transiently, such treatment needs to be concurrent with the institution of myelosuppressive agents.[48,60] Hydroxyurea (HU), at a dose of 2–4 g daily can work to suppress platelet production in a matter of days, though administration should be closely monitored, given risk of myelosuppression. Extended use of pheresis is not an effective method of controlling thrombocytosis, likely because of the rapid rate of production of platelets. Also complicating the use of emergent plateletpheresis is the fact that there is poor correlation between platelet number and onset or resolution of thrombotic events[61] and therefore there is no ideal endpoint, once the procedure has been undertaken.

Asymptomatic/Low Risk Patients

There are no convincing data that asymptomatic, low risk patients need to initiate cytoreductive therapy[10,26,41,62]—specifically patients under the age of 60 years without a prior vascular event. A small study, which followed age- and sex-matched individuals with and without ET, found no increase in the rate of thrombosis, bleeding or other morbidities over relatively short periods of time (i.e., 4–9 years).[47] That being said, all patients should clearly be educated regarding smoking cessation, controlling hypertension and mitigating—MPN-unrelated risks for cerebrovascular, cardiac, or venous thrombosis.

There are two possible exceptions to the watch-and-wait recommendation in asymptomatic patients. The first is in asymptomatic patients with a platelet count greater than about 1.0–1.5 × 10^9/L, which is considered a risk factor for bleeding. Recommendations in such a population include either starting cytoreductive therapy[41] or testing for acquired von Willebrand's disease with a ristocetin cofactor assay and beginning cytoreductive therapy if the activity level is reduced.[26] The second exception is that some practitioners start patients on low-dose aspirin as primary prophylaxis for venous thromboembolism (VTE) or arterial events. There is no randomized data to support this practice, however, and data are extrapolated from a study of PV patients. The European Collaboration on Low-dose Aspirin in Polycythemia Vera (ECLAP) study, a large Italian population of primarily low risk PV patients randomized 518 individuals to aspirin (100 mg) or placebo.[44] With a mean follow-up of 3 years, results favored the intervention arm, where there were fewer vascular complications. This study provides some evidence that aspirin in low risk MPN patients may prevent vascular complications, but this has not been tested in the population of asymptomatic, low risk ET (rather than PV) patients. Aspirin is not without risk, however, and some authors have made a point that the ECLAP study should not be used to justify treating ET patients with aspirin.[46] Bleeding occurs in particular in patients with a WHO classification of early-PMF, rather than ET,[62] and in patients with severe functional platelet defects or with acquired vWF deficiency. For this reason, recommendations on aspirin therapy should be undertaken on a case-by-case basis in asymptomatic, low-risk and is likely contraindicated in patients with risks for bleeding, for example, platelet count over 1,000 × 10^9/L.

Vasomotor Symptoms

Low-dose aspirin is effective at treating some of the vasomotor disturbances in patients with ET, including erythromelalgia, ocular disturbances, migraines and even seizures.[63-65] Patients with progression of erythromelalgia to frank gangrene likely warrant rapid cytoreductive therapy in addition to aspirin.

High Risk Patients

As outlined above, high-risk patients in ET include those with a history of prior hemorrhage, thrombosis, or age greater than 60 years. In these patients, cytoreductive therapy is indicated. The goals are to reduce the risk of additional arterial or venous thrombosis and to minimize symptoms. There is no treatment currently able to prevent myelofibrotic or leukemic transformation. In the later part of the last century, HU—a ribonucleotide reductase inhibitor–became the drug of choice in patients with ET requiring therapy. This is largely because other options, including radioactive phosphorus and busulfan had been demonstrated to be leukemogenic. Such has not been proven for HU, though concerns about stem cell damage and subsequent development of AML after therapy may still be considered, especially when treating a younger patient. Currently evidence supports HU as a first choice[10,26,41,66] in many patients, while interferon (INF)-based therapies have gained acceptance as a reasonable alternative in younger patients.

Data from a randomized study demonstrated that HU is more effective than placebo in preventing thrombosis in patients with high risk ET.[67] In this Italian study, more than 114 patients above the age of 40 were randomized to HU versus no cytoreductive therapy. Over a median follow-up of 27 months, there were significantly more thrombotic events in the placebo arm (10.7% patient-year vs. 1.6% patient-year; p = 0.003). These data established HU as a first-line agent for this condition. The dose administered was 15 mg/kg daily and was thereafter adjusted for a goal platelet count of less than 600,000/mL and a WBC of greater than 4,000/mm^3. In patients with a prior history of arterial clotting or with vasomotor symptoms, aspirin was also administered.

As noted above, concerns have been raised about the possible leukemogenic potential of HU. In particular, a French study published in 1998, identified 17 cases of MDS or AML in a population of 357 patients with ET.[68] Additional studies have not validated this finding, however. A Mayo Clinic analysis of this association summarized 13 studies of leukemic transformation in ET, in total including more than 3,000 patients.[69] Some studies suggested that HU added to another agent was implicated as a risk factor for leukemia, while HU was implicated in another of the analyzed studies. Further analysis of the French study[68] suggested that advanced age more closely associated with the 17p deletions rather than HU.[70] Many experts believe that the leukemic potential in this condition lies with the aberrations in the stem cell niche, rather than in the effect of therapy. Nevertheless, some advise caution in younger, high-risk patients, those with cytogenetic abnormalities and in patients previously treated with radiophosphorus or alkylators. Finally, HU is teratogenic, so typically alternative therapies such as INF are selected in women who desire fertility.[71,73]

Skin, hair, and nail changes have been recorded among those taking HU. Lower extremity ulcerations may reflect vasculitis, and represent an indication for permanent cessation of the medication. In addition, individuals with resistance to or intolerance of HU[73]—defined by an International Working Group as either a platelet count greater than 600 × 10^9/L after 3 months of at least 2 g/day of HU (2.5 g/day in patients with a body weight over 80 kg); a platelet count greater than 400 × 10^9/L and WBC less than 2.5 × 10^9/L or Hb less than 10 g/dL at any dose of HU; the presence of leg ulcers or other unacceptable mucocutaneous manifestations at any dose of HU; and HU-related fever. In cases of HU resistance or intolerance, patients should be managed with second-line therapy.

Anagrelide is an imidazoquinoline compound that inhibits the maturation of megakaryocytes, and represents a second-line option for the treatment of ET. The recommended initial dose is 0.5 mg orally two to four times daily. The dose should be increased by 0.5 mg/week to control thrombocytosis, but should generally not exceed 10 mg/day or 2 mg/dose. A randomized controlled trial, published in 2005 however, changed practice, as anagrelide was previously used as a frontline therapy.[74] In this study, 809 patients with high risk ET received low-dose aspirin plus either anagrelide or HU. After a median follow-up of 39 months, patients in the anagrelide arm had higher rates of arterial thrombosis, bleeding and MF. Since that time, anagrelide has lost favor as a frontline agent and is generally considered only after HU failure. Although equivalent control of the platelet count was achieved with both agents, HU also controlled leukocytosis, possibly explaining a mechanism for arterial thrombosis risk reduction, since patients in both groups had a platelet goal of 600 × 10^9/L or less. In addition, the combination of anagrelide and low-dose aspirin was associated with a higher incidence of bleeding episodes and some practioners discourage concomitant therapy with aspirin and anagrelide. The drug is not considered leukemogenic, but there is some evidence that treatment with this medication can cause an increase in reticulin fibrosis.[75] Common side-effects include palpitations and headache with rare patients reporting edema or even a reversible congestive heart failure. These 2005 data may come under reconsideration, however. In 2013, the ANAHYDRET (anagrelide vs hydroxyurea in patients with essential thrombocythemia) study was published, providing additional clinical experience on anagrelide use? This study was powered to show noninferiority in a randomization of 259 previously untreated, high risk patients with ET to anagrelide or HU. After 6 years of follow-up, the authors report no difference in event-free survival for ET-related events. They confirmed an increase rate of palpitations and tachycardia in the anagrelide arm and increased myelosuppression in the hydrea arm. Transformation to MF occurred in three patients, two in the anagrelide arm and one in the HU arm.[76]

An additional treatment option in second line, in younger high risk patients and in individuals pursuing fertility, is INF-α or pegylated (PEG) INF-α. Results in several cohort studies indicate that INF-α, at average doses of about 3 million IU daily, can induce remission (platelet counts <600 × 10^9/L) in about 90% of patients.[77] The cytokine therapy suppresses megakaryocyte-colony formation and can be effective within the first several months of therapy. The medication, which has to be injected, is cumbersome and has toxicities, especially in older patients, including flu-like symptoms during induction therapy, such as fever, bone and muscle pain, fatigue, lethargy and depression. It does not cross the placenta and has been used for therapy during pregnancy though there is very little evidence in this setting and pros and cons should be discussed in depth with the patient. A once weekly formulation of the drug, PEG-IFN-α, has also been tested in ET.[78,79] One of these studies, a prospective phase II trial by researchers at the MD Anderson included 39 patients with ET.[79] The complete response rate was about 76%, as measured by normalization of platelet counts (without additional therapy) and absence of thrombotic events. Most responses were achieved within the first 3 months of therapy. In practice, patients are started at a variety of doses, with some practitioners using the MD Anderson dose of 90 μg weekly and others starting lower than that and escalating to control counts.[78] No data are available on whether IFN therapy delays or prevents the evolution to MF or AL. To answer the question of whether IFN therapy or HU is preferable in the frontline treatment of ET, large randomized trials are ongoing.

CONCLUSION

The clinical trajectory of patients with ET is one of clinical heterogeneity—with some patients living largely unaffected for years, and other patients experiencing significant morbidity and occasionally mortality from the arterial or vascular events that punctuate the condition. Our current therapies are aimed at preventing vascular morbidity—hopefully in the future our therapeutic strategies will evolve toward delaying the transformation to AL or MF.

REFERENCES

1. Levine RL, Gilliland DG. Myeloproliferative disorders. *Blood.* 2008;112(6):2190-8.
2. Melo JV, Goldman JM. Hematologic Malignancies: Myeloproliferative Disorders, illustrated edition. Berlin, New York: Springer; 2007.p.xi, 354.
3. Dameshek W. Some speculations on the myeloproliferative syndromes. *Blood.* 1951;6(4): 372-5.
4. Baxter EJ, Scott LM, Campbell PJ, et al. Acquired mutation of the tyrosine kinase JAK2 in human myeloproliferative disorders. *Lancet.* 2005;365(9464):1054-61.
5. James C, Ugo V, Le Couedic JP, et al. A unique clonal JAK2 mutation leading to constitutive signalling causes polycythaemia vera. *Nature.* 2005;434(7037):1144-8.
6. Kralovics R, Passamonti F, Buser AS, et al. A gain-of-function mutation of JAK2 in myeloproliferative disorders. *N Engl J Med.* 2005;352(17):1779-90.
7. Levine RL, Wadleigh M, Cools J, et al. Activating mutation in the tyrosine kinase JAK2 in polycythemia vera, essential thrombocythemia, and myeloid metaplasia with myelofibrosis. *Cancer Cell.* 2005;7(4):387-97.

8. Levine RL, Heaney M. New advances in the pathogenesis and therapy of essential thrombocythemia. *Hematology Am Soc Hematol Educ Program.* 2008:76-82.
9. Soriano G, Heaney M. Polycythemia vera and essential thrombocythemia: new developments in biology with therapeutic implications. *Curr Opin Hematol.* 2013;20(2):169-75.
10. Tefferi A. Myeloproliferative neoplasms 2012: the John M. Bennett 80th birthday anniversary lecture. *Leukemia Res.* 2012;36(12):1481-9.
11. Mesa RA, Silverstein MN, Jacobsen SJ, et al. Population-based incidence and survival figures in essential thrombocythemia and agnogenic myeloid metaplasia: an Olmsted County Study, 1976-1995. *Am J Hematol.* 1999;61(1):10-5.
12. Chuncharunee S, Archararit N, Ungkanont A, et al. Etiology and incidence of thrombotic and hemorrhagic disorders in Thai patients with extreme thrombocytosis. *J Med Assoc Thai.* 2000;83(Suppl 1):S95-100.
13. Jensen MK, de Nully Brown P, Nielsen OJ, et al. Incidence, clinical features and outcome of essential thrombocythaemia in a well defined geographical area. *Eur J Haematol.* 2000; 65(2):132-9.
14. Vardiman JW, Thiele J, Arber DA, et al. The 2008 revision of the World Health Organization (WHO) classification of myeloid neoplasms and acute leukemia: rationale and important changes. *Blood.* 2009;114(5):937-51.
15. Johansson P, Kutti J, Andreasson B, et al. Trends in the incidence of chronic Philadelphia chromosome negative (Ph-) myeloproliferative disorders in the city of Goteborg, Sweden, during 1983-99. *J Intern Med.* 2004;256(2):161-5.
16. Girodon F, Bonicelli G, Schaeffer C, et al. Significant increase in the apparent incidence of essential thrombocythemia related to new WHO diagnostic criteria: a population-based study. *Haematologica.* 2009;94(6):865-9.
17. Nguyen HM, Kiladjian JJ. Is there a role for the use of IFN-α in primary myelofibrosis? *Hematology Am Soc Hematol Educ Program.* 2012;2012:567-70.
18. Vainchenker W, Delhommeau F, Constantinescu SN, et al. New mutations and pathogenesis of myeloproliferative neoplasms. *Blood.* 2011;118(7):1723-35.
19. Palandri F, Ottaviani E, Salmi F, et al. JAK2 V617F mutation in essential thrombocythemia: correlation with clinical characteristics, response to therapy and long-term outcome in a cohort of 275 patients. *Leuk Lymphoma.* 2009;50(2):247-53.
20. Cho YU, Chi HS, Lee EH, et al. Comparison of clinicopathologic findings according to JAK2 V617F mutation in patients with essential thrombocythemia. *Inter J Hematol.* 2009;89(1):39-44.
21. Carobbio A, Thiele J, Passamonti F, et al. Risk factors for arterial and venous thrombosis in WHO-defined essential thrombocythemia: an international study of 891 patients. *Blood.* 2011;117(22):5857-9.
22. Passamonti F, Thiele J, Girodon F, et al. A prognostic model to predict survival in 867 World Health Organization-defined essential thrombocythemia at diagnosis: a study by the International Working Group on Myelofibrosis Research and Treatment. *Blood.* 2012;120(6):1197-201.
23. Lussana F, Caberlon S, Pagani C, et al. Association of V617F Jak2 mutation with the risk of thrombosis among patients with essential thrombocythaemia or idiopathic myelofibrosis: a systematic review. *Thromb Res.* 2009;124(4):409-17.
24. Nangalia J, Massie CE, Baxter EJ, Nice FL, Gundem G, Wedge DC et al. Somatic CALR mutations in myeloproliferative neoplasms with nonmutated JAK2. *N Engl J Med.* 2013;369:2391-405.
25. Klampfi T, Gisslinger H, Harutyunyan AS, Nivarthi H, Rumi E, Milosevic JD, et al. Somatic mutations of calreticulin in myeloproliferative neoplasms. N Engl J Med. 2013;369:2379-90.
26. Tefferi A. Polycythemia vera and essential thrombocythemia: 2012 update on diagnosis, risk stratification, and management. *Am J Hematol.* 2012;87(3):285-93.
27. Barbui T, Thiele J, Passamonti F, et al. Survival and disease progression in essential thrombocythemia are significantly influenced by accurate morphologic diagnosis: an international study. *J Clin Oncol.* 2011;29(23):3179-84.

28. Barbui T, Barosi G, Grossi A, et al. Practice guidelines for the therapy of essential thrombocythemia. A statement from the Italian Society of Hematology, the Italian Society of Experimental Hematology and the Italian Group for Bone Marrow Transplantation. *Haematologica.* 2004;89(2):215-32.
29. Bazzan M, Tamponi G, Schinco P, et al. Thrombosis-free survival and life expectancy in 187 consecutive patients with essential thrombocythemia. *Ann Hematol.* 1999;78(12):539-43.
30. Kessler CM, Klein HG, Havlik RJ. Uncontrolled thrombocytosis in chronic myeloproliferative disorders. *Br J Haematol.* 1982;50(1):157-67.
31. Rozman C, Giralt M, Feliu E, et al. Life expectancy of patients with chronic nonleukemic myeloproliferative disorders. *Cancer.* 1991;67(10):2658-63.
32. Passamonti F, Rumi E, Pungolino E, et al. Life expectancy and prognostic factors for survival in patients with polycythemia vera and essential thrombocythemia. *Am J Med.* 2004;117(10):755-61.
33. Wolanskyj AP, Schwager SM, McClure RF, et al. Essential thrombocythemia beyond the first decade: life expectancy, long-term complication rates, and prognostic factors. *Mayo Clin Proc.* 2006;81(2):159-66.
34. Hultcrantz M, Kristinsson SY, Andersson TM, et al. Patterns of survival among patients with myeloproliferative neoplasms diagnosed in Sweden from 1973 to 2008: a population-based study. *J Clin Oncol.* 2012;30(24):2995-3001.
35. World Health Organization classification of tumors of hematopoietic and lymphoid tissues. Lyon, France: IARC; 2008.
36. Passamonti F, Randi ML, Rumi E, et al. Increased risk of pregnancy complications in patients with essential thrombocythemia carrying the JAK2 (617V>F) mutation. *Blood.* 2007;110(2):485-9.
37. Singh N, Kumar S, Roy KK, et al. Successful maternal and fetal outcome in a rare case of essential Thrombocythemia with pregnancy using Interferon alpha. *Platelets.* 2012;23(4):319-21.
38. Valera MC, Parant O, Vayssiere C, et al. Essential thrombocythemia and pregnancy. *Eur J Obstet Gynecol Reprod Biol.* 2011;158(2):141-7.
39. Kiladjian JJ, Cervantes F, Leebeek FW, et al. The impact of JAK2 and MPL mutations on diagnosis and prognosis of splanchnic vein thrombosis: a report on 241 cases. *Blood.* 2008;111(10):4922-9.
40. Smalberg JH, Arends LR, Valla DC, et al. Myeloproliferative neoplasms in Budd-Chiari syndrome and portal vein thrombosis: a meta-analysis. *Blood.* 2012;120(25):4921-8.
41. Finazzi G, Barbui T. Risk-adapted therapy in essential thrombocythemia and polycythemia vera. *Blood Rev.* 2005;19(5):243-52.
42. Harrison CN, Gale RE, Machin SJ, et al. A large proportion of patients with a diagnosis of essential thrombocythemia do not have a clonal disorder and may be at lower risk of thrombotic complications. *Blood.* 1999;93(2):417-24.
43. Jantunen R, Juvonen E, Ikkala E, et al. The predictive value of vascular risk factors and gender for the development of thrombotic complications in essential thrombocythemia. *Ann Hematol.* 2001;80(2):74-8.
44. Marchioli R, Finazzi G, Landolfi R, et al. Vascular and neoplastic risk in a large cohort of patients with polycythemia vera. *J Clin Oncol.* 2005;23(10):2224-32.
45. Campbell PJ, MacLean C, Beer PA, et al. Correlation of blood counts with vascular complications in essential thrombocythemia: analysis of the prospective PT1 cohort. *Blood.* 2012;120(7):1409-11.
46. Barbui T, Finazzi MC, Finazzi G. Front-line therapy in polycythemia vera and essential thrombocythemia. *Blood Rev.* 2012;26(5):205-11.
47. Tefferi A, Fonseca R, Pereira DL, et al. A long-term retrospective study of young women with essential thrombocythemia. *Mayo Clin Proc.* 2001;76(1):22-8.
48. Hoffman R. Hematology: Basic Principles and Practice. 5th ed. Philadelphia, PA: Churchill Livingstone/Elsevier; 2009. p. xxvii, 2523.

49. Michiels JJ, Berneman Z, Schroyens W, et al. The paradox of platelet activation and impaired function: platelet-von Willebrand factor interactions, and the etiology of thrombotic and hemorrhagic manifestations in essential thrombocythemia and polycythemia vera. *Semin Thromb Hemost.* 2006;32(6):589-604.
50. Kessler CM. Propensity for hemorrhage and thrombosis in chronic myeloproliferative disorders. *Semin Hematol.* 2004;41(2 Suppl 3):10-4.
51. Landolfi R, Cipriani MC, Novarese L. Thrombosis and bleeding in polycythemia vera and essential thrombocythemia: pathogenetic mechanisms and prevention. *Best Pract Res Clin Haematol.* 2006;19(3):617-33.
52. Murakawa M, Okamura T, Tsutsumi K, et al. Acquired von Willebrand's disease in association with essential thrombocythemia: regression following treatment. *Acta Haematologica.* 1992;87(1-2):83-7.
53. Raman BK, Sawdyk M, Saeed SM. Essential thrombocythemia with acquired von Willebrand's disease. *Am J Clin Pathol.* 1987;88(1):102-6.
54. Rolf N, Suttorp M, Budde U, et al. Essential thrombocythaemia in a teenage girl resulting in acquired von Willebrand syndrome with joint haemorrhage and menorrhagia. *Thromb Haemost.* 2010;103(6):1272-4.
55. Schafer AI. Thrombocytosis. *N Engl J Med.* 2004;350(12):1211-9.
56. Ruggeri M, Finazzi G, Tosetto A, et al. No treatment for low-risk thrombocythaemia: results from a prospective study. *Br J Haematol.* 1998;103(3):772-7.
57. Greist A. The role of blood component removal in essential and reactive thrombocytosis. *Ther Apher.* 2002;6(1):36-44.
58. Schafer AI. Bleeding and thrombosis in the myeloproliferative disorders. *Blood.* 1984;64(1):1-12.
59. Taft EG, Babcock RB, Scharfman WB, Tartaglia AP. Plateletpheresis in the management of thrombocytosis. *Blood.* 1977;50(5):927-33.
60. Duvall D. Therapeutic cytapheresis: too many platelets, too many white blood cells. *J Clin Apher.* 2011;26(1):47-52.
61. Di Nisio M, Barbui T, Di Gennaro L, et al. The haematocrit and platelet target in polycythemia vera. *Br J Haematol.* 2007;136(2):249-59.
62. Finazzi G, Carobbio A, Thiele J, et al. Incidence and risk factors for bleeding in 1104 patients with essential thrombocythemia or prefibrotic myelofibrosis diagnosed according to the 2008 WHO criteria. *Leukemia.* 2012;26(4):716-9.
63. Michiels JJ. Platelet-mediated microvascular inflammation and thrombosis in thrombocythemia vera: a distinct aspirin-responsive arterial thrombophilia, which transforms into a bleeding diathesis at increasing platelet counts. *Pathologie Biol.* 2003;51(3):167-75.
64. Michiels JJ, Berneman Z, Schroyens W, et al. Platelet-mediated erythromelalgic, cerebral, ocular and coronary microvascular ischemic and thrombotic manifestations in patients with essential thrombocythemia and polycythemia vera: a distinct aspirin-responsive and coumadin-resistant arterial thrombophilia. *Platelets.* 2006;17(8):528-44.
65. Michiels JJ, van Genderen PJ, Lindemans J, et al. Erythromelalgic, thrombotic and hemorrhagic manifestations in 50 cases of thrombocythemia. *Leuk Lymphoma.* 1996;22(Suppl 1):47-56.
66. Barbui T, Finazzi G. When and how to treat essential thrombocythemia. *N Engl J Med.* 2005;353(1):85-6.
67. Cortelazzo S, Finazzi G, Ruggeri M, et al. Hydroxyurea for patients with essential thrombocythemia and a high risk of thrombosis. *N Engl J Med.* 1995;332(17):1132-6.
68. Sterkers Y, Preudhomme C, Lai JL, et al. Acute myeloid leukemia and myelodysplastic syndromes following essential thrombocythemia treated with hydroxyurea: high proportion of cases with 17p deletion. *Blood.* 1998;91(2):616-22.
69. Gangat N, Wolanskyj AP, McClure RF, et al. Risk stratification for survival and leukemic transformation in essential thrombocythemia: a single institutional study of 605 patients. *Leukemia.* 2007;21(2):270-6.

70. Liu TC, Suri R. Multiple factors in the transformation of essential thrombocythemia to acute leukemia or myelodysplastic syndrome. *Blood.* 1998;92(4):1465-6.
71. Griesshammer M, Struve S, Barbui T. Management of Philadelphia negative chronic myeloproliferative disorders in pregnancy. *Blood Rev.* 2008;22(5):235-45.
72. Harrison CN, Robinson SE. Myeloproliferative disorders in pregnancy. *Hematol Oncol Clin N Am.* 2011;25(2):261-75, vii.
73. Barosi G, Besses C, Birgegard G, et al. A unified definition of clinical resistance/intolerance to hydroxyurea in essential thrombocythemia: results of a consensus process by an international working group. *Leukemia.* 2007;21(2):277-80.
74. Harrison CN, Campbell PJ, Buck G, et al. Hydroxyurea compared with anagrelide in high-risk essential thrombocythemia. *N Engl J Med.* 2005;353(1):33-45.
75. Hultdin M, Sundstrom G, Wahlin A, et al. Progression of bone marrow fibrosis in patients with essential thrombocythemia and polycythemia vera during anagrelide treatment. *Med Oncol.* 2007;24(1):63-70.
76. Gisslinger H, Gotic M, Holowiecki J, et al. Anagrelide compared with hydroxyurea in WHO-classified essential thrombocythemia: the ANAHYDRET Study, a randomized controlled trial. *Blood.* 2013;121(10):1720-8.
77. Lengfelder E, Griesshammer M, Hehlmann R. Interferon-alpha in the treatment of essential thrombocythemia. *Leuk Lymphoma.* 1996;22(Suppl 1):135-42.
78. Gowin K, Thapaliya P, Samuelson J, et al. Experience with pegylated interferon alpha-2a in advanced myeloproliferative neoplasms in an international cohort of 118 patients. *Haematologica.* 2012;97(10):1570-3.
79. Quintas-Cardama A, Kantarjian H, Manshouri T, et al. Pegylated interferon alfa-2a yields high rates of hematologic and molecular response in patients with advanced essential thrombocythemia and polycythemia vera. *J Clin Oncol.* 2009;27(32):5418-24.

CHAPTER

5 Polycythemia Vera

Jonathan M Gerber, Alison R Moliterno

INTRODUCTION

Plethora has been observed in individuals since antiquity. The first published report of a disease of overproduction of red cells in the absence cardiopulmonary disease, erythremia, is attributed to Vaquez in his 1892 case report. William Oslcr reported four cases of his own in addition to reviewing five other published cases,[1] recognized splenomegaly as an associated feature, coined the term Polycythemia vera (PV), and promoted the concept that PV represented a distinct clinical entity through lectures and his textbook. By 1920, hundreds of cases had been reported and the disease entity extended to include elevations of white cells and platelets in addition to red cells. The primary nature of the bone marrow's overproduction was compared to that of leukemia, and both chronic myelogenous leukemia and PV were "looked upon as neoplasms of the hemopoietic tissue".[2] Over the first 50 years of the disease reporting, the variation of clinical presentation, blood and bone marrow pathology and natural history became evident, as were similarities to both agnogenic myeloid metaplasia and chronic granulocytic leukemia.[3] William Dameshek theorized that these entities might be driven by a shared stimulus intrinsic to the marrow itself, and coined the term myeloproliferative disorders (MPDs),[4] a classification that included erythroleukemia.

Given the phenotypic variability within PV, the Polycythemia Vera Study Group (PVSG) developed a set of diagnostic criteria for entrance into their studies, and this criteria, incorporating major criteria of elevated red cell mass, oxygen saturation threshold, splenomegaly and minor criteria of thrombocytosis, leukocytosis, leukocyte alkaline phosphatase, and serum B_{12} became a tool with which to distinguish PV from secondary forms of erythrocytosis.[3,5] These criteria, if met, led one to a high confidence of identifying PV; not fulfilling the criteria however did not exclude PV.

PATHOGENESIS

Progress in understanding the cause of PV was intimately tied to discoveries in the regulation of erythropoiesis, stem cell physiology, signal transduction, cancer genetics, and gene resequencing technology. While hypoxia was excluded as a stimulus in PV,[6] the dissection of normal erythropoiesis, however, was critical to the understanding the pathophysiology of PV. Excess erythropoietin as stimulus source was excluded given very low erythropoietin levels in PV patients.[7,8] However, the seminal observations of erythropoietin independent erythroid colony formation,[9] growth factor hypersensitivity,[10] and the influence of tyrosine kinase inhibitors to abolish this aberrant growth[11] established that this growth advantage was an intrinsic capacity present in progenitor cells, and pointed to an intracellular stimulus that amplified or recapitulated erythroid, megakaryocyte, and myeloid signal transduction pathways.

At the same time, advances in cancer genetics informed the MPD classification. The identification of the Philadelphia (Ph) chromosome as specific to chronic myelogenous leukemia (CML) and not to the rest of the MPD class was critical in generating another exclusion criterion for PV.[12,13] Moreover, the Ph chromosome lesion ultimately was proven to be the marrow stimulus to generate the disease CML via the gene product of the translocation, breakpoint cluster region (BCR)-Abelson leukemia virus (ABL),[14] confirming the causal association of an acquired genetic lesion in the generation of human cancer. Clonality assays applied to PV showed that like CML, patients' hematopoiesis was clonal, and was clonal not only in red cells and white cells but also B lymphocytes, indicating that this stimulus was active in a multipotent stem cell.[15] Unlike CML, however, chromosomal studies in PV patients did not identify a highly prevalent structural rearrangement or defect that could point to a causative genetic lesion.

Acquired Somatic Mutations of Janus Kinase 2 (JAK2)

Given the assembled observations, it is not unexpected that a causative lesion generating the pathobiology of PV would reside in a tyrosine kinase critical to erythropoietin, thrombopoietin, and granulocyte colony-stimulating factor (G-CSF) signal transduction. Advances in deoxyribonucleic acid (DNA) sequencing technology led several investigators to resequence the JAK2 gene in PV patients due to its specific activity in primary PV cells,[16] due to its identity as a tyrosine kinase,[17-19] or due to its location in the chromosome 9p loss of heterozygosity region highly prevalent in PV.[20,21]

All of the 2005 reports found not only the same allele, JAK2 V617F (a change of valine to phenylalanine at the 617 position), but also found variation in the relative amounts of the mutant allele compared to the wild-type allele across PV patients, and that in roughly 30% of PV patients the wild-type JAK2 allele could not be detected at all. Moreover, the greater the sensitivity of the assay used to detect V617F, the higher the prevalence of JAK2 V617F in a PV cohort, indicating that relative amounts of JAK2 V617F could be quite low in PV, and that the sensitivity of the assay would need to approach 1% in order to reliably capture all JAK2 V617F positive cases. Thus studies using Sanger sequencing technology, which typically is sensitive only to 10% of a particular allele, reported the prevalence of JAK2 V617F in PV to be only 74%. Higher sensitivity assays, applied to either the same PV cohort[17] or different PV cohorts[22-24] found the prevalence of JAK2 V617F to be greater than 95% of PV cases (Table 5-1).

Soon after the reports of V617F came the findings of lesions in other regions of the JAK2 gene in JAKV617F-negative PV cases, which were identified in roughly 3% of large PV cohorts[25,26] and in a far lower prevalence in patients with patients classified clinically as idiopathic erythrocytosis.[24,27] The clinical manifestations of these cases uniformly include erythrocytosis, while to a lesser degree other aspect of JAK2 V617F positive PV, such as splenomegaly, leukocytosis, and thrombocytosis. Taken together, the vast majority of patients with a PV phenotype will harbor an acquired somatic mutation in the JAK2 gene. A small fraction of PV patients remain molecularly undefined, either due to assay sensitivity issues, or due to lesions in the JAK2 gene or other genes that are not targeted by current clinical or research assays.

Janus kinase 2 mutations are found in more than 97% of PV patients but JAK2 V617F is also highly prevalent in patients with essential thrombocytosis (ET) and primary myelofibrosis (PMF). How a shared mutation in JAK2 V617F can lead to these myeloproliferative neoplasm (MPN) phenotypes is an important question, and hypothetical mechanisms include variation in gene dosage, host genetic

Table 5-1 Prevalence of Janus Kinase 2 V617F (A Change of Valine to Phenylalanine at the 617 Position) in Polycythemia Vera (PV)

Reference	*Number V617F+*	*Total PV studied*	*% V617F+*	*Technique*
James 2005[16]	40	45	89	Sanger
Baxter 2005[17]	50	73	68	Sanger
Levine 2005[18]	121	164	74	Sanger
Jones 2005[22]	58	72	81	ARMS
Kralovics 2005[21]	83	128	65	Sanger
Wang 2008[23]	27	33	82	Pyrosequencing
Zhao 2005[19]	20	24	83	Sanger
Total	**399**	**539**	**74**	
Reference	*Number V617F+*	*Total PV studied*	*% V617F+*	*Technique*
Baxter 2005[17]	71	73	97	Allele Specific
Williams 2007[24]	147	157	94	Allele Specific
Wang 2008[23]	103	104	99	ARMS-modified
Total	**321**	**334**	**96**	

ARMS, amplification refractory mutation system.

background, progenitor cell clonal dominance, and the influence of additional acquired somatic lesions (vide infra). Credence to the concept that JAK2 mutations are causative lesions in PV are as follows: high prevalence in PV, recapitulation of PV disease in JAK2 V617F transgenic murine models,[28] gene-dosage effect of JAK2 V617F on PV phenotype,[29] and hematologic remissions corresponding to molecular remissions.[30,31]

JAK2 V617F Gene Dosage in the MPN

JAK 2 V617F is an acquired mutation where a single nucleotide substitution of thymidine for guanidine results in the amino acid substitution of phenylalanine for valine at position 617 within the JH2 (pseudokinase domain) regulatory domain, a region with a purported autoinhibitory effect on the kinase activity. The JAK2 gene is located on chromosome 9p24. Years prior to the JAK2 mutation discovery a genome wide screen in PV identified a recurrent genomic lesion characterized by copy neutral loss of heterozygosity of chromosome 9p resulting in uniparental disomy (UPD).[20] While the bounds of the region encompassing the 9p UPD varied among PV cases and contained many genes, virtually all of the cases contained the JAK2 gene. Within myeloid diseases, 9p UPD associates closely with mutation of the JAK2 gene, such that virtually all cases with 9p UPD harbor a mutation of the JAK2 gene; conversely, a high proportion of individuals with a JAK2 mutation have 9p UPD, either at diagnosis during follow-up. Thus, because of a high prevalence of UPD involving the JAK2 gene associated with JAK2 V617F, JAK2 V617F can exist in a homozygous genotype. The sequence of events appears to be the acquisition of JAK2 V617F, followed by the development of 9p UPD and subsequently homozygosity of JAK2 V617F. This model is supported by the observations that in the majority of PV patients, hematopoietic colonies with JAK2 wild-type, JAK2 V617F heterozygous, and JAK2 V617F homozygous clonal genotypes coexist.

Unlike CML, in which the majority of cells carry the BCR-ABL oncogene at diagnosis, in PV, not all progenitor cells may carry JAK2 V617F. Moreover, a PV patient is typically mosaic at the progenitor level, with wild-type, JAK2 V617F heterozygous and JAK2 V617F homozygous clones participating in hematopoiesis at any one time.[32-34] Because of the variability in the number of cells that carry the mutation and the number of JAK2 V617F alleles harbored in each cell, there is marked variability in the JAK2 V617F gene dosage across MPN patient cohorts, whether ascertained in marrow progenitors or peripheral blood cells. Thus the gene dosage of JAK2 V617F becomes not just a categorical variable but a continuous, quantitative variable, in which a large dynamic range of JAK2 V617F allele percentages, or allele burden, has been reported. Moreover, there is time dependence to both the acquisition of 9p UPD, and to the expansion of various clones, such that allele burdens may increase over time.

EPIDEMIOLOGY

The 20th century reports of PV describe PV as a disease of older males, with a median age at presentation of 60 years and a male predominance.[35,36] In contrast to CML, where the identification of BCR-ABL oncogene did not dramatically alter the ascertainment of the disease, the discovery of JAK2 mutations has the potential to alter the ascertainment, and therefore the epidemiology of PV. JAK2 V617F in many individuals is latent and may be asymptomatic or a-phenotypic for undisclosed periods of time, as evidenced by its detection in large unselected population surveys[37] or even as the result of personalized genome sequencing (www.bloomberg.com/news/2012-02-15/harvard-mapping-my-dna-turns-scary-as-threatening-gene-emerges.html) in individuals not yet identified as having an MPN. PV is often preceded by isolated thrombocytosis or erythrocytosis by years to decades before the panmyelosis of PV is fully realized.[24] Thus, prior to molecular testing for JAK2 V617F, some patients might not have fulfilled PVSG or World Health Organization (WHO) diagnostic criteria, or even considered to have a clonal MPN. On the other hand, entities that have clinical features of PV (i.e., obstructive sleep apnea, Chuvash polycythemia) can be effectively ruled out by a negative JAK2 mutation analysis, and a more accurate assessment of PV epidemiology is possible. Thus one would anticipate that the age at JAK2 V617F positive MPN diagnosis may be lower in the post-JAK2 era compared to the pre-JAK2 era due to both sensitive molecular ascertainment and revised diagnostic criteria.

RISK FACTORS

Like CML, PV historically was perceived as a sporadic disease without well-defined lifestyle or environmental exposure risk factors, or associated cancer predisposition syndromes. The JAK2 V617F discovery has informed both germline and environmental risk factor analyses. Genome wide association studies have identified a haplotype within the JAK2 gene that appears to be overrepresented in both JAK2 V617F-positive MPN patients, and also in JAK2 V617F-negative patients.[38-40] The JAK2 haplotype is in a noncoding region of the JAK2 gene, thus the mechanism behind this association is not immediately apparent. JAK2 V617F testing has facilitated the identification of a cluster of PV cases in a region of the United States where there has been a concern about environment hazards, suggesting that a unique toxic exposure may influence risk of developing PV.[41,42] In contrast to CML, familial clustering in PV has been observed for decades, suggesting a germline risk as an additional factor for susceptibility.[43,44]

Reports of large MPN cohorts phenotyped and genotyped in the post-2005 discovery era indicate that JAK2 V617F-positive PV patients comprise a diverse age at onset, with JAK2 V617F-positive PV presenting as early as the 1st decade, and as late as the 10th decade, with median ages differing depending on the cohort described.[45]

Modern, post-JAK2 V617F discovery cohorts indicate that females outnumber males in PV,[46,47] and that females comprise the majority of PV patients diagnosed below the age of 40 years (75%), whereas a gender differences are not as pronounced in PV cohorts diagnosed after the age of 50 years.[48] Female predominance at a younger age is atypical for cancer in general (cancer rates increase with age and males have higher cancer rated than females), and for hematologic malignancies in particular. Males outnumber females in both acute myelogenous leukemia (AML) and myelodysplastic syndrome (MDS),[49] and in other chronic MPN, such as chronic myelomonocytic leukemia, PMF, CML, and hypereosinophilic syndrome associated with aberrations of the platelet-derived growth factor receptor alpha gene, male predominance is the rule.[50] Figure 5-1 shows the age and gender distribution at diagnosis of 273 JAK2 mutation positive PV patients from the Johns Hopkins Hospital. In this prospective, post-2005 cohort, women outnumber men at every age, although this gender gap is most pronounced in patients diagnosed below the age of 50 years. The excess of younger women with PV is highly atypical for myeloid disease, and suggests a unique risk factor for either acquisition or elaboration of the JAK2 mutation that is specifically applicable to young females.

DIFFERENTIAL DIAGNOSIS

Polycythemia vera may present with isolated erythrocytosis, without extramedullary disease, or panmyelosis. Before JAK2 V617F, discriminating PV from secondary erythrocytosis relied heavily on the interpretation of serum erythropoietin levels and oxygen saturation studies, neither of which could be entirely relied upon.[45] Given the high prevalence of JAK2 mutations in PV, currently the diagnosis of PV should be seriously questioned in erythrocytosis patients who are negative for JAK2 mutations. In those patients, efforts to define high-affinity hemoglobins, lesions in hypoxia-sensing pathways or erythropoietin-sensing should be pursued.[51]

Polycythemia vera commonly presents with erythrocytosis and thrombocytosis. Moreover, PV frequently develops after many years (at times decades) of ET. In these circumstances, JAK2 V617F testing can be helpful in distinguishing clinical phenotypes, as the finding of JAK2 V627F homozygosity (allele burdens >55%) favors a diagnosis of PV over ET. However, JAK2 V617F allele burdens less than 55% are compatible with either ET or PV, and in this circumstance, red cell mass testing particularly is critical in establishing one entity from another.[52-54]

NATURAL HISTORY

The natural history of PV is centered on two main complications: thrombosis and transformation to higher grade myeloid disease. These two broad categories conspire to shorten the lifespan of PV patients compared to control populations.[55] However, unlike CML in which disease transformation is both inevitable, and on

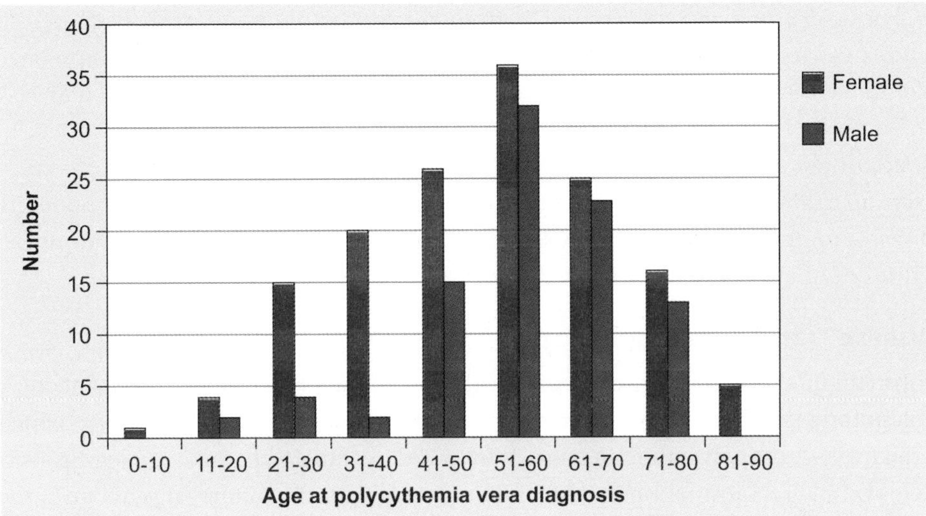

Figure 5-1 A modern era polycythemia vera (PV) cohort stratified by age at diagnosis and by gender. 239 Janus kinase 2 (JAK2) mutation positive PV patients were evaluated at the Johns Hopkins Hospital between 2005 and 2012, 148 (62%) of whom were female. The median age at PV diagnosis of 53 (range 8–88) in female PV patients was significantly lower compared to the median age of 58 years (range 15–78) in males ($p = 0.012$, Mann Whitney Rank Sum).

a fairly uniform time-course, PV demonstrates marked variability in the rate of these complications, with many patients experiencing several decades of PV, uncomplicated by either thrombosis or transformation, while others experience both, at times simultaneously and early on in their PV. Unlike CML, in PV, host genetics, gender, lifestyle, treatment, and comorbidities exert a large influence of the risks of these complications.[45,56-58]

Thrombosis

Nearly 20% of PV patients may experience a thrombotic event over the course of their disease.[45,48] Thrombotic events in many cases herald the diagnosis of PV, or may even precede the diagnosis by several years. Thrombotic events occur on the arterial and venous circulation, microvascular, or thromboembolic, such as transient ischemic attacks, myocardial infarction, deep venous thromboses, or pulmonary embolism. Alternatively, atypical circulations and events unique to PV include the portal and hepatic systems, cerebral venous sinus, and splenic veins.[59-63]

Thrombosis historically was a major cause of mortality in PV, and was cited as the most common cause of death when natural histories were first reported, and was subsequently well documented during the initial PVSG trials. Recognition of elevation in the hematocrit as a critical risk factor for thrombosis, particularly on the venous circulation, had led to the recommendations for lowering hematocrit to below 45% to avoid this complication, a recommendation recently validated in a prospective randomized controlled trial.[64] Multivariate analyses in addition have identified the white cell count, platelet count, and the traditional vascular risk factors (age, hypertension, prior thrombotic events, diabetes, and hyperlipidemia) as important risks for thrombotic events in PV. The JAK2 V617F mutation seems to exert an influence on thrombosis risk, either indirectly through its effect on white cell count, or even more directly on mechanisms, such as platelet activation and white cell/platelet interactions.[65]

Disease Transformation

Polycythemia vera may run a course of uncomplicated decades requiring only phlebotomy, or may follow a progressive, malignant course similar to CML in which a relatively short polycythemic phase is followed by transformation to myelofibrosis, followed by transformation to AML, all occurring within a matter of years from the original PV diagnosis. Like CML, time and genomic instability may interact to drive transformation forward, but unlike CML, this is neither inevitable nor predictable in PV, and suggests additional risk factors for transformation beyond disease classification.

Post-polycythemic vera myelofibrosis (post-PVMF) is defined as the development of anemia (hemoglobin below 10 g/dL), osteosclerosis of the marrow, and usually prominent extramedullary hematopoiesis. The post-PVMF phase of the disease clinically and molecularly resembles de novo PMF, with expansion of circulating stem cells, high JAK2 allele burdens in the stem cells as well as neutrophils, and the association of chromosome changes, such as 20q deletion, 13q deletion, trisomy 9, and mutation of the additional sex combs-like protein 1 (ASXL1) gene.[66-68] The nonrandom chromosomal changes that are present in greater than 60% of post-PVMF patients, and their similar prevalence in de novo PMF, suggests that these lesions drive myelofibrosis physiology and alter the cellular context of JAK2 V617F signaling.[69] Red cell production, unheeded in JAK2 V617F-positive PV, becomes impaired when these additional lesions develop and come to dominate the stem cell pool.[67] Despite the unwanted development of post-PVMF, this phase may extend years to even decades, unlike the accelerated phase of CML, which historically was less than 2 years. Recent studies of post-PVMF indicated that about 15% of patients developed myelofibrosis at a median of 10 years after PV diagnosis that this percentage increased to almost 50% after 20 years, and that subset of PV patients who had lower JAK2 V617F allele burdens had a significantly lower risk of this outcome compared to the subset with higher allele burdens.[46,70]

Acute myelogenous leukemia arising directly out of chronic phase PV is unusual, estimated to occur in up to 4% of PV patients, whereas AML evolving from post-PVMF is more common, occurring in as many as 20% of MF patients.[46,71] The leukemia-accelerating effects of radioactive phosphorus and the alkylator pipobroman on the natural history of PV was and remains sobering,[45,72] and reveals the power of good intentioned myelosuppressive therapy to unleash genomic unstability with miserable outcomes. Moreover, this experience in PV calls any potentially genotoxic therapy into question regarding safety, especially given the long-term exposure to any therapy that some PV patients will require, and the need for therapy in elderly PV patients. Traditional risk factors for AML development include older age, P23 or alkylator therapy, post-PVMF, and hemoglobin below 10 g/dL.[72] Surprisingly, however, a substantial fraction of the leukemias arising from JAK2 V617F-positive PV are themselves JAK2 V617F negative.[73-75] Whether high JAK2 V617F allele burdens impart a risk of leukemia due to JAK2 V617F homozygosity driving genomic instability in the stem cell pool directly, as is the case with CML,[76] or whether the genetic process underlying the acquisition of two copies of the JAK2 mutation also serves to drive leukemia in residual JAK2 wild-type stem cell clones are both possible, and probably likely biologies.[77,78]

THERAPY

Conventional therapeutic goals for PV have included reducing the expanded blood volume to achieve a more normal blood volume physiology with positive effects on blood viscosity, blood pressure and blood flow. Phlebotomy achieves these goals, and reduces thrombotic risks associated with uncontrolled blood volume. Phlebotomy alone will not control white cell count or platelet count, and generally does not prevent the development of extramedullary hematopoiesis. Myelosuppressive agents will serve these ends to some extent, although therapeutic targets for white cell count and platelet count are lacking, and choice of agent is also complicated by side-effect profiles and long-term toxicity concerns. Antiplatelet therapy is important in thrombotic risk reduction, and has been shown to be safe and beneficial.[36,64]

Hematologic remission and molecular remission have long been concepts in CML, but are more recent to PV given the lack of a measureable and quantitative clonal molecular lesion. The JAK2 V617F discovery has now revolutionized approach to therapy in PV, as JAK2 V617F serves as a clonal marker with which to track molecular response to therapy, and molecular remissions can be added as a therapeutic goal. The JAK2 discovery has enabled the study of clonal burdens in prospective clinical trials, allowing for more concrete endpoints, evaluation of response and estimation of minimal residual disease. The use of JAK2 allele burden monitoring in recent interferon trials not only has identified molecular remissions in PV, but also indicated the time course of these responses.[30,31] JAK2 itself now serves a therapeutic target for treatment of PV. As interferon trials mature, and as JAK2 inhibitor trials in PV emerge, the categories of response—clinical, hematologic, and molecular—will be integrated. Post-JAK2 discovery therapeutic goals will now focus on prevention of disease transformation, prevention of extramedullary disease, and potentially full hematologic and molecular remission, as we have realized in targeted tyrosine kinase inhibitor therapy for CML.

CONCLUSION

The identification of JAK2 mutations in PV has revealed its somatic basis, has redefined its epidemiology and has greatly informed its natural history. The latency and gene dosage aspects of JAK2 mutations in PV introduce variability such that every aspect of PV—its acquisition, its natural history, and likely its response to therapy—is influenced by this variability. At the same time, the post-JAK2 discovery era has shown us the remarkable variation that host genetics, gender, and environment bring to bear on these same aspects and represent contributions not previously recognized in clonal myeloid malignancies. The elucidation of the relationships and the mechanisms underpinning the phenotypic variability in PV will enhance our ability to prevent, treat and ultimately cure PV, and will be highly applicable to understanding and treating other myeloid malignancies.

REFERENCES

1. Osler W. Chronic cyanotic polycythaemia with enlarged spleen. *Br Med J.* 1904;1(2246):121-2.
2. Minot GR, Buckman TE. Erythremia (polycythemia rubra vera). *Am J Med Sci.* 1923;166:469-89.
3. Videbaek A. Polycythaemia vera. Course and prognosis. *Acta Med Scand.* 1950;138(3):179-87.
4. Dameshek W. Some speculations on the myeloproliferative syndromes. *Blood.* 1951;6(4): 372-5.
5. Wasserman LR. The management of polycythaemia vera. *Br J Haematol.* 1971;21(4):371-6.
6. Berk L, Burchenal JH. Oxygen saturation of sternal marrow blood with special reference to pathogenesis of polycythemia vera. *Proc Soc Exp Biol Med.* 1948;69(2):316-20.
7. Adamson JW, Finch CA. Erythropoietin and the polycythemias. *Ann N Y Acad Sci.* 1968; 149(1):560-3.
8. Erslev AJ, Caro J, Kansu E, et al. Plasma erythropoietin in polycythemia. *Am J Med.* 1979; 66(2):243-7.
9. Prchal JF, Axelrad AA. Letter: Bone-marrow responses in polycythemia vera. *N Engl J Med.* 1974;290(24):1382.
10. Dai CH, Krantz SB, Means RT, et al. Polycythemia vera blood burst-forming units-erythroid are hypersensitive to interleukin-3. *J Clin Invest.* 1991;87(2):391-6.
11. Ugo V, Marzac C, Teyssandier I, et al. Multiple signaling pathways are involved in erythropoietin-independent differentiation of erythroid progenitors in polycythemia vera. *Exp Hematol.* 2004;32(2):179-87.
12. Nowell PC, Hungerford DA. Chromosome studies on normal and leukemic human leukocytes. *J Natl Cancer Inst.* 1960;25:85-109.
13. Rowley JD. Letter: A new consistent chromosomal abnormality in chronic myelogenous leukaemia identified by quinacrine fluorescence and Giemsa staining. *Nature.* 1973; 243(5405):290-3.
14. Kurzrock R, Gutterman JU, Talpaz M. The molecular genetics of Philadelphia chromosome-positive leukemias. *N Engl J Med.* 1988;319(15):990-8.
15. Adamson JW, Fialkow PJ, Murphy S, et al. Polycythemia vera: stem-cell and probable clonal origin of the disease. *N Engl J Med.* 1976;295(17):913-6.

16. James C, Ugo V, Le Couédic JP, et al. A unique clonal JAK2 mutation leading to constitutive signalling causes polycythaemia vera. *Nature.* 2005;434(7037):1144-8.
17. Baxter EJ, Scott LM, Campbell PJ, et al. Acquired mutation of the tyrosine kinase JAK2 in human myeloproliferative disorders. *Lancet.* 2005;365(9464):1054-61.
18. Levine RL, Wadleigh M, Cools J, et al. Activating mutation in the tyrosine kinase JAK2 in polycythemia vera, essential thrombocythemia, and myeloid metaplasia with myelofibrosis. *Cancer Cell.* 2005;7(4):387-97.
19. Zhao R, Xing S, Li Z, et al. Identification of an acquired JAK2 mutation in polycythemia vera. *J Biol Chem.* 2005;280(24):22788-92.
20. Kralovics R, Guan Y, Prchal JT. Acquired uniparental disomy of chromosome 9p is a frequent stem cell defect in polycythemia vera. *Exp Hematol.* 2002;30(3):229-36.
21. Kralovics R, Passamonti F, Buser AS, et al. A gain-of-function mutation of JAK2 in myeloproliferative disorders. *N Engl J Med.* 2005;352(17):1779-90.
22. Jones AV, Kreil S, Zoi K, et al. Widespread occurrence of the JAK2 V617F mutation in chronic myeloproliferative disorders. *Blood.* 2005;106(6):2162-8.
23. Wang YL, Vandris K, Jones A, et al. JAK2 mutations are present in all cases of polycythemia vera. *Leukemia.* 2008;22(6):1289.
24. Williams DM, Kim AH, Rogers O, et al. Phenotypic variations and new mutations in JAK2 V617F-negative polycythemia vera, erythrocytosis, and idiopathic myelofibrosis. *Exp Hematol.* 2007;35(11):1641-6.
25. Scott LM, Tong W, Levine RL, et al. JAK2 exon 12 mutations in polycythemia vera and idiopathic erythrocytosis. *N Engl J Med.* 2007;356(5):459-68.
26. Scott LM. The JAK2 exon 12 mutations: a comprehensive review. *Am J Hematol.* 2011; 86(8):668-76.
27. Percy MJ, Scott LM, Erber WN, et al. The frequency of JAK2 exon 12 mutations in idiopathic erythrocytosis patients with low serum erythropoietin levels. *Haematologica.* 2007;92(12):1607-14.
28. Xing S, Wanting TH, Zhao W, et al. Transgenic expression of JAK2V617F causes myeloproliferative disorders in mice. *Blood.* 2008;111(10):5109-17.
29. Vannucchi AM, Antonioli E, Guglielmelli P, et al. Prospective identification of high-risk polycythemia vera patients based on JAK2(V617F) allele burden. *Leukemia.* 2007;21(9):1952-9.
30. Kiladjian JJ, Cassinat B, Chevret S, et al. Pegylated interferon-alfa-2a induces complete hematologic and molecular responses with low toxicity in polycythemia vera. *Blood.* 2008;112(8):3065-72.
31. Kiladjian JJ, Mesa RA, Hoffman R. The renaissance of interferon therapy for the treatment of myeloid malignancies. *Blood.* 2011;117(18):4706-15.
32. Moliterno AR, Williams DM, Rogers O, et al. Phenotypic variability within the JAK2 V617F-positive MPD: roles of progenitor cell and neutrophil allele burdens. *Exp Hematol.* 2008;36(11):1480-6.
33. Dupont S, Massé A, James C, et al. The JAK2 617V>F mutation triggers erythropoietin hypersensitivity and terminal erythroid amplification in primary cells from patients with polycythemia vera. *Blood.* 2007;110(3):1013-21.
34. Godfrey AL, Chen E, Pagano F, et al. JAK2V617F homozygosity arises commonly and recurrently in PV and ET, but PV is characterized by expansion of a dominant homozygous subclone. *Blood.* 2012;120(13):2704-7.
35. Berlin NI. Diagnosis and classification of the polycythemias. *Semin Hematol.* 1975;12(4):339-51.
36. Landolfi R, Marchioli R, Kutti J, et al. Efficacy and safety of low-dose aspirin in polycythemia vera. *N Engl J Med.* 2004;350(2):114-24.
37. Nielsen C, Birgens HS, Nordestgaard BG, et al. Diagnostic value of JAK2 V617F somatic mutation for myeloproliferative cancer in 49 488 individuals from the general population. *Br J Haematol.* 2013;160(1):70-9.
38. Olcaydu D, Harutyunyan A, Jäger R, et al. A common JAK2 haplotype confers susceptibility to myeloproliferative neoplasms. *Nat Genet.* 2009;41(4):450-4.

39. Jones AV, Chase A, Silver RT, et al. JAK2 haplotype is a major risk factor for the development of myeloproliferative neoplasms. *Nat Genet.* 2009;41(4):446-9.
40. Pietra D, Casetti I, Da Vià MC, et al. JAK2 GGCC haplotype in MPL mutated myeloproliferative neoplasms. *Am J Hematol.* 2012;87(7):746-7.
41. Seaman V, Jumaan A, Yanni E, et al. Use of molecular testing to identify a cluster of patients with polycythemia vera in eastern Pennsylvania. *Cancer Epidemiol Biomarkers Prev.* 2009;18(2):534-40.
42. Seaman V, Dearwent SM, Gable D, et al. A multidisciplinary investigation of a polycythemia vera cancer cluster of unknown origin. *Int J Environ Res Public Health.* 2010;7(3):1139-52.
43. Ranjan A, Penninga E, Jelsig AM, et al. Inheritance of the chronic myeloproliferative neoplasms. A systematic review. *Clin Genet.* 2013;83(2):99-107.
44. Landgren O, Goldin LR, Kristinsson SY, et al. Increased risks of polycythemia vera, essential thrombocythemia, and myelofibrosis among 24,577 first-degree relatives of 11,039 patients with myeloproliferative neoplasms in Sweden. *Blood.* 2008;112(6):2199-204.
45. Tefferi A, Rumi E, Finazzi G, et al. Survival and prognosis among 1545 patients with contemporary polycythemia vera: an international study. *Leukemia,* 2013;27(9):1874-81.
46. Passamonti F, Rumi E, Pietra D, et al. A prospective study of 338 patients with polycythemia vera: the impact of JAK2 (V617F) allele burden and leukocytosis on fibrotic or leukemic disease transformation and vascular complications. *Leukemia.* 2010;24(9):1574-9.
47. Hernández-Boluda JC, Pereira A, Cervantes F, et al. A polymorphism in the XPD gene predisposes to leukemic transformation and new nonmyeloid malignancies in essential thrombocythemia and polycythemia vera. *Blood.* 2012;119(22):5221-8.
48. Stein BL, Saraf S, Sobol U, et al. Age-related differences in disease characteristics and clinical outcomes in polycythemia vera. *Leuk Lymphoma.* 2012;54(9):1989-95.
49. Maynadié M, Girodon F, Manivet-Janoray I, et al. Twenty-five years of epidemiological recording on myeloid malignancies: data from the specialized registry of hematologic malignancies of Cote d'Or (Burgundy, France). *Haematologica.* 2011;96(1):55-61.
50. Cools J, DeAngelo DJ, Gotlib J, et al. A tyrosine kinase created by fusion of the PDGFRA and FIP1L1 genes as a therapeutic target of imatinib in idiopathic hypereosinophilic syndrome. *N Engl J Med.* 2003;348(13):1201-14.
51. McMullin MF. Diagnosis and management of congenital and idiopathic erythrocytosis. *Ther Adv Hematol.* 2012;3(6):391-8.
52. Cassinat B, Laguillier C, Gardin C, et al. Classification of myeloproliferative disorders in the JAK2 era: is there a role for red cell mass? *Leukemia.* 2008;22(2):452-3.
53. Kiladjian JJ. The spectrum of JAK2-positive myeloproliferative neoplasms. *Hematology Am Soc Hematol Educ Program.* 2012;2012:561-6.
54. Alvarez-Larrán A, Ancochea A, Angona A, et al. Red cell mass measurement in patients with clinically suspected diagnosis of polycythemia vera or essential thrombocythemia. *Haematologica.* 2012;97(11):1704-7.
55. Bonicelli G, Abdulkarim K, Mounier M, et al. Leucocytosis and thrombosis at diagnosis are associated with poor survival in polycythaemia vera: a population-based study of 327 patients. *Br J Haematol.* 2012;160(2):251-4.
56. Zangari M, Fink L, Tolomelli G, et al. Could hypoxia increase the prevalence of thrombotic complications in polycythemia vera? *Blood Coagul Fibrinolysis.* 2013;24(3):311-6.
57. Stein BL, Moliterno AR. Primary myelofibrosis and the myeloproliferative neoplasms: the role of individual variation. *JAMA.* 2010;303(24):2513-8.
58. Segal JB, Moliterno AR. Platelet counts differ by sex, ethnicity, and age in the United States. *Ann Epidemiol.* 2006;16(2):123-30.
59. Stein BL, Rademaker A, Spivak JL, et al. Gender and vascular complications in the JAK2 V617F-positive myeloproliferative neoplasms. *Thrombosis.* 2011;2011:874146.
60. Westbrook RH, Lea NC, Mohamedali AM, et al. Prevalence and clinical outcomes of the 46/1 haplotype, Janus kinase 2 mutations, and ten-eleven translocation 2 mutations in Budd-

Chiari syndrome and their impact on thrombotic complications post liver transplantation. *Liver Transpl.* 2012;18(7):819-27.

61. Kiladjian JJ, Cervantes F, Leebeek FW, et al. The impact of JAK2 and MPL mutations on diagnosis and prognosis of splanchnic vein thrombosis: a report on 241 cases. *Blood.* 2008;111(10):4922-9.
62. Valla D, Casadevall N, Lacombe C, et al. Primary myeloproliferative disorder and hepatic vein thrombosis. A prospective study of erythroid colony formation in vitro in 20 patients with Budd-Chiari syndrome. *Ann Intern Med.* 1985;103(3):329-34.
63. Pemmaraju N, Hamilton JP, Cameron AM, et al. Abdominal venous thrombosis presenting in myeloproliferative neoplasm with JAK2 V617F mutation: a case report. *J Med Case Rep.* 2012;6(1):102.
64. Marchioli R, Finazzi G, Specchia G, et al. Cardiovascular events and intensity of treatment in polycythemia vera. *N Engl J Med.* 2013;368(1):22-33.
65. Falanga A, Marchetti M. Thrombotic disease in the myeloproliferative neoplasms. *Hematology Am Soc Hematol Educ Program.* 2012;2012:571-81.
66. Tam CS, Abruzzo LV, Lin KI, et al. The role of cytogenetic abnormalities as a prognostic marker in primary myelofibrosis: applicability at the time of diagnosis and later during disease course. *Blood.* 2009;113(18):4171-8.
67. Stein BL, Williams DM, O'Keefe C, et al. Disruption of the ASXL1 gene is frequent in primary, post-essential thrombocytosis and post-polycythemia vera myelofibrosis, but not essential thrombocytosis or polycythemia vera: analysis of molecular genetics and clinical phenotypes. *Haematologica.* 2011;96(10):1462-9.
68. Carbuccia N, Murati A, Trouplin V, et al. Mutations of ASXL1 gene in myeloproliferative neoplasms. *Leukemia.* 2009;23(11):2183-6.
69. Scott LM, Rebel VI. JAK2 and genomic instability in the myeloproliferative neoplasms: a case of the chicken or the egg? *Am J Hematol.* 2012;87(11):1028-36.
70. Alvarez-Larrán A, Bellosillo B, Martínez-Avilés L, et al. Postpolycythaemic myelofibrosis: frequency and risk factors for this complication in 116 patients. *Br J Haematol.* 2009; 146(5):504-9.
71. Cervantes F, Tassies D, Salgado C, et al. Acute transformation in nonleukemic chronic myeloproliferative disorders: actuarial probability and main characteristics in a series of 218 patients. *Acta Haematol.* 1991;85(3):124-7.
72. Finazzi G, Caruso V, Marchioli R, et al. Acute leukemia in polycythemia vera: an analysis of 1638 patients enrolled in a prospective observational study. *Blood.* 2005;105(7):2664-70.
73. Rinaldi CR, Rinaldi P, Gemei M, et al. JAK2V617F mutation persists in blasts and mature cells of transformed JAK2V617F-positive-myeloproliferative neoplasia: a European Leukemia Net (ENL) study. *Am J Hematol.* 2010;85(5):383-6.
74. Theocharides A, Boissinot M, Girodon F, et al. Leukemic blasts in transformed JAK2-V617F-positive myeloproliferative disorders are frequently negative for the JAK2-V617F mutation. *Blood.* 2007;110(1):375-9.
75. Beer PA, Delhommeau F, LeCouédic JP, et al. Two routes to leukemic transformation after a JAK2 mutation-positive myeloproliferative neoplasm. *Blood.* 2010;115(14):2891-900.
76. Grossmann V, Kohlmann A, Zenger M, et al. A deep-sequencing study of chronic myeloid leukemia patients in blast crisis (BC-CML) detects mutations in 76.9% of cases. *Leukemia.* 2011;25(3):557-60.
77. Beer PA, Jones AV, Bench AJ, et al. Clonal diversity in the myeloproliferative neoplasms: independent origins of genetically distinct clones. *Br J Haematol.* 2009;144(6):904-8.
78. Kralovics R, Teo SS, Li S, et al. Acquisition of the V617F mutation of JAK2 is a late genetic event in a subset of patients with myeloproliferative disorders. *Blood.* 2006;108(4):1377-80.

CHAPTER 6

Primary, Post-PV, and Post-ET Myelofibrosis: Clinical Features, Prognosis, and Conventional Therapy

Jagoda K Jasielec, Olatoyosi Odenike

INTRODUCTION

Primary myelofibrosis (PMF) is a clonal stem cell disorder characterized by marrow fibrosis and extramedullary hematopoiesis. Historically, PMF has been frequently referred to as chronic idiopathic myelofibrosis (MF), agnogenic myeloid metaplasia, MF with myeloid metaplasia, and idiopathic MF.[1] The term MF in this chapter is utilized to encompass PMF, as well as MF that develops as a complication of polycythemia vera (PV) and essential thrombocytosis (ET), so called post-PV and post-ET MF, respectively, since these latter entities result in a clinical phenotype that is ultimately indistinguishable from established PMF.[2] Significant efforts have been made in recent years to standardize the diagnostic criteria for the disease[3,4] and these issues are discussed in a separate chapter.

Myelofibrosis can closely mimic other chronic myeloproliferative neoplasms (MPNs), all of which can be associated with varying degrees of marrow fibrosis and extramedullary hematopoiesis. This disorder, however, has the worst prognosis of the MPNs. Currently, there is no standard approach to the treatment of MF and most therapies are directed toward alleviation of symptoms related to the disease and its complications. Allogeneic stem cell transplant (SCT) is the only potentially curative treatment option and will be discussed in detail in chapter 7 .

This chapter focuses on the epidemiology, clinical features, prognosis, and conventional treatment options for the disorder, including the recently approved agent, ruxolitinib.

EPIDEMIOLOGY

Myelofibrosis is a rare disorder with an estimated incidence of 0.5–1.5 per 100,000.[5,6] It is a disease of older adults, with a median age at diagnosis of 67 years.[5] In individuals with PV, the 15-year cumulative risk of developing post-PV MF is approximately 6%, compared to patients with ET in whom the risk of developing post-ET MF approximates 4% over the same time period.[7] Reported median survivals are variable and range from 4 years to 7 years from the time of diagnosis.[8,9] Progressive bone marrow failure, transformation into acute leukemia, thrombosis, and cardiovascular complications are amongst the major causes of death.[10,11]

CLINICAL FEATURES

In approximately 15–30% of patients, MF may be asymptomatic at the time of diagnosis. The diagnosis is often made during an evaluation of splenomegaly or abnormal blood counts.[12,13] In symptomatic patients, the typical symptoms include fatigue, weight loss, night sweats, musculoskeletal pain, and fever.[14] These constitutional symptoms are believed to be mediated by an abnormal cytokine release associated with the clonal myeloproliferation in MF.[15] Approximately 30% of patients will have marked splenomegaly (spleen >10 cm below left costal margin) at the time of diagnosis, which may result in early satiety, abdominal fullness, and left upper quadrant abdominal pain, often from splenic infarction or perisplenitis.[16] Enlargement of the spleen and liver are due to extramedullary hematopoiesis associated with MF and are a prominent feature of the disease. In more advanced disease, foci of extramedullary hematopoiesis may occur in almost any organ, including the lymph nodes, pleura, lung, pericardium, gastrointestinal, or genitourinary tracts, as well as the central nervous system, and the skin.[17-20] In one small series, the most commonly involved areas other than the liver and the spleen are the vertebral column, retroperitoneum, lungs, or pleura.[19]

Patients with MF have an increased risk of arterial and venous thrombotic events compared to the general population and this risk is estimated to be approximately 2 per 100 patient-years.[21,22] In one study, the risk of cardiovascular events in MF was associated with increased age, higher white blood cell (WBC), count and positive Janus kinase 2 (*JAK2*) mutation status, while in another report a prior history of thrombosis was the only predictive variable.[22,23] In addition, MF is associated with increased risk of intra-abdominal thrombosis. For example, hepatic vein thrombosis, or Budd-Chiari syndrome can be a feature of early-phase disease and can sometimes be the presenting symptom.[24,25] In addition, portal hypertension leading to variceal bleeding and portal vein thrombosis are common complications of hepatosplenomegaly in MF patients.[26,27] A higher incidence of pulmonary hypertension has also been detected in patients with MF and while often under recognized, it has been associated with reduced survival.[28-30]

LABORATORY FINDINGS

The most common uniform laboratory abnormality is anemia, which is multifactorial and may be secondary to ineffective hematopoiesis, splenic sequestration, bleeding, and hemolysis.[12] The characteristic features on the peripheral blood smear include leukoerythroblastosis, anisocytosis, poikilocytosis, and dacrocytes, or teardrop-shaped red blood cells. The WBC and platelet (PLT) counts may be variable. Leukocytosis and thrombocytosis occur at diagnosis in approximately 11–13% of patients.[12,31] Thrombocytosis is commonly observed in prefibrotic PMF, an entity that may be difficult to distinguish from ET. Thrombocytopenia occurs in about one-third of individuals with established MF at the time of diagnosis[14] and is seen more frequently as the disease progresses. Myeloblasts may be seen in the peripheral smear, and usually account for less than 5% of the circulating white cells in the chronic phase of the disease. Molecular analysis of the peripheral blood and/or bone marrow may reveal the presence of the *JAK2* V617F mutation, which occurs in approximately 50% of patients with MF, and is useful in establishing the clonal nature of the disease.[32-34]

A bone marrow examination is a crucial part of the initial evaluation. A bone marrow aspirate may often be difficult to obtain, yielding a "dry-tap". If obtainable, the most frequent findings on an aspirate are granulocytic and megakaryocytic hyperplasia. Increased fibrosis is a hallmark feature on a bone marrow biopsy and is, best visualized with silver and trichrome stains for reticulin and mature collagen, respectively. Furthermore, the bone marrow may be either hypo- or hypercellular with prominent megakaryocytic hyperplasia and osteosclerosis. In prefibrotic MF, the bone marrow is hypercellular and reticulin fibrosis may initially be absent, but will increase during the disease course, finally resulting in collagen fibrosis and osteosclerosis.[35,36]

The diagnosis of MF is currently based on the 2008 World Health Organization (WHO) criteria which include clinical, morphologic, cytogenetic, and molecular assessments.[37] The diagnosis requires meeting all three major and at least two minor criteria, as outlined in a separate chapter of this book. The diagnosis of post-PV and post-ET MF is based on the International Working Group for Myclofibrosis Research and Treatment (IWG-MRT) criteria,[38] also outlined in a separate chapter.

EVOLUTION OF PROGNOSTIC MODELS

Since MF is a largely heterogeneous disease, with highly variable survival rates, prognostic models (Tables 6.1 and 6.2) have evolved to provide tools for risk stratification. This is essential to enable individualization of management of the disease, as well as to ensure uniformity of reporting of outcomes of clinical trials conducted in this disease. The majority of earlier models were based on relatively small numbers of patients. For example, the Lille model was developed based on a multivariate analysis of survival of 195 patients diagnosed with PMF between 1962 and 1992 and identified hemoglobin (Hb) of less than 10 g/dL and WBC of less than 4×10^9/L or greater than 30×10^9/L as poor prognostic factors.[31] Individuals with MF were stratified into three prognostic groups: (1) low (zero), (2) intermediate (one), and (3) high (both) factors, corresponding to median survival of 93 months, 26 months, and 13 months, respectively.[31] However, this model was based on a relatively small cohort of patients, was only applicable at the time of diagnosis, and furthermore, did not clearly separate intermediate and high-risk patients, as later demonstrated by subsequent studies.

Table 6-1 Prognostic Scoring Systems for Myelofibrosis

Prognostic variables	*Lille*	*IPPS*	*DIPPS*	*DIPPS-plus*
Age	–	+	+ (Age adjusted)	+ (Age adjusted)
Constitutional symptoms	–	+	+	+
Red cell transfusion requirement	–	–	–	+
Hemoglobin (<10 g/dL)	+	+	+	+
White blood cell count	+ (<4 × 109/L or >30 × 109/L)	+ (>25 × 109/L)	+ (>25 × 109/L)	+ (>25 × 109/L)
Thrombocytopenia (<100 × 109/L)	–	–	–	+
Peripheral blasts (≥1%)	–	+	+	+
Unfavorable karyotype*	–	–	–	+

IPSS, International Prognostic Scoring System; DIPSS, Dynamic International Prognostic Scoring System; +, prognostic variable present; –, prognostic variable absent.

*Complex karyotype or abnormalities including +8, -7/7q, i(17q), -5/5q, 12p-, inv(3), or 11q23 rearrangements.

Table 6-2 Prognostic Risk Categories and Survival

	IPSS		*DIPSS*		*DIPSS-plus*	
Risk group	Number of predictors	Median survival (years)	Number of adverse points	Median survival (years)	Number of adverse points	Median survival (years)
Low	0	11.3	0	Not reached	0	15.4
Intermediate-1	1	7.9	1–2	14.2	1	6.5
Intermediate-2	2	4.0	3–4	4	2–3	2.9
High	≥3	2.3	5–6	1.5	4–6	1.3

IPSS, International Prognostic Scoring System; DIPSS, Dynamic International Prognostic Scoring System

A more discriminate prognostic system, otherwise known as the International Prognostic Scoring System (IPSS) was then proposed in 2008 by the International Working Group for Myelofibrosis Research and Treatment (IWG-MRT). Based on a multivariate analysis of 1,054 patients diagnosed with MF between 1980 and 2007, the group identified five factors as predictors of shortened survival. These included: age greater than 65 years, presence of constitutional symptoms, Hb level less than 10 g/dL, leukocyte count greater than 25 × 10^9/L, and 1% or more circulating blasts.

It categorized patients into four risk groups based on the presence of zero (low risk), one (intermediate risk-1), two (intermediate risk-2), or greater than or equal to three (high risk) factors, with corresponding median survivals of 135 months, 95 months, 48 months, and 27 months, respectively.[11] This model was later revised into the Dynamic International Prognostic Scoring System (DIPPS) to account for the acquisition of adverse risk factors over time, as well as age. This showed that the acquisition of anemia over time affects survival with a hazard ratio double than that of other parameters and allowed the assignment of a greater weight to anemia with two points, instead of one, as in the previous model.[39]

Three additional, non-IPSS risk factors were then added to the DIPSS score to develop the DIPSS-plus score and include cytogenetics [complex karyotype, or abnormalities including +8, −7/7q-, i(17q)-, 5/5q-, 12p-, inv(3), or 11q23 rearrangements],[40] need for red cell transfusions[41] and thrombocytopenia.[42] These additional factors were incorporated to refine the DIPSS and create the DIPSS-plus risk model which stratifies patients into low (zero adverse points), intermediate-1 (one adverse point), intermediate-2 (two or three adverse points), and high (four to six adverse points) groups with respective median survivals of 15.4 years, 6.5 years, 2.9 years, and 1.3 years, respectively.[43] Younger patients, under the age of 60 years were found to have a better prognosis with corresponding median survivals of 20 years, 14.3 years, 5.3 years, and 1.7 years, respectively.[16]

Interestingly, in general, the presence or absence of *JAK2* V617F has not been associated with an effect on survival or leukemic transformation rates.[11,44,45]

The survival and prognostic factors in post-PV and post-ET MF are not yet well-defined. The IPSS model excluded patients with previous diagnosis of ET and PV although clinically, the IPSS-based system is often applied to these patients. In a relatively small series of 68 patients with post-PV MF, Hb less than 10 g/dL, PLT count less than 100×10^9/L, and leukocyte greater than 30×10^9/L were useful to predict survival at any time from the diagnosis of MF,[46] but models based on larger cohorts are needed.

TREATMENT APPROACH

At the present time, an allogeneic SCT is the only known cure for patients with MF; this treatment approach will be discussed in detail in chapter. Despite the fact that transplant-related mortality has decreased since the introduction of reduced intensity conditioning approaches, and has allowed the application of SCT to a greater number of patients with MF, this modality of therapy is still limited in applicability due to the older age of patients, associated comorbid conditions, and donor availability. Therefore, for most patients with MF, therapy is largely palliative, and is focused on alleviating the signs and symptoms of disease, and the bone marrow failure state associated with the disorder. This treatment approach will be discussed in another chapter. In this chapter, we will outline the conventional treatment approaches, including therapies focused on the improvement of splenomegaly, anemia, and constitutional symptoms.

It is important to note that until recently, there was no standardized criteria to assess response to therapy in MF and compare outcomes reported in the context of clinical trials. The first of such efforts were made by the European Myelofibrosis Network (EUMNET) where five clinicohematologic criteria were defined based on scoring of responses by an international expert panel.[47] Subsequently, the IWG-MRT outlined its own set of criteria which identified three response categories: (1) complete response (CR), (2) partial response (PR), and (3) clinical improvement (CI) and unlike the EUMNET criteria, also included histologic remission.[48]

Treatment of Anemia in Myelofibrosis

Several therapeutic agents have been evaluated for the treatment of anemia in MF, including erythropoietin, androgens, danazol, thalidomide (Thal), and newer analogs.

Erythropoiesis Stimulating Agents

Erythropoietin or darbopoeitin has relatively limited efficacy in MF-associated anemia. Although, they have produced improvement in Hb level in some patients; in most cases, this was limited to patients who did not require transfusion support[49,50] and those with inappropriately low serum erythropoietin levels.[49] Patients with an appropriate erythropoietin level for the degree of anemia, for example, had no response to darbopoeitin[51] and in another small study of 20 patients, erythropoietin levels of less than 125 U/L were associated with a favorable response.[49] The median duration of response was anywhere from 5 months to 12 months.[51] In addition, there have been reports of exacerbation of splenomegaly with these agents, possibly due to the stimulation of erythropoiesis in extramedullary sites as well.[52] Therefore the use of erythropoiesis-stimulating agents should be limited in general, to patients with inappropriately low erythropoietin levels. A recent report has also suggested an association between erythropoietin use and leukemic transformation in MF,[53] although this has not yet been confirmed by other groups.

Androgens

Androgen treatment has been shown to improve anemia in some patients with MF. Several androgen preparations have been studied including fluoxymesterone,[54] oxymetholone, and a synthetic androgen, danazol, which is now the most commonly used. The response rate to androgen therapy varies between 29% and 57%[54,55] and interestingly, in one series, the response rate to fluoxymesterone was significantly lower in patients with chromosomal abnormalities, as compared to a normal karyotype.[55] An overall response rate (ORR) to danazol defined as decrease in transfusion requirement or transfusion independence is also highly variable[56-58] and reported to be approximately 37% in the largest series, with a median time to response of 5 months.[57] Lack of transfusion dependence and higher Hb levels pretreatment were associated with a better response.[57] Danazol is generally well tolerated. It is important to note, however, that men who are treated with androgen therapy should be screened for prostate cancer and all patients should undergo regular monitoring of liver function tests. In addition, female patients taking danazol should be warned about the virulizing side effects.

Immunomodulatory Agents

Several immunomodulatory agents have been evaluated in the treatment of MF (Table 6.3). Single agent Thal showed beneficial responses in 20–40% of patients, including improvement in constitutional symptoms, reduction in splenic size, as well as hematologic improvements, including transfusion independence.[59-62] However, the drug was overall poorly tolerated at the initial doses utilized, leading to a high rate of discontinuation due to side effects including drowsiness, constipation, fatigue, paresthesias, and neutropenia.[63] In a single institution phase II trial with combination of low-dose Thal (50 mg/day) with a 3 month prednisone (Pred) taper (starting dose of 0.5 mg/kg daily), a 62% improvement in anemia and 19% improvement in splenomegaly was reported. This regimen was better tolerated than those used in the earlier studies.[64] The authors subsequently reported a long-term follow-up of this trial, in addition to two other Thal-based trials with Thal-cyclophosphamide and Thal-etanercept, and responses were reported based on IWG-MRT response criteria. With a total of 50 patients in all three trials, zero achieved a CR, one had a PR, and 14 patients achieved CI, including 10 with improvement in anemia, three in splenomegaly, and one in both. The median duration of response was 8.5 months with a median survival of 36 months. Although this was not a randomized trial, the overall experience suggested that patients who received Thal-cyclophosphamide had greater toxicity, inferior response rates, and shorter duration of response.[65]

Lenalidomide (Len) has also been evaluated in several phase II studies for treatment of patients with MF. In two similarly designed phase II clinical trials of 68 symptomatic patients who received single agent Len, the ORRs were 22%, 33%, and 50% for anemia, splenomegaly, and thrombocytopenia, respectively, based on response criteria-specific for the trial. Eight out of 46 patients with baseline Hb of less than 10 g/dL achieved normalization of Hb levels, or major anemia response. In addition, four of these patients achieved a resolution of leukoerythroblastosis and two of the four had a decrease in bone marrow fibrosis.[67]

In a subsequent single institution study, 40 patients were treated with a combination of Len and a 3-month Pred taper. With a median follow-up of 22 months, based on IWG-MRT response criteria, three patients (7.5%) had achieved

Table 6-3 Selected Clinical Trials with Immunomodulatory Agents in Myelofibrosis

Reference	*Treatment*	*Patients (n)*	*Duration of therapy*	*Response*	*Comments*
Barosi et al., 2002[59]	Thal starting at 100 mg/day (patients treated on five separate phase II clinical trials)	62	79% had at least 4 weeks of therapy	29% had improvement in hemoglobin (Hb), 38% in thrombocytopenia, and 41% with high-grade splenomegaly achieved reduction in splenic size	Used uniform response criteria; 66% discontinued therapy before 6 months due to toxicity
Elliot et al., 2002[61]	Thal 200 mg/day with escalation to maximum 1,000 mg/day	15	NA	3/15 had improvement in anemia, 12/15 in thrombocytopenia, and 3/9 in splenomegaly	MTD 200 mg/day Leukocytosis in two patients developed worsening leukocytosis and three patients thrombocytosis
Thomas et al., 2006[62]	Thal 200 mg/day, escalation weekly to 800 mg/day as tolerated	44	3 months	41% objective response; 21% hematologic improvement; 31% reduction in splenomegaly	MTD dose 400 mg/day
Marchetti et al., 2004[63]	Thal 50 mg/day, with escalation to 400 mg daily as tolerated	63	NA	22% improvement in anemia and thrombocytopenia; 39% became transfusion independent 19% had decrease in splenomegaly by > 50%	51% drop out rate at 6 months of therapy due to occurrence of adverse events; median of MTD 100 mg daily
Mesa et al., 2003[64]	Thal 50 mg/day plus 3-month prednisone (Pred) taper	21	NA	13/21 patients had improvement in anemia, 6/8 in thrombocytopenia, and 4/21 in splenomegaly	Better tolerated with 95% patients completing 2 month of planned therapy
Thapaliya et al., 2011[65,*]	Long-term follow-up of 3 trials: Thal/Pred (TP), Thal/cyclophosphamide (TPC) and Thal/etanercept (PET)	50	NA	No patients achieved CR, one achieved PR (TP arm) and CI was seen in one, four and 11 patients on TPC, PET, TP arms, respectively	95% on TP, 73% Thal-etanercept, 57% on Thal-cyclophosphamide completed 3 months of therapy; hematologic toxicity greatest in Thal-cyclophosphamide trial

Contd...

Contd...

Barosi et al., 2001[66]	Thal 200 mg/day, with escalation to maximum 400 mg/day	21	NA	Hematologic improvement was seen in 43% of patients treated for anemia, 66.6% in those treated for thrombocytopenia. Splenomegaly reduced in four patients (30%)	Maximum tolerated dose (MTD) 100–200 mg/day On 13 patients completed >1 months of therapy and included in analysis; 90% discontinued before 6 months due to somnolence, fatigue, neuropathy, and neutropenia
Tefferi et al., 2006[67]	Len 10 mg/day [5 mg/day if platelet (PLT) <100 × 109/L] Report on two separate phase II trials	68	5–6 months	22% had improvement in anemia, 50% in thrombocytopenia and 33% in splenomegaly; two patients had improvement in marrow fibrosis	Grade 3 and 4 neutropenia in 31% patients, thrombocytopenia in 19%; ~50% of patients received planned three to six cycles of therapy in one trial and 50% were on therapy at 5-month follow-up
Quintas-Cardama et al., 2009[68,*]	Len 10 mg/day (5 mg/day if baseline PLT count <100 × 109/L) in combination with Pred taper	40	NA	7.5% PR, 23% CI, overall response rate (ORR) 30% for anemia and 42% splenomegaly	Grade 3 to 4 neutropenia (58%), anemia (42%) and thrombocytopenia (13%)
Mesa et al., 2010[69,*]	Len 10 mg/day (5 mg/day if baseline PLT count <100 × 109/L) in combination with Pred taper	42	3–6 months	ORR 23%, CI in anemia 19%, CI in splenomegaly 10%	Grade 3 and 4 hematologic toxicity on 88%; no change in marrow fibrosis observed
Tefferi et al., 2009[70,*]	Pom 2 mg/day plus placebo, Pom 2 mg/day plus Pred, Pom 0.5 mg/day plus Pred, Pred plus placebo	84	~3 months	ORR in the four treatment arms were 23%, 16%, 36%, and 19%, respectively	Grade 3 and 4 hematologic toxicities were rare; Pom 0.5 plus Pred was best tolerated with 36% of patient continuing greater than three cycles; no effect on splenomegaly
Begna et al., 2011[71,*]	Pom 0.5–3 mg/day ±Pred	94	7 months	ORR for anemia 27%; 17/34 patients had improvement in thrombocytopenia	91% discontinued at 2 years; no improvement in splenomegaly

CR, complete response; PR, partial response, CI, clinical improvement; NA, not available; Thal, Thalidomide; Len, Lenalidomide; Pom, Pomalidomide; MTD, maxium tolerated dose

*Assessment of response based on International Working Group-Myeloproliforative Neoplasma Research and Treatment (IWG-MRT) criteria.

a PR and nine (23%) had CI. The ORRs were approximately 30% for anemia and 42% for splenomegaly. The median time to response was 12 weeks and median duration of response was 18 months.[68] All eight *JAK2* V617F-positive responders had some decrease in the mutant allele burden with a greater than 50% reduction in four.[68]

In an Eastern Cooperative Oncology Group (ECOG) multicenter phase II trial of 42 MF patients treated with Len plus a 3-month Pred taper, with a median of six cycles of therapy, 10 (23%) patients achieved CI, 29 (69%) had stable disease (SD), and three (7%) progressed based on IWG-MRT criteria.[69] Although some investigators reported a decrease in marrow fibrosis in responders to Len,[67,68] this was not uniformly observed in all studies.[69] It is also notable that three patients with MF associated with del5q treated with Len had cytogenetic improvement (complete in one patient, partial in two), as well as a reduction in the bone marrow *JAK2* V617F allele burden in two out of three patients (from 80% to 8% and 4% to <1%, respectively).[72] Therefore, Len may be a reasonable first choice in patients with del5q MF. The most common grade 3 and 4 toxicities associated with Len use were neutropenia and thrombocytopenia, as well as peripheral neuropathy with prolonged use.

Pomalidomide (Pom), a third-generation immunomodulatory agent is being evaluated in MF. In a phase II multicenter clinical trial, 84 patients with MF were randomized to receive either Pom 2 mg daily plus placebo, Pom 2 mg daily plus Pred, Pom 0.5 mg daily plus Pred, or Pred alone. Based on IWG-MRT criteria, the best response rate was demonstrated in the low-dose Pom and Pred arm. The response rates were observed based on improvements in anemia with no effect on spleen size. The median time to response in all arms was 2 months with median response duration of 6.5 months.[70] A phase I/II trial of Pom in 19 patients with MF established 3 mg daily given in 21 of 28 days as the maximum tolerated dose (MTD), with myelosuppression being dose-limiting. The authors also observed that most of the responses observed occurred after dose reduction to 0.5 mg daily, thus validating the concept of improved tolerability and potentially enhanced efficacy with lower doses of this agent.[73]

In another phase II study of low-dose Pom plus Pred in 58 patients with MF-associated anemia, 10 (17%) patients achieved an IWG-MRT CI based on improvement in anemia. There was no impact on improvement of splenomegaly. In addition, in that study, anemia response was observed only in the presence of *JAK2* V617F but was independent of the allele burden. A subsequent report of the long-term outcome of 94 patients enrolled at a single institution and treated on two consecutive Pom trials revealed absence of marked splenomegaly, presence of the JAK2 V617F mutation, and absence of greater than or equal to 5% circulating blasts as positive predictors of response. Overall, anemia response rate was 27% by

IWG-MRT criteria and median duration of response was 16 months.[71,74] Currently, a phase III double-blind, placebo-controlled study of pomalidomide in persons with myeloproliferative-neoplasm-associated myelofibrosis and RBC-transfusion-dependence myelofibrosis and RBC-transfusion-dependent (NCT01178281) patients is underway.

Treatment of the Myeloproliferative Manifestations of Myelofibrosis, Including Splenomegaly

Hydroxyurea

Hydroxyurea is an effective first-line therapy for the hyperproliferative manifestations of MF and has been shown to reduce both PLT and WBC counts in doses as low as 500 mg daily.[75-77] In one series of 40 patients treated with hydroxyurea, 40% achieved CI based on IGW-MRT criteria; the majority of these were improvement in splenomegaly. Overall, according to EUMNET criteria, 82% had improvement in constitutional symptoms, 50% in pruritis, 40% in splenomegaly, and 12.5% in anemia, with a median duration of response of 1 year.[77] Hydroxyurea dose necessary to maintain a response was variable, and ranged from 500 mg to 2 g daily. The most common toxicity was the accentuation of anemia which occurred in approximately 18 out of 40 patients.[77] It is postulated that patients with MF are particularly sensitive to this agent and it is recommended that the drug is started at low doses, followed by incremental doses as tolerated. In another study of 69 patients with MF treated with hydroxyurea, alone or in combination with other agents, the response rate based on IWG-MRT criteria was 28%, with 4% achieving a PR and 23% CI. In addition, on a multivariate analysis of 33 patients with known *JAK2* V617F mutation status, the presence of the mutation was associated with an increased response to hydroxyurea (48% vs. 8% response in mutation positive versus negative cases).[78] There is no significant evidence at this time, however, to suggest that hydroxyurea significantly alters the natural history of this disease, and although one group found a significant reduction in bone marrow fibrosis in patients on hydroxyurea,[79] this has not been confirmed by other studies.

Cladribine

Cladribine is a nucleoside analog with significant activity in hairy cell leukemia. The agent is quite myelosuppressive and has been used at low doses for hepatomegaly, thrombocytosis, and leukocytosis associated with MF.[80]

Melphalan

Low-dose oral melphalan, 2.5 mg three times a week with progressive increase up to a maximum of 2.5 mg daily, has also been evaluated in 104 patients with symptomatic MF after pretreatment with 2 months of danazol (200 mg/day) or Pred (0.25 mg/kg/day).[81] Responses, which were assessed by protocol-specific criteria, including improvement in splenic size, leukocytosis, and thrombocytosis were noted in 67% of the 99 evaluable patients and normalization of clinical and hematologic parameters in 40%, at a median time of 6.7 months.[81] Reversible hematologic toxicities, including moderate neutropenia is the most common complication of melphalan treatment, and may often prevent initiation or necessitate cessation of treatment. With median treatment duration of 21.7 months, transformation to blast phase of the disease was observed in 20% of evaluable patients. The authors observed that the rates of leukemia transformation were higher in patients who had been previously splenectomized or had received prior therapies for MF before enrollment on this study.

Interferon Alpha

In general, interferon alpha is not commonly used for symptomatic treatment in MF due to poor tolerability and significant myelosuppression, particularly in advanced MF. Interferon alpha was evaluated in a series of 54 patients with myeloproliferative disorders including PV, ET, and PMF, and found to improve the myeloproliferative features of these diseases including hyperleukocytosis and splenomegaly.[82] Treatment was discontinued due to toxicity in 7 out of 54 patients.[82] In a retrospective report from the GEM (Groupe d'Etudes des Myelofibroses; French Intergroup for MF) of pegylated interferon alpha-2a in 18 patients with MF, responses were assessed by the EUMNET criteria, and included improvement in leukocytosis, thrombocytosis and anemia.[83]

More recently, recombinant interferon (either recombinant interferon alpha-2b 500,000 to 3 million units three times weekly, or pegylated recombinant interferon alpha-2a 45 μg or 90 μg weekly) was prospectively evaluated in 17 patients with low- to intermediate-risk MF. Out of 17 patients, two achieved a complete remission, seven partial remission, one CI, four SD, and three progressive disease based on IWG-MRT criteria with a median time to response of 1 year.[84] Out of 15 bone marrow follow-up studies, four patients had improvement in bone marrow morphology, including improvement in marrow architecture, reticulin and collagen fibrosis, and megakaryocytic atypia. It is important to note that eligibility was restricted to patients with MF and significant residual hematopoiesis and patients with grade 3 and 4 reticulin fibrosis were excluded from the study. In this select patient population, the drug was better tolerated than previously reported, with the most common toxicities being grade 1 and 2 fatigue, asthenia, and hematologic toxicities. These findings are intriguing, and suggest the need for additional investigation of this agent in early MF, prior to the development of significant hematopoietic failure.

Ruxolitinib

Since the discovery of the JAK *V617F* mutation in 2005, multiple JAK inhibitors have been developed with the anticipation that they will be more effective than current therapies in the treatment of the Philadelphia chromosome negative MPNs especially MF, where novel therapies are desperately needed.[85,86] Ruxolitinib, or INCB01424 was the first JAK inhibitor evaluated in clinical trials and the only one that is currently approved for use in intermediate- and high-risk MF.[87-89] Ruxolitinib is an adenosine triphosphate (ATP) mimetic tyrosine kinase inhibitor with selective activity against JAK1 and JAK2 kinases. The IC_{50} (50% inhibitory concentration) of ruxolitinib for the JAK kinases is 2.7 nmol/L, 4.5 nmol/L, and 322 nmol/L for JAK1, JAK2, and JAK3 kinases, respectively.[90] In murine models of MF, ruxolitinib use caused reduction in splenomegaly, decreased inflammatory cytokines, and preferential elimination of neoplastic cells, as well as prolonged survival.[90] In a phase I/II study of 153 MF patients treated at a starting dose of 15 mg per orally (PO) twice daily, 52% had a relatively rapid reduction in splenomegaly according to IWG-MRT criteria and the majority of patients enrolled had a significant improvement in constitutional symptoms. A median reduction in spleen volume on magnetic resonance imaging (MRI) of 33% was found to correlate with a 52% reduction in spleen length by palpation.[87] As expected, given the central role of the JAK2 kinase in hematopoietic signaling, the dose-limiting toxicity of ruxolitinib was thrombocytopenia and the dose was individually titrated in each patient based on PLT counts. The authors concluded that a 15 mg twice daily starting dose, followed by individualized dose titration was the safest dosing regimen.[87]

Ruxolitinib was then concurrently evaluated in two separate phase III clinical trials, the results of which led to its approval by the Food and Drug Administration (FDA) in November of 2011.[88,89] In the first, Controlled Myelofibrosis Study with Oral JAK Inhibitor Treatment (COMFORT I), conducted in the United States, approximately 300 patients with MF were randomized to receive either ruxolitinib or placebo with primary endpoint of reduction in spleen size, defined as greater than 35% decline in spleen volume as measured by MRI at 24 weeks. The protocol allowed unblinding of study-drug assignments and crossover from placebo to ruxolitinib for predefined worsening of splenomegaly.[88]

In the second clinical trial (COMFORT II), conducted in Europe, the primary end-point was the same (but was assessed at 48 weeks) and patients were randomized to ruxolitinib versus best available therapy, which included supportive care and cytoreductive agents.[89] Similar provisions were made in COMFORT II for discontinuation from the randomized treatment phase of the study and entry into an extension phase for protocol specified worsening of splenomegaly. Eligibility for these trials included IPSS intermediate-2 or high-risk disease, PLT counts over 100×10^9/L and palpable splenomegaly greater than or equal to 5 cm below the costal margin. Starting dose of ruxolitinib was tailored to baseline PLT count, with patients who had a PLT count of 100–200 × 10^9/L starting at 15 mg twice daily, and those with PLT counts over 200 × 10^9/L starting at 20 mg twice daily. Both trials demonstrated that ruxolitinib had a significant effect on spleen reduction.

The primary end-point was reached in 41.9% and 28% of patients enrolled in the ruxolitinib arm of the COMFORT I and COMFORT II trials respectively, compared to 0.7% in the placebo arm of COMFORT I and 0% in the best available therapy arm of COMFORT II. Responses were independent of *JAK2* mutation status.[88,89] In addition, about 46% of patients reported at least a 50% decrease in their total symptom score, which may be attributed, at least in part, to the decrease of inflammatory cytokines in the ruxolitinib group.[88] There was a trend toward a survival advantage in the treatment group at a median follow-up of 51 weeks in COMFORT I.[88]

The most common adverse effects of ruxolitinib were hematologic events, including grade 3 or 4 anemia and thrombocytopenia, in 45% and 13% of patients, respectively.[88] There was no significant effect on improvement of cytopenias, or improvement in the allele burden in *JAK2* mutant MF, nor was there major histomorphologic changes observed in follow-up bone marrow biopsy specimens. These findings suggest that *JAK* inhibition with ruxolitinib may have limited effects in significantly modifying the natural history of the disease;[89] however, longer follow-up is necessary. The placebo/controlled trial (COMFORT-I) did demonstrate a modest survival advantage for the ruxolitinib arm, which has not yet been reported for the COMFORT-II trial. Follow-up reports on the effects of ruxolitinib on MF-associated symptoms in the context of the COMFORT-I trial have confirmed the significant activity of this agent with regard to alleviating MF-associated symptomatology.[90] There are other *JAK* inhibitors, reviewed in a separate chapter, currently being evaluated in clinical trials on the premise of a potential greater selectivity for inhibition of *JAK2* relative to the other *JAK* kinases, and/or an improved toxicity profile with regard to myelosuppression.

Splenectomy

Splenectomy may be an option for palliation of symptoms in carefully selected patients with MF, although it has no impact on disease survival.[91] The most common indications for a splenectomy in one of the largest retrospective studies included mechanical symptoms related to massive splenomegaly, anemia, portal hypertension, and thrombocytopenia.[92]

Of a total of 314 patients who underwent an open splenectomy at the Mayo Clinic between 1976 and 2004, 97% achieved CI, (83% for portal hypertension, 70% for anemia, 56% for thrombocytopenia and almost all had relief of mechanical symptoms) with a median duration of response of 1 year.[92] Perioperative complications occurred in 27.7% of patients and most commonly included infections, bleeding, and thrombosis. Nine percent of patients died within 45 days of surgery and 6.7% of deaths were attributable to surgical complications. Patients with presplenectomy thrombocytopenia as defined by PLT counts less than 100,000/L were found to have decreased perioperative and overall survival.[92] Similarly, an older retrospective review showed that almost all splenectomy patients achieved improvement in painful splenomegaly and portal hypertension, but only approximately half had improvements in thrombocytopenia and anemia.[91]

Potential long-term complications of splenectomy in patients with MF include progressive hepatomegaly and thrombocytosis. Post-splenectomy hepatomegaly may occur in 12–29% of patients, and in some results in hepatic failure.[92,93] Hepatic enlargement is thought to be secondary to a shift of extramedullary hematopoiesis to the hepatic sinusoids[94] with a variable time course, occurring up to several years after the procedure. Unfortunately, there are no reliable preoperative predictors for this complication. Post-splenectomy thrombocytosis has been reported in approximately 22–24% of patients and was associated with both thrombotic and hemorrhagic events, as well as decreased survival.[92,95,96] Thrombocytosis may occur shortly after the surgery and necessitate postoperative apheresis and cytoreductive therapy. Increased rate of leukemic transformations has also been described in splenectomized patients;[95,97] however, this association is not entirely clear due to many confounding variables in the studies reported. Leukemic transformation was also associated with increasing splenic mass and thrombocytopenia, suggesting that patient who requires a splenectomy may have more advanced disease, and therefore a greater likelihood of leukemic transformation.

With the advent of therapy with *JAK* inhibitors and the significant associated effects on alleviating splenomegaly, splenectomy will likely to be reserved for patients with significant symptomatic splenomegaly who fail to respond to, or progress on therapy with ruxolitinib and/or other experimental *JAK* inhibitors.

Splenic Radiation

Splenic radiation was historically performed in patients with symptomatic splenomegaly and may still be of benefit in palliating symptoms in a carefully selected group of patients who fail to respond to therapy with JAK inhibitors, and are too frail to undergo splenectomy. The response rates to splenic radiation with symptomatic decrease in splenomegaly range anywhere from 59% to over 90% in the largest observational studies.[98-101] The response duration is usually transient, lasting on average 3–10 months[100,101] and many patients receive repeat courses of treatment.[100,102] The median dose of radiation used is variable.

In a study of 23 patients treated at the Mayo Clinic, the median dose of radiation per course was 277 cGy, given over 7.5 fractions where all patients had improvement in symptoms with 30–70% reduction in spleen size.[100] The most common toxicities associated with splenic radiation are significant cytopenias,[100-102] occasionally resulting in fatal sepsis and hemorrhage.[100] In addition, patients who underwent a subsequent splenectomy postradiation had a higher complication rate, including increased rate of bleeding and increased risk of mortality.[100] Therefore, splenic radiation is generally reserved for symptomatic patients with splenomegaly without significant cytopenias and in those in whom a subsequent splenectomy is not an option or is not desired.

Radiation Therapy to Other Sites of Disease

Palliative radiotherapy has also been successful in alleviating symptoms related to foci of extramedullary hematopoiesis. The experience and outcomes reported in the literature is limited largely to case reports as summarized in table 6.4. Radiotherapy has been administered to the paraspinal and intraspinal foci, bone, the abdomen for ascites, the liver, and the lungs to relieve pulmonary hypertension.[103-106] Similarly as in cases of splenic irradiation, radiation therapy to the liver resulted in a transient response with resulting significant cytopenias.[104]

Table 6-4 Radiotherapy for Palliating Extramedullary Hematopoiesis in Patients with Myelo-Fibrosis (MF)

Sites	*Reference*	*Patients (n)*	*Dose*	*Fractions*	*Response*
Liver	Riesterer et al. 2008[107]	1	200	1	Case report: Therapy repeated every 3 months to control symptoms
	Tefferi et al 2001[104]	14	150	6	• 35% transient reduction in hepatomegaly • Significant cytopenias
Abdomen	Leinweber et al. 1991[108]	1	1,000	10	• Gradual improvement in ascites over 5 months
	Koch et al. 2003[19]	4	200	7	• Most responded with improvement in ascites • Significant cytopenias
Lungs	Weinschenker et al. 2002[109]	1	200	4	• Improvement in dyspnea and effusions
	Koch et al. 2003[19]	2	125	5	• Improvement in pulmonary hypertension in 75%
	Steensma et al. 2002[103]	4	100	1	
Paraspinal/ infraspinal	Koch et al. 2003[19]	4	100–1,000	1–5	• Four out of five patients had a prompt response
Bone	Neben-Wittich et al. 2010[105]	5	100–600	1	• Four out of five patients had improvement in pain • Response lasted from 1 month to 2 years

CONCLUSION

Although noteworthy progress has been made in the diagnosis and risk stratification of patients with MF, much remains to be understood about the biology of the disease, and therefore targeted therapies with the potential to significantly alter the natural history of the disease remain elusive. Existing therapeutic approaches remain largely palliative. At the present time, *JAK* inhibitors are a promising class of agents for patients with MF, but have not been effective in improving the bone marrow failure state associated with this disease. Ongoing efforts to decipher the molecular pathogenesis of this group of diseases may lead to additional insights and targets that will hopefully translate into improved treatment approaches for patients with these disorders.

REFERENCES

1. Odenike O. Myelofibrosis with myeloid metaplasia: where is the biology leading us? *Semin Oncol.* 2005;32:357-8.
2. Mesa RA, Verstovsek S, Cervantes F, et al. Primary myelofibrosis (PMF), post polycythemia vera myelofibrosis (post-PV MF), post essential thrombocythemia myelofibrosis (post-ET MF), blast phase PMF (PMF-BP): Consensus on terminology by the international working group for myelofibrosis research and treatment (IWG-MRT). *Leuk Res.* 2007;31:737-40.
3. Vardiman JW, Thiele J, Arber DA, et al. The 2008 revision of the World Health Organization (WHO) classification of myeloid neoplasms and acute leukemia: rationale and important changes. *Blood.* 2009;114:937-51.
4. Tefferi A, Vardiman JW. Classification and diagnosis of myeloproliferative neoplasms: the 2008 World Health Organization criteria and point-of-care diagnostic algorithms. *Leukemia.* 2008;22:14-22.
5. Mesa RA, Silverstein MN, Jacobsen SJ, et al. Population-based incidence and survival figures in essential thrombocythemia and agnogenic myeloid metaplasia: an Olmsted County Study, 1976-1995. *Am J Hematol.* 1999;61:10-5.
6. McNally RJ, Rowland D, Roman E, et al. Age and sex distributions of hematological malignancies in the U.K. *Hematol Oncol.* 1997;15:173-89.
7. Passamonti F, Rumi E, Pungolino E, et al. Life expectancy and prognostic factors for survival in patients with polycythemia vera and essential thrombocythemia. *Am J Med.* 2004;117:755-61.
8. Cervantes F, Pereira A, Esteve J, et al. Identification of 'short-lived' and 'long-lived' patients at presentation of idiopathic myelofibrosis. *Br J Haematol.* 1997;97:635-40.
9. Tefferi A, Huang J, Schwager S, et al. Validation and comparison of contemporary prognostic models in primary myelofibrosis: analysis based on 334 patients from a single institution. *Cancer.* 2007;109:2083-8.
10. Mesa RA, Li CY, Ketterling RP, et al. Leukemic transformation in myelofibrosis with myeloid metaplasia: a single-institution experience with 91 cases. *Blood.* 2005;105:973-7.
11. Cervantes F, Dupriez B, Pereira A, et al. New prognostic scoring system for primary myelofibrosis based on a study of the International Working Group for Myelofibrosis Research and Treatment. *Blood.* 2009;113:2895-901.
12. Visani G, Finelli C, Castelli U, et al. Myelofibrosis with myeloid metaplasia: clinical and haematological parameters predicting survival in a series of 133 patients. *Br J Haematol.* 1990;75:4-9.
13. Varki A, Lottenberg R, Griffith R, et al. The syndrome of idiopathic myelofibrosis. A clinicopathologic review with emphasis on the prognostic variables predicting survival. *Medicine (Baltimore).* 1983;62:353-71.

14. Tefferi A: Myelofibrosis with myeloid metaplasia. *N Engl J Med.* 2000;342:1255-65.
15. Tefferi A, Vaidya R, Caramazza D, et al. Circulating interleukin (IL)-8, IL-2R, IL-12, and IL-15 levels are independently prognostic in primary myelofibrosis: a comprehensive cytokine profiling study. *J Clin Oncol.* 2011;29:1356-63.
16. Tefferi A, Lasho TL, Jimma T, et al. One thousand patients with primary myelofibrosis: the mayo clinic experience. *Mayo Clin Proc.* 2012;87:25-33.
17. Mizoguchi M, Kawa Y, Minami T, et al. Cutaneous extramedullary hematopoiesis in myelofibrosis. *J Am Acad Dermatol.* 1990;22:351-5.
18. Loewy G, Mathew A, Distenfeld A. Skin manifestation of agnogenic myeloid metaplasia. Am *J Hematol.* 1994;45:167-70.
19. Koch CA, Li CY, Mesa RA, et al. Nonhepatosplenic extramedullary hematopoiesis: associated diseases, pathology, clinical course, and treatment. *Mayo Clin Proc.* 2003;78:1223-33.
20. Georgiades CS, Neyman EG, Francis IR, et al. Typical and atypical presentations of extramedullary hemopoiesis. *AJR Am J Roentgenol.* 2002;179:1239-43.
21. Cervantes F, Alvarez-Larran A, Arellano-Rodrigo E, et al. Frequency and risk factors for thrombosis in idiopathic myelofibrosis: analysis in a series of 155 patients from a single institution. *Leukemia.* 2006;20:55-60.
22. Barbui T, Carobbio A, Cervantes F, et al. Thrombosis in primary myelofibrosis: incidence and risk factors. *Blood.* 2010;115:778-82.
23. Elliott MA, Pardanani A, Lasho TL, et al. Thrombosis in myelofibrosis: prior thrombosis is the only predictive factor and most venous events are provoked. *Haematologica.* 2010;95:1788-91.
24. Cobo F, Cervantes F, Garcia-Pagan JC, et al. [Budd-Chiari syndrome associated with chronic myeloproliferative syndromes: analysis of 6 cases]. *Med Clin (Barc).* 1996;107:660-3.
25. Valla D, Casadevall N, Lacombe C, et al. Primary myeloproliferative disorder and hepatic vein thrombosis. A prospective study of erythroid colony formation in vitro in 20 patients with Budd-Chiari syndrome. *Ann Intern Med.* 1985;103:329-34.
26. Valla D, Casadevall N, Huisse MG, et al. Etiology of portal vein thrombosis in adults. A prospective evaluation of primary myeloproliferative disorders. *Gastroenterology.* 1988;94: 1063-9.
27. Abu-Hilal M, Tawaker J. Portal hypertension secondary to myelofibrosis with myeloid metaplasia: a study of 13 cases. *World J Gastroenterol.* 2009;15:3128-33.
28. Garcia-Manero G, Schuster SJ, Patrick H, et al. Pulmonary hypertension in patients with myelofibrosis secondary to myeloproliferative diseases. *Am J Hematol.* 1999;60:130-5.
29. Dingli D, Utz JP, Krowka MJ, et al. Unexplained pulmonary hypertension in chronic myeloproliferative disorders. *Chest.* 2001;120:801-8.
30. Cortelezzi A, Gritti G, Del Papa N, et al. Pulmonary arterial hypertension in primary myelofibrosis is common and associated with an altered angiogenic status. *Leukemia.* 2008;22:646-9.
31. Dupriez B, Morel P, Demory JL, et al. Prognostic factors in agnogenic myeloid metaplasia: a report on 195 cases with a new scoring system. *Blood.* 1996;88:1013-8.
32. Barosi G, Bergamaschi G, Marchetti M, et al. JAK2 V617F mutational status predicts progression to large splenomegaly and leukemic transformation in primary myelofibrosis. *Blood.* 2007;110:4030-6.
33. Tefferi A. Novel mutations and their functional and clinical relevance in myeloproliferative neoplasms: JAK2, MPL, TET2, ASXL1, CBL, IDH and IKZF1. *Leukemia.* 2010;24:1128-38.
34. Abdel-Wahab O, Pardanani A, Patel J, et al. Concomitant analysis of EZH2 and ASXL1 mutations in myelofibrosis, chronic myelomonocytic leukemia and blast-phase myeloproliferative neoplasms. *Leukemia.* 2011;25:1200-2.
35. Thiele J, Kvasnicka HM, Fischer R. Histochemistry and morphometry on bone marrow biopsies in chronic myeloproliferative disorders-aids to diagnosis and classification. *Ann Hematol.* 1999;78:495-506.

36. Thiele J, Kvasnicka HM. Myelofibrosis in chronic myeloproliferative disorders--dynamics and clinical impact. *Histol Histopathol.* 2006;21:1367-78.
37. Tefferi A, Thiele J, Orazi A, et al. Proposals and rationale for revision of the World Health Organization diagnostic criteria for polycythemia vera, essential thrombocythemia, and primary myelofibrosis: recommendations from an ad hoc international expert panel. *Blood.* 2007;110:1092-7.
38. Barosi G, Mesa RA, Thiele J, et al. Proposed criteria for the diagnosis of post-polycythemia vera and post-essential thrombocythemia myelofibrosis: a consensus statement from the International Working Group for Myelofibrosis Research and Treatment. *Leukemia.* 2008; 22:437-8.
39. Passamonti F, Cervantes F, Vannucchi AM, et al. A dynamic prognostic model to predict survival in primary myelofibrosis: a study by the IWG-MRT (International Working Group for Myeloproliferative Neoplasms Research and Treatment). *Blood.* 2010;115:1703-8.
40. Caramazza D, Begna KH, Gangat N, et al. Refined cytogenetic-risk categorization for overall and leukemia-free survival in primary myelofibrosis: a single center study of 433 patients. *Leukemia.* 2011;25:82-8.
41. Tefferi A, Mesa RA, Pardanani A, et al. Red blood cell transfusion need at diagnosis adversely affects survival in primary myelofibrosis-increased serum ferritin or transfusion load does not. *Am J Hematol.* 2009;84:265-7.
42. Patnaik MM, Caramazza D, Gangat N, et al. Age and platelet count are IPSS-independent prognostic factors in young patients with primary myelofibrosis and complement IPSS in predicting very long or very short survival. *Eur J Haematol.* 2010;84:105-8.
43. Gangat N, Caramazza D, Vaidya R, et al. DIPSS plus: a refined Dynamic International Prognostic Scoring System for primary myelofibrosis that incorporates prognostic information from karyotype, platelet count, and transfusion status. *J Clin Oncol.* 2011;29:392-7.
44. Tefferi A, Lasho TL, Huang J, et al. Low JAK2V617F allele burden in primary myelofibrosis, compared to either a higher allele burden or unmutated status, is associated with inferior overall and leukemia-free survival. *Leukemia.* 2008;22:756-61.
45. Guglielmelli P, Barosi G, Specchia G, et al. Identification of patients with poorer survival in primary myelofibrosis based on the burden of JAK2V617F mutated allele. *Blood.* 2009;114:1477-83.
46. Passamonti F, Rumi E, Caramella M, et al. A dynamic prognostic model to predict survival in post-polycythemia vera myelofibrosis. *Blood.* 2008;111:3383-7.
47. Barosi G, Bordessoule D, Briere J, et al. Response criteria for myelofibrosis with myeloid metaplasia: results of an initiative of the European Myelofibrosis Network (EUMNET). *Blood.* 2005;106:2849-53.
48. Tefferi A, Barosi G, Mesa RA, et al. International Working Group (IWG) consensus criteria for treatment response in myelofibrosis with myeloid metaplasia, for the IWG for Myelofibrosis Research and Treatment (IWG-MRT). *Blood.* 2006;108:1497-503.
49. Cervantes F, Alvarez-Larran A, Hernandez-Boluda JC, et al. Erythropoietin treatment of the anaemia of myelofibrosis with myeloid metaplasia: results in 20 patients and review of the literature. *Br J Haematol.* 2004;127:399-403.
50. Huang J, Tefferi A. Erythropoiesis stimulating agents have limited therapeutic activity in transfusion-dependent patients with primary myelofibrosis regardless of serum erythropoietin level. *Eur J Haematol.* 2009;83:154-5.
51. Cervantes F, Alvarez-Larran A, Hernandez-Boluda JC, et al. Darbepoetin-alpha for the anaemia of myelofibrosis with myeloid metaplasia. *Br J Haematol.* 2006;134:184-6.
52. Rodriguez JN, Martino ML, Dieguez JC, et al. rHuEpo for the treatment of anemia in myelofibrosis with myeloid metaplasia. Experience in 6 patients and meta-analytical approach. *Haematologica.* 1998;83:616-21.
53. Huang J, Li CY, Mesa RA, et al. Risk factors for leukemic transformation in patients with primary myelofibrosis. *Cancer.* 2008;112:2726-32.

54. Brubaker LH, Briere J, Laszlo J, et al. Treatment of anemia in myeloproliferative disorders: a randomized study of fluoxymesterone v transfusions only. *Arch Intern Med.* 1982;142:1533-7.
55. Besa EC, Nowell PC, Geller NL, et al. Analysis of the androgen response of 23 patients with agnogenic myeloid metaplasia: the value of chromosomal studies in predicting response and survival. *Cancer.* 1982;49:308-13.
56. Cervantes F, Hernandez-Boluda JC, Alvarez A, et al. Danazol treatment of idiopathic myelofibrosis with severe anemia. *Haematologica.* 2000;85:595-9.
57. Cervantes F, Alvarez-Larran A, Domingo A, et al. Efficacy and tolerability of danazol as a treatment for the anaemia of myelofibrosis with myeloid metaplasia: long-term results in 30 patients. *Br J Haematol.* 2005;129:771-5.
58. Levy V, Bourgarit A, Delmer A, et al. Treatment of agnogenic myeloid metaplasia with danazol: a report of four cases. *Am J Hematol.* 1996;53:239-41.
59. Barosi G, Elliott M, Canepa L, et al. Thalidomide in myelofibrosis with myeloid metaplasia: a pooled-analysis of individual patient data from five studies. *Leuk Lymphoma.* 2002;43:2301-7.
60. Canepa L, Ballerini F, Varaldo R, et al. Thalidomide in agnogenic and secondary myelofibrosis. *Br J Haematol.* 2001;115:313-5.
61. Elliott MA, Mesa RA, Li CY, et al. Thalidomide treatment in myelofibrosis with myeloid metaplasia. *Br J Haematol.* 2002;117:288-96.
62. Thomas DA, Giles FJ, Albitar M, et al. Thalidomide therapy for myelofibrosis with myeloid metaplasia. *Cancer.* 2006;106:1974-84.
63. Marchetti M, Barosi G, Balestri F, et al. Low-dose thalidomide ameliorates cytopenias and splenomegaly in myelofibrosis with myeloid metaplasia: a phase II trial. *J Clin Oncol.* 2004;22:424-31.
64. Mesa RA, Steensma DP, Pardanani A, et al. A phase 2 trial of combination low-dose thalidomide and prednisone for the treatment of myelofibrosis with myeloid metaplasia. *Blood.* 2003;101:2534-41.
65. Thapaliya P, Tefferi A, Pardanani A, et al. International working group for myelofibrosis research and treatment response assessment and long-term follow-up of 50 myelofibrosis patients treated with thalidomide-prednisone based regimens. *Am J Hematol.* 2011;86:96-8.
66. Barosi G, Grossi A, Comotti B, et al. Safety and efficacy of thalidomide in patients with myelofibrosis with myeloid metaplasia. *Br J Haematol.* 2001;114:78-83.
67. Tefferi A, Cortes J, Verstovsek S, et al. Lenalidomide therapy in myelofibrosis with myeloid metaplasia. *Blood.* 2006;108:1158-64.
68. Quintas-Cardama A, Kantarjian HM, Manshouri T, et al. Lenalidomide plus prednisone results in durable clinical, histopathologic, and molecular responses in patients with myelofibrosis. *J Clin Oncol.* 2009;27:4760-6.
69. Mesa RA, Yao X, Cripe LD, et al. Lenalidomide and prednisone for myelofibrosis: Eastern Cooperative Oncology Group (ECOG) phase 2 trial E4903. *Blood.* 2010;116:4436-8.
70. Tefferi A, Verstovsek S, Barosi G, et al. Pomalidomide is active in the treatment of anemia associated with myelofibrosis. *J Clin Oncol.* 2009;27:4563-9.
71. Begna KH, Mesa RA, Pardanani A, et al. A phase-2 trial of low-dose pomalidomide in myelofibrosis. *Leukemia.* 2011;25:301-4.
72. Tefferi A, Lasho TL, Mesa RA, et al. Lenalidomide therapy in del(5)(q31)-associated myelofibrosis: cytogenetic and JAK2V617F molecular remissions. *Leukemia.* 2007;21:1827-8.
73. Mesa RA, Pardanani AD, Hussein K, et al. Phase1/-2 study of Pomalidomide in myelofibrosis. *Am J Hematol.* 2010;85:129-30.
74. Begna KH, Pardanani A, Mesa R, et al. Long-term outcome of pomalidomide therapy in myelofibrosis. *Am J Hematol.* 2012;87:66-8.
75. Lofvenberg E, Wahlin A. Management of polycythaemia vera, essential thrombocythaemia and myelofibrosis with hydroxyurea. *Eur J Haematol.* 1988;41:375-81.
76. Manoharan A. Management of myelofibrosis with intermittent hydroxyurea. *Br J Haematol.* 1991;77:252-4.

77. Martinez-Trillos A, Gaya A, Maffioli M, et al. Efficacy and tolerability of hydroxyurea in the treatment of the hyperproliferative manifestations of myelofibrosis: results in 40 patients. *Ann Hematol.* 2010;89:1233-7.
78. Sirhan S, Lasho TL, Hanson CA, et al. The presence of JAK2V617F in primary myelofibrosis or its allele burden in polycythemia vera predicts chemosensitivity to hydroxyurea. *Am J Hematol.* 2008;83:363-5.
79. Lofvenberg E, Wahlin A, Roos G, et al. Reversal of myelofibrosis by hydroxyurea. *Eur J Haematol.* 1990;44:33-8.
80. Faoro LN, Tefferi A, Mesa RA. Long-term analysis of the palliative benefit of 2-chlorodeoxy-adenosine for myelofibrosis with myeloid metaplasia. *Eur J Haematol.* 2005;74:117-20.
81. Petti MC, Latagliata R, Spadea T, et al. Melphalan treatment in patients with myelofibrosis with myeloid metaplasia. *Br J Haematol.* 2002;116:576-81.
82. Gilbert HS. Long term treatment of myeloproliferative disease with interferon-alpha-2b: feasibility and efficacy. *Cancer.* 1998;83:1205-13.
83. Ianotto JC, Kiladjian JJ, Demory JL, et al. PEG-IFN-alpha-2a therapy in patients with myelofibrosis: a study of the French Groupe d'Etudes des Myelofibroses (GEM) and France Intergroupe des syndromes Myeloproliferatifs (FIM). *Br J Haematol.* 2009;146:223-5.
84. Silver RT, Vandris K, Goldman JJ. Recombinant interferon-alpha may retard progression of early primary myelofibrosis: a preliminary report. *Blood.* 2011;117:6669-72.
85. Verstovsek S. Therapeutic potential of JAK2 inhibitors. *Hematology Am Soc Hematol Educ Program.* 2009:636-42.
86. Kralovics R, Passamonti F, Buser AS, et al. A gain-of-function mutation of JAK2 in myeloproliferative disorders. *N Engl J Med.* 2005;352:1779-90.
87. Verstovsek S, Kantarjian H, Mesa RA, et al. Safety and efficacy of INCB018424, a JAK1 and JAK2 inhibitor, in myelofibrosis. *N Engl J Med.* 2010;363:1117-27.
88. Verstovsek S, Mesa RA, Gotlib J, et al. A double-blind, placebo-controlled trial of ruxolitinib for myelofibrosis. *N Engl J Med.* 2012;366:799-807.
89. Harrison C, Kiladjian JJ, Al-Ali HK, et al. JAK inhibition with ruxolitinib versus best available therapy for myelofibrosis. *N Engl J Med.* 2012;366:787-98.
90. Quintas-Cardama A, Vaddi K, Liu P, et al. Preclinical characterization of the selective JAK1/2 inhibitor INCB018424: therapeutic implications for the treatment of myeloproliferative neoplasms. *Blood.* 2010;115:3109-17.
91. Mesa RA, Gotlib J, Gupta V, et al. Effect of Ruxolitinib Therapy on Myelofibrosis-Related Symptoms and Other Patient-Reported Outcomes in COMFORT-I: A Randomized, Double-Blind, Placebo-Controlled Trial. *J Clin Oncol.* 2013;31:1285-92.
92. Benbassat J, Gilon D, Penchas S. The choice between splenectomy and medical treatment in patients with advanced agnogenic myeloid metaplasia. *Am J Hematol.* 1990;33:128-35.
93. Mesa RA, Nagorney DS, Schwager S, et al. Palliative goals, patient selection, and perioperative platelet management: outcomes and lessons from 3 decades of splenectomy for myelofibrosis with myeloid metaplasia at the Mayo Clinic. *Cancer.* 2006;107:361-70.
94. Towell BL, Levine SP. Massive hepatomegaly following splenectomy for myeloid metaplasia. Case report and review of the literature. *Am J Med.* 1987;82:371-5.
95. Lopez-Guillermo A, Cervantes F, Bruguera M, et al. Liver dysfunction following splenectomy in idiopathic myelofibrosis: a study of 10 patients. *Acta Haematol.* 1991;85:184-8.
96. Barosi G, Ambrosetti A, Buratti A, et al. Splenectomy for patients with myelofibrosis with myeloid metaplasia: pretreatment variables and outcome prediction. *Leukemia.* 1993;7:200-6.
97. Brenner B, Nagler A, Tatarsky I, et al. Splenectomy in agnogenic myeloid metaplasia and postpolycythemic myeloid metaplasia. A study of 34 cases. *Arch Intern Med.* 1988;148:2501-5.
98. Barosi G, Ambrosetti A, Centra A, et al. Splenectomy and risk of blast transformation in myelofibrosis with myeloid metaplasia. Italian Cooperative Study Group on Myeloid with Myeloid Metaplasia. *Blood.* 1998;91:3630-6.

99. Silverstein MN. Control of hypersplenism and painful splenomegaly in myeloid metaplasia by irradiation. *Int J Radiat Oncol Biol Phys.* 1977;2:1221-2.
100. Slanina J, Vondraczek A, Wannenmacher M. [Symptomatic irradiation therapy of the spleen in advanced osteomyelosclerosis]. *Dtsch Med Wochenschr.* 1986;111:1144-50.
101. Elliott MA, Chen MG, Silverstein MN, et al. Splenic irradiation for symptomatic splenomegaly associated with myelofibrosis with myeloid metaplasia. *Br J Haematol.* 1998;103:505-11.
102. Bouabdallah R, Coso D, Gonzague-Casabianca L, et al. Safety and efficacy of splenic irradiation in the treatment of patients with idiopathic myelofibrosis: a report on 15 patients. *Leuk Res.* 2000;24:491-5.
103. McFarland JT, Kuzma C, Millard FE, et al. Palliative irradiation of the spleen. *Am J Clin Oncol.* 2003;26:178-83.
104. Steensma DP, Hook CC, Stafford SL, et al. Low-dose, single-fraction, whole-lung radiotherapy for pulmonary hypertension associated with myelofibrosis with myeloid metaplasia. *Br J Haematol.* 2002;118:813-6.
105. Tefferi A, Jimenez T, Gray LA, et al. Radiation therapy for symptomatic hepatomegaly in myelofibrosis with myeloid metaplasia. *Eur J Haematol.* 2001;66:37-42.
106. Neben-Wittich MA, Brown PD, Tefferi A. Successful treatment of severe extremity pain in myelofibrosis with low-dose single-fraction radiation therapy. *Am J Hematol.* 2010;85:808-10.
107. Riesterer O, Gmur J, Lutolf U. Repeated and preemptive palliative radiotherapy of symptomatic hepatomegaly in a patient with advanced myelofibrosis. *Onkologie.* 2008;31:325-7.
108. Leinweber C, Order SE, Calkins AR. Whole-abdominal irradiation for the management of gastrointestinal and abdominal manifestations of agnogenic myeloid metaplasia. *Cancer.* 1991;68:1251-4.
109. Weinschenker P, Kutner JM, Salvajoli JV, et al. Whole-pulmonary low-dose radiation therapy in agnogenic myeloid metaplasia with diffuse lung involvement. *Am J Hematol.* 2002;69:277-80.

CHAPTER 7 Hematopoietic Stem Cell Transplant in Myelofibrosis

Irum Khan, Damiano Rondelli

INTRODUCTION

Myelofibrosis (MF) is a clonal disorder that results in expansion of abnormal hematopoietic cells, cytopenias, bone marrow fibrosis and angiogenesis,[1] and extramedullary hematopoiesis. The disease can occur de novo [primary myelofibrosis (PMF)] or be secondary to a pre-existing myeloproliferative neoplasm, such as polycythemia vera (PV) or essential thrombocythemia (ET) and polycythemia vera myelofibrosis or essential thrombocythemia myelofibrosis (PV-MF or ET-MF). Together, these entities are referred to as MF. MF is clinically heterogeneous, ranging from an indolent disease persisting for up to a decade to an aggressive course with a median survival of 1–2 years.[2] Therapy for MF has historically used chemotherapeutic agents, immunomodulatory drugs, or biological-response modifiers. Increased insight into the biologic underpinnings of PMF has led to the recent development and approval of Janus kinase (JAK) inhibitors.

Although these interventions may improve the symptoms associated with the disease, they do not alter the natural history of the disease. Moreover, palliative strategies are not satisfactory for intermediate-2 or high-risk patients less than 55 years of age, whose median expected survival is less than 3 years. The only possible curative treatment is allogeneic hematopoietic stem cell transplantation (ASCT). However, this option is offered only to patients less than 65 years of age and in overall good health, provided that a compatible donor is available. In addition, because of the risks associated with this procedure, it is currently offered mainly to patients with advanced disease.

The adoption of reduced intensity conditioning regimens (RIC) will make ASCT available to a broader population of patients. Moreover, optimal positioning of JAK inhibitor therapy in transplant-eligible patients is an exciting area of research.

ROLE OF HEMATOPOIETIC STEM CELL TRANSPLANT IN MYELOFIBROSIS

Patients with PMF have a significantly increased number of circulating hematopoietic CD34+ progenitors in the peripheral blood[3,4] compared to normal individuals. Investigators were able to harvest mobilized progenitor cells and perform autologous hematopoietic stem cell transplants in 27 patients after conditioning chemotherapy. This procedure resulted in some improvement of splenomegaly and reduced transfusion requirements,[5] but the study did not have adequate follow-up.

Allogeneic hematopoietic stem cell transplant is currently the only curative therapy for patients with MF. The effect of transplant relies on the cytoreductive activity of the preparative regimen in the marrow[6] and extramedullary sites,[7] and an immunological effect mediated by T-lymphocytes in the graft against clonal hematopoietic cells. This graft-versus-tumor effect was initially demonstrated in a study showing a 5 year survival of 54% for patients receiving an unmanipulated human leukocyte antigen (HLA) matched related graft compared to 26% for those receiving a T-cell-depleted graft or a graft coming from an alternative donor.[8] Further proof of a graft-versus-myelofibrosis effect was obtained with the successful use of donor lymphocyte infusion (DLI) therapy in patients relapsing after transplant.[9] The curative effect of transplant is demonstrated by a complete normalization of marrow fibrosis,[10] restoration of normal hematopoiesis, and reduction of splenomegaly to within normal limits over 12–24 months following donor cell infusion.[11]

A recent large retrospective study demonstrated the safety and efficacy of allogeneic transplant in secondary myelofibrosis. Two-hundred fifty consecutive patients with an initial diagnosis of PV, or ET underwent transplantation due to progression to myelofibrosis (n = 193) or acute myeloid leukemia (n = 57). With a median follow-up from transplantation of 13 months, 3 year-overall survivor (OS) and relapse incidence were 55% and 32%, respectively.[12]

CONDITIONING REGIMEN

Conventional myeloablative conditioning (MAC) regimens for ASCT for PMF resulted in an overall 3-year survival of 33–53%[8,13-15] with considerable non-relapse mortality (NRM) of 27–48%. Kerbuay et al.[16] demonstrated that targeting busulfan levels between 800 ng/mL and 900 ng/mL in combination with cyclophosphamide led to a higher probability of survival than other regimens. However, for the population subset more than 45 years of age, the 5-year OS was only 14%. This transplant-related toxicity precluded ASCT for most patients with PMF who have a median age of presentation of 67 years. Deeg et al.[15] reported intermediate- and high-risk patients were likely to have increased relapse-related and NRM. Patients with a low Lille score had an 80% overall survival rate at 3 years after transplantation, whereas patients with intermediate or high-risk scores had 45% and 25% 3-year OS, respectively.

This led to the introduction of reduced intensity conditioning (RIC) regimens with the potential reduction in NRM making allogeneic transplantation accessible to older patients and those with more advanced disease. In the early 2000s, several retrospective studies showed successful engraftment with stable full-donor hematopoietic

Table 7-1 Retrospective Experience of Transplant in Myelofibrosis

Reference	*Study period*	*Regimen*	*Number*	*Age*	*Acute GVHD Grades II-IV*	*TRM*	*Overall survival*
Myeloablative conditioning							
Guardiola[8]	1979–1997	TBI (n = 35) other (n = 20)	55	42 (54–53)	60%	27% at 1 year	47% at 5 years
Deeg[15]	1980–2002	Bu/Cy (n = 44) TBI (n=12)	56	43 (10–66)	68%	32% at 1 year	58% at 3 years
Daly[13]	1990–2002	Cy/TBI (n=23) Bu/Cy (n = 2)	25	48 (45–50)	52%	48% at 1 year	41% at 2 years
Kerbauey[16]	unknown	Bu/Cy (n = 80) TBI based (n = 15) RIC (n = 9)	104	49 (18–70)	64%	35% at 5 years	61% at 7 years
Ballen[28]	1989–2002	Bu/Cy (n=80) TBI (n=15) RIC (n=60) Multiple	289	47 (18–73)	MSD 43% MUD 40%	MSD 22% MUD 42% At day 100	MSD 39% MUD31% at 5 years
Reduced intensity conditioning							
Rondelli[20]	NR	Multiple	21	54 (27–68)	33%	10% at 1 year	85% at 2.5 years
Bacigalupo[33]	1994–2007	Thiotepa-Cy-melphalan	46	51 (24–67)	NR	24% at 5 years	45% at 5 years
Alchalby[48]	1999–2009	Flu-Bu (n = 156)	162	56 (32–73)		22% at 1 year	62% at 5 years
Studies of RIC and MAC							
Patriarca[24]	1986–2006	MAC (n = 48): Bu-Cy in 24/48 RIC (n = 52): Thiotepa-Cy in 24, Flu/Bu in 14,Flu/Mel in 6	100	49 (21–68)	41%	35% at 1 year	42% at 3 years

Contd...

Contd...

Lissandre[25]	1999–2009	MAC (n = 15) RIC (n = 24)	39	49 (15–65)	69%	30% at 3 years	60% at 3 years
Abelsson[21]	1982–2009	MAC (n = 40) RIC (n = 52)	92	46 for MAC (5–63) 55 for RIC (22–66)	23%	32% for MAC,24% for RIC at 2 years	49% for MAC, 55% for RIC at 5 years
Robin[29]	1997–2008	MAC (n = 46): RIC (n = 101)	147	53 (20–68)	43%	39% at 4 years	39% at 4 years
Merup[22]	1982–2004	MAC (n = 17): Cy/TBI in 10, Bu/Cy in 7 RIC (n = 10): Flu/Bu in 8,Flu/Cy/Mel in 2	27	48 (5–62)	26%	30% for MAC; 10% for RIC at 55 months	70% at 55 months
Gupta[23]	1998–2005	MAC (n = 23): Cy/TBI in 22, Bu/Cy in 1 RIC (n = 23) Flu/Bu in 16, Flu/TBI 200 in 6, Flu/Mel in 1	46	47 for MAC (31–60) 54 for RIC (38–74)	78% with MAC versus 18% with RIC at day 100	39% for MAC; 23% for RIC at 1 year	48% for MAC; 68% for RIC at year

GVHD, graft-versus-host disease; TRM, transplant-related mortality; TBI, total body irradiation; Bu, busulfan; Cy, cyclophosphamide; Flu, fludarabine; Mel, melphalan; MAC, myeloablative conditioning; RIC, reduced intensity conditioning; MSD, matched sibling donor; MUD, matched unrelated donor.

chimerism[17-20] and reversal of marrow fibrosis with RIC transplants in older patients. These studies used matched sibling as well as matched unrelated donors (MUD). Conditioning regimens included mostly fludarabine-based regimens. A retrospective study of 21 patients by the Myeloproliferative Disorders-Research Consortium (MPD-RC) observed an OS of 85% and event-free-survival of 76% with a median follow-up of 31 months, despite a median patient age of 54 years and all patients with intermediate/high-risk disease according to Lille score system.[20]

There have been several retrospective comparisons using MAC versus RIC in MF (Table 7-1). Ninety-two patients with MF in chronic phase underwent ASCT in nine Nordic transplant centers. MAC was given to 40 patients, and RIC was used in 52 patients. When adjustment for age differences was made, the survival of the patients treated with RIC was significantly better ($p = 0.003$). Patients treated with RIC experienced significantly less acute acute graft-versus-host disease (GVHD) compared with patients treated with MAC ($p < 0.001$).[21] The Swedish experience comparing MAC with RIC at 6 transplant centers ($n = 27$) showed treatment-related mortality (TRM) was 10% in the RIC group and 30% in the myeloablative group after a median follow-up of 55 months.[22] In a review of 46 patients who underwent MAC or RIC over a 7-year period, Gupta et al.[23] reported a reduced risk of GVHD, more rapid engraftment and reduced hospitalization within the first 100 days with RIC. No difference in relapse rate or rate of histological regression was noted. There was a trend toward improved disease free-survival (DFS) and OS in the RIC group at median follow-up of 50 months. Retrospective studies from the Italian transplant registry (GITMO)[24] and four major French transplant centers[25] failed to demonstrate any improvement in survival or NRM using RIC over MAC. However, these studies may have been flawed by selection bias and were conducted over several decades.

This ambivalence in the retrospective data led to a pilot study using RIC with busulfan (10 mg/kg), fludarabine (180 mg/m^2), and antithymocyte globulin (ATG) followed by allogeneic stem cell transplantation from related ($n = 8$) and unrelated donors ($n = 13$) in 21 MF patients, median age of 53 years.[26] Hematological response was seen in 100% and after a median follow-up of 22 months, the 3-year estimated OS and DFS was 84% [95% confidence interval (CI): 67–100%]. This was followed by a phase II multicenter prospective trial conducted by the European group for Blood and Marrow Transplantation (EBMT)[11] using a busulfan (10 mg/kg)/fludarabine (180 mg/m^2)-based RIC regimen followed by allogeneic stem cell transplantation from related ($n = 33$) or unrelated donors ($n = 70$). GVHD grades 2–4 occurred in 27% and chronic GVHD in 43% of patients. Cumulative incidence of NRM at 1 year was 16% but significantly higher in HLA-mismatched case. The cumulative incidence of relapse at 3 years was 22% (95% CI, 13–31%) and was influenced by Lille score and splenectomy. The estimated 5-year event-free survival (EFS) and OS were 51% and 67%, respectively.

The MPD-RC undertook another prospective phase II study in the United States and Europe using a reduced intensity regimen with fludarabine/melphalan (FluMel) in related or FluMel + ATG in unrelated ASCT in patients with MF. Of 66 patients, 63 were at intermediate/high-risk according to Lille score system. Interim results, after a median follow-up for survivors of 24 months, showed that NRM was 18% in matched related transplants and 53% in the unrelated group. Median survival time has not been reached in the related transplant group and is 7 months in the unrelated group (hazard ratio 4.2, 95% CI: 1.7–10.1, $p < 0.001$).[27]

Allogeneic stem cell transplantation with fully myeloablative conditioning is an accepted therapeutic option for young patients (<45 years). NRM with RIC regimens, especially with matched related donors (MRD), is in the range of 15–20% and the risk of relapse in most studies does not exceed that seen with myeloablative conditioning. These observations suggest that the majority of patients with MF should be prepared with RIC regimens.

SELECTION OF DONOR

Several studies have reported similar outcomes in patients undergoing an ASCT from an HLA MRD and MUD,[11,15,16] while outcomes of transplants from mismatched donors were significantly inferior. These conclusions are different from the MPD-RC prospective study reported above and from the retrospective data of the Center for International Blood and Marrow Transplant Research reported by Ballen et al.[28] who showed a 5-year NRM of 27% in MRD and 43% in MUD ASCT. Gruppo Italiano Trapianto di Midollo Osseo (GITMO) data also revealed a reduction in transplant-related mortality associated with the choice of a MRD.[24] The Société Française de Greffe de Moelle et de Thérapie Cellulaire (SFGM-TC) registry including patients with MF transplanted between 1997 and 2008 showed engraftment probability and OS to be significantly inferior in non-sibling donors compared to matched siblings.[29] The contradictory results from these different studies are attributable to small sample sizes, retrospective design and patient and conditioning regimen heterogeneity.

ROLE OF SPLENECTOMY

Splenomegaly is virtually a pathognomonic feature of MF and leads to many symptoms including pain, early satiety, splenic infarcts, and sequestration causing anemia and thrombocytopenia. Significant splenomegaly at the time of transplant may adversely impact time to engraftment,[30,31] prompting the question of whether or not splenectomy should be performed prior to transplant. Enthusiasm for this procedure is limited as a review of over 300 should be performed patients who underwent splenectomy between 1976 and 2004 revealed a 27.7% risk of perioperative complications including infection, thrombosis, or bleeding, 21 of which (6.7% of all patients) were fatal.[32] Conflicting results have been reported on the benefit of

Table 7-2 Prognostic Fators Affecting Transplant Outcome

Variable	Hazard ratio	Study
DIPPS • Age 65 years • WBC >25 × 109/L • Hb <10 g/dL • Peripheral blood blasts >1% • Constitutional symptoms	• High risk DIPSS was associated with a fourfold increased risk of post-transplant mortality and threefold increase in non-relapse mortality • High DIPSS associated with increased RFS (HR 1.3) and overall survival (HR 1.4)	Scott et al.[34] Ditschkowski et al.[52]
High platelet count in PV/ET	• High platelet count associated with increased survival post-transplant	Kerbauy et al.[16]
Advanced Lille score	• Intermediate and high scores associated with 3-fold and 5-fold increased risk respectively of relapse	Kroger et al.[11]
Abnormal karyotype	Decrease in relapse-free survival (HR = 2.2)	Ditschkowski et al.[52]
No pharmacologic pretreatment	Improved overall survival (HR = 2.7)	Ditschkowski et al.[52]
Chronic GVHD	Reduced risk of death: HR 0.2 3-year overall survival higher in patients with than without chronic GVHD	Ditschkowski et al.[52] Kroger et al.[11]
HLA-mismatched donor	Decrease in overall survival (HR = 3)	Kroger et al.[11]
Non HLA-identical sibling	Decrease in overall survival (HR = 1.86)	Robin et al.[29]
Age >55 years	Decrease in survival (HR = 2.7)	Kroger et al.[11]
JAK2 V617F wild type	Decrease in survival (HR = 2.02)	Alchalby et al.[49]
Constitutional symptoms	Decrease in survival (HR = 2.8)	Alchalby et al.[49]
Non-chronic phase disease	Decrease in survival (HR = 1.8)	Robin et al.[29]
Spleen size greater than 22 cm	Relative risk of death = 2.71	Bacigalupo et al.[33]
>20 RBC transfusions	Relative risk of death = 4.43	Bacigalupo et al.[33]
Time from diagnosis to SCT	Long interval was predictor of increased transplant-related mortality	Patriarca et al.[24]
Grade III marrow fibrosis	5-year survival of 55% with grade I- II marrow fibrosis, and 38% with grade III	Guardiola et al.[8]
Targeted busulfan level (800–900 ng/mL)	Improved overall survival	Deeg et al.[15] Kerbauy et al.[16]

DIPPS, Dynamic International Prognostic Scoring System; WBC, white blood cell; Hb, hemoglobin; HR, high risk; PV/ET, polycythemia vera/essential thrombocythemia; GVHD, graft-versus-host disease; HLA, human leukocyte antigen; RBC, red blood cell; RFS, recurrence free survival; HR, Hazard ratio; SCT, stem cell transprantation.

splenectomy should be performed prior to transplantation. The European Group for Blood and Marrow Transplantation study reported a threefold increased risk of relapse after splenectomy, although it is argued that this may have been a reflection of more advanced disease.[11] In contrast, an Italian study has recently reported a reduced risk of relapse in patients with marked splenomegaly who were underwent splenectomy before ASCT.[33] Review of the data from the Fred Hutchinson Cancer Center[34] showed that after adjustment for Dynamic International Prognostic Scoring System (DIPSS) score and the hematopoietic cell transplant comorbidity index (HCT-CI), patients who had a splenectomy were at significantly lower risk for mortality compared with patients who had not (HR = 0.44). Retrospective data from the Center for International Blood and Bone marrow Transplant Research (CIBMTR)[28] and 2 other studies[16,35] failed to show an effect of splenectomy on progression-free survival (PFS) or OS. Postulated setbacks of splenectomy in the setting of ASCT include a worsened severity of GVHD due to altered immunomodulation[36] and an excess risk of AML transformation.[32,37]

In the absence of any intervention for splenomegaly, successful engraftment can still occur. A study of 10 patients with extensive splenomegaly who underwent RIC-hematopoietic stem cell transplantation (HSCT) demonstrated a progressive reduction of splenomegaly within 12 months post-transplant and this paralleled the reduction of marrow fibrosis.[31] Given the absence of strong favorable evidence and inherent operative risks, at this time routine splenectomy is not advocated prior to transplant. Recently, post-transplant splenectomy has been studied as a way to manage delayed engraftment in patients with splenomegaly and MF.[38] The discovery of novel targeted agents, such as JAK-inhibitors or mammalian target of rapamycin (mTOR) inhibitors, whose effect will be discussed at the end of this chapter, may mitigate the problem of extensive splenomegaly prior to transplant in a large number of patients.

VALIDITY OF CURRENT PROGNOSTIC SCORING SYSTEMS IN PREDICTING POST-TRANSPLANT OUTCOMES

Given the marked heterogeneity in the clinical course of MF, it has been very important to identify prognostic indicators to predict which patients would derive maximal benefit from a procedure as inherently risky as ASCT. The Lille scoring system was based on hemoglobin (Hb) less than 10g/dL, leukopenia [white blood cell (WBC) $<4 \times 10^9$/L] or leukocytosis (WBC $>30 \times 10^9$/L) classifying patients as low (no risk factors), intermediate or high-risk (>1 risk factor)[39] with the latter two groups undergoing consideration for ASCT. The Lille prognostic score had several major limitations: it was developed on a very limited number of patients, was based on patients characteristics at diagnosis and not at the time of possible transplant, was tested only in primary and not in secondary MF, and did not include age or cytogenetics among risk factors.

This system was replaced by the International Prognostic Scoring System (IPSS) which encompassed five independent risk factors: age more than 65 years, WBC more than 25 × 10^9/L, Hb less than 10 g/dL, peripheral blood blasts more than 1% and constitutional symptoms.[2] Development of anemia had twice the adverse impact on survival and was therefore weighted more heavily in the DIPSS.[40] DIPSS was then further modified to include red cell transfusion dependency, platelet count less than 100 × 10^9/L, and unfavorable karyotype (i.e., complex karyotype or sole or two abnormalities that include +8, –7/7q–, i(17q), inv(3), –5/5q–, 12p–, or 11q23 rearrangement). This DIPSS-plus model utilizes the presence of 0, 1, "2 or 3," and more than or equal four adverse factors to define low, intermediate-1, intermediate-2, and high-risk disease with median survivals of approximately 15.4, 6.5, 2.9, and 1.3 years, respectively.[41] Although the current prognostic system is comprehensive and has been validated on large groups of patients, all the retrospective and prospective clinical trials addressing stem cell transplantation in MF reported to date have been based on the older Lille scoring system.

Recently, the DIPSS was retrospectively applied to a cohort of transplant patients in two separate analyses from Germany[14] and Seattle[34] with similar results. The German study showed that using the DIPSS for risk stratification, low-risk patients had significantly better OS (p = 0.014, hazard ratio 1.4) and relapse-free survival (p = 0.02, Hazard ratio 1.3) compared to the other risk groups of patients. Analysis of OS stratified by DIPSS-Plus scores demonstrated even better results for each risk group. In the latter study, 170 patients, median 51.5 years of age, underwent ASCT from related (n = 86) or unrelated donors (n = 84) at the Fred Hutchinson Cancer Center. After a median follow-up of 5.9 years, the median survivals have not been reached for DIPSS low and intermediate-1 groups, and were 7 and 2.5 years for intermediate-2 and high-risk patients, respectively.

FACTORS AFFECTING TRANSPLANT OUTCOME

Progress in ASCT over the past 2 decades has led to markedly improved outcomes[42,43] with improved long-term survival and reduced treatment related mortality from the late 80s/early 90s to the first decade of this century. Advances are mostly related to the development of novel preparative regimens at reduced intensity, improved antimicrobial prophylaxis, and improved GVHD prophylaxis. A number of nondisease factors such as age, donor type, and comorbidities may also impact the outcome of transplant in MF[44] (Table 7-2).

In initial studies with myeloablative conditioning regimens, patient age at the time of transplantation represented an important prognostic factor; with a 5-year survival of only 14% in PMF patients older than 45 years, as compared with 62% of younger patients.[45] Retrospective studies both from the Nordic[21] and the Australia/New Zealand[46] co-operative groups confirmed the adverse prognostic impact of age on the outcome of ASCT.

Interestingly a study of 30 patients aged 60–78 years with primary or secondary MF treated with a range of conditioning regimen intensities revealed a 3-year OS of 45% and PFS of 40%. This suggests that with careful patient selection, ASCT can be considered for the elderly.[47]

Although transplant-related mortality has significantly decreased with reduced intensity preparative agents, multiple factors have been considered as independent prognostic factors for outcomes. Alchalby et al.[48] initially showed that patients with wild-type *JAK2*-V617F had an inferior survival after ASCT but this could not be corroborated in other studies. In a following study, Cox multivariate analysis performed on 150 homogeneously treated patients[49] showed JAK2 status, constitutional symptoms and age more than 57 years independently predicted poor survival after reduced intensity conditioning (RIC-HSCT). The recently discovered calreticulin (CALR) mutation[50] seen in 30% of MF cases has demonstrated predictive potential in transplant outcomes. Patients with mutated CALR had a better OS after ASCT than with wild-type CALR (4-year OS 82 vs. 56%, respectively, $p = 0.043$). More specifically, patients with mutated CALR had the best prognosis, patients with JAK2 or MPL mutations had an intermediate prognosis and triple negative patients had the worst prognosis.[51]

Another study of 46 patients undergoing RIC-HSCT demonstrated that spleen size more than 22 cm, transfusion history more than 20 units packed red blood cells (pRBCs), and a donor other than a matched sibling donor (MSD) (e.g., matched/mismatched unrelated or mismatched related) predicted an adverse outcome.[33] Analysis of the French stem cell transplant registry[29] showed that factors favorably affecting engraftment were splenectomy before HCT, HLA-matched sibling donor, and peripheral stem cell use as source of stem cells and absence of pretransplant thrombocytopenia. The German experience showed the incidence of relapse to be significantly higher in the absence of chronic GVHD ($p = 0.006$), and in the setting of pretransplant pharmacotherapy ($p = 0.001$).[52]

Leukemic transformation (LT) is often a catastrophic event in MF and chances of success with chemotherapy are dismal, with a median survival of 2.7 months.[53] The French group demonstrated that non-chronic phase MF is an adverse prognostic marker in a multivariate analysis for OS. Transplant at the time of LT also has poor outcome, however, in a small series of 13 patients transplanted in blast phase, 49% patients were alive after a median follow-up of 31 months.[54]

There is increasing interest in the role of ASCT early in the course of the disease, especially in younger patients, when the post-transplant OS rates are significantly better than in more advanced stage of disease. This is substantiated by the GITMO experience where longer interval between diagnosis and transplant negatively impacted survival after HSCT.[24]

COMPLICATIONS OF HSCT

Hepatotoxicity

The most common etiologies of abnormal liver function tests after HCT are hepatic GVHD, drug-induced hepatitis, and iron overload,[55] whereas severe hepatotoxicity (AST >1500 U/L) is mediated mainly by veno-occlusive disease (VOD) and hypoxia.[56] According to a recent study, patients with MF are at higher risk of early hepatotoxicity after ASCT compared to matched controls (n = 53) undergoing transplant for alternate indications.[57] A history of portal hypertension, biopsy-proven hepatic iron overload, or splanchnic vein thrombosis strongly predicted moderate/severe hyperbilirubinemia ($p = 0.02$) and moderate/severe hyperbilirubinemia or transaminitis was associated with inferior survival at 12 months ($p = 0.02$). In light of these risk factors and their impact on survival, some groups are screening for portal hypertension prior to transplant and risk stratification for VOD is recommended prior to transplant. While it is known that iron overload is associated with increased treatment-related mortality after ASCT,[58,59] a pilot study showed that attempts to correct this with chelation in the peritransplant period had difficulty accruing patients due to intolerability.[60]

Graft Versus Host Disease

The incidence of GVHD must be interpreted in the context of the conditioning regimen, T-cell depletion, donor type, and source of stem cells. Rates of acute GVHD ranged from 40–50%[8,13,27] with MAC or RIC. The Fred Hutchinson Cancer Center MAC experience revealed a 68% incidence of acute GVHD.[14] Use of RIC with T-cell depletion with ATG appears to lower the rate of acute grade II-IV GVHD to 27%.[11] Several retrospective comparisons have provided conflicting results about the role of RIC in reducing acute GVHD. Gupta et al. reported a day 100 cumulative incidence of a GVHD of 78% in the MAC-HSCT group versus 18% in the RIC-HSCT recipients, most likely because 70% of the RIC patients received ATG or alemtuzumab. The Nordic data showed 72% of patients undergoing RIC to be free of GVHD compared to 24% of those undergoing MAC-ASCT.[21] However, this was not confirmed by the British study[35] where a GVHD occurred in 29% and 38% of patients in the myeloablative and RIC groups, respectively, even though 70% RIC patient underwent T-cell depletion. Chronic GVHD was reported in 40–59% of cases and predicted for improved OS[11,15,20] underscoring the importance of the graft-versus-tumor effect of allogeneic transplant. In a retrospective study of 73 patients relapse incidence was significantly higher in the absence of chronic GVHD ($p = 0.006$).[52]

Regarding GVHD prophylaxis, a prospective experience at City of Hope showed that tacrolimus/sirolimus ± methotrexate was superior to cyclosporine/mycophenolate mofetil (CsA/MMF) ± methotrexate. The estimated 2-year OS for the CsA/MMF cohort was 55.6% (CI 36.0–71.3), and for the tacrolimus/sirolimus cohort it was 92.9% (63.3–98.8) ($p = 0.047$). The probability of grade III or IV acute GVHD was 60% for the CsA/MMF patients, and 10% for the tacrolimus/sirolimus group ($p = 0.0102$).[61]

Incidence of GVHD in some studies of MF[8,15,16,27] exceeds that in other hematologic malignancies. This has been postulated to be due to elevated proinflammatory cytokines enhancing dendritic cell activation of T cells. An interesting observation in this regard is that the JAK2 inhibitor CP-690550 abrogated acute GVHD related mortality in murine models, this effect was largely related to the suppression of donor CD4 T-cell-mediated interferon-gamma production.[62] Moreover, ruxolitinib has also been shown to reduce the levels of proinflammatory cytokines in MF patients dramatically.[63] It remains to be seen what effect ruxolitinib and other JAK inhibitors will have on the cytokines mediating GVHD.

Graft Failure

Concern about graft failure caused initial reluctance to carry out transplantations in patients with MF. Previous data showed that graft failure was a problem only in 5–25% of patients, particularly those who received transplants from "alternative" (other than MSD) donors.[27,28] The MPD-RC prospective study, however, reported a high rate of rejection in patients transplanted with unrelated donors and conditioned with fludarabine/melphalan and ATG.[55]

MONITORING POST-TRANSPLANT MINIMAL RESIDUAL DISEASE

In addition to its diagnostic and possible prognostic role, the *JAK2 V617F* mutation can also be used as a marker for minimal residual disease (MRD) post-ASCT. A study using real-time polymerase chain reaction (RT-PCR) demonstrated that of 15 JAK2-positive patients analyzed, three patients relapsed shortly after JAK2 gene mutation was detected for the first time after transplant.[64] Kroger et al.[65] demonstrated 78% of patients with the JAK2 mutation undergoing a RIC-ASCT achieved a molecular response after a median 89 days following transplant. This achievement of molecular response 6 months after ASCT predicted for a reduced risk of relapse (5% vs. 35%).[48] There is controversy surrounding the prognostic value of the JAK2 allele burden in PMF. Low levels of the mutation seem to predict a worse survival with a higher risk for bone marrow failure.[66] However, in the setting of an allogeneic transplant, allele burden early after transplantation is an important predictive parameter in monitoring patients. Allele burden on day 28 post transplantation discriminates two prognostic groups, with patients having more than 1% being at significant higher risk for relapse and having an inferior OS.[67]

Other molecular markers that have been studied in primary and secondary MF that could be utilized as markers of MRD after transplantation include the MPL W515L/K mutation.[68,69]

ROLE OF DONOR LEOKOCYTIC INFUSIONS OR SECOND ALLOGRAFT IN POST-TRANSPLANT RELAPSE

The efficacy of donor leukocyte infusions (DLI) was previously established in chronic myeloid leukemia with molecular remissions achieved in 67% of patients.[70] An immunologic graft-versus-myelofibrosis effect was also observed upon DLI in MF.[9,71]

The timing of DLI, whether as pre-emptive or salvage therapy, is debatable. In a series of 17 patients[72] where DLI was used pre-emptively in 8 patients and as salvage in 9, complete molecular response rate was superior in the pre-emptive group (68% vs. 44%).

The role of lymphodepleting chemotherapy prior to DLI has been explored.[73] In preclinical models, lymphodepletion potentiates T-cell expansion and function by a number of mechanisms including decreasing competition for cytokines and growth,[74] elimination of regulatory T cells,[75] and enhancement of antigen-presenting cell function.[76]

In a study on their experience with relapsed MF published by the German group,[77] 17 patients underwent a second HSCT at a median of 17 months (range, 11–77) from the first allograft due to relapse (n = 13), graft-rejection (n = 3), and transformation to blast phase (n = 1). Fifteen patients were transplanted with cells from alternative donors, and two patients from the same donor. The response rate was 80% and 1-year OS and PFS were 82% and 70%, respectively. The 1-year cumulative NRM and cumulative relapse incidence were only 6% and 24%, respectively. In the 13 patients who previously received DLI, the use of the second HSCT after a median of 5 months (range, 2–13) from the last DLI-application did not seem to increase the acute and chronic GVHD rates.

USE OF JANUS KINASE INHIBITORS PRIOR TO TRANSPLANTATION

With the advent of JAK inhibitors into the clinical armamentarium there will be increasing debate on whether and when to refer a patient with MF for transplant. In fact, JAK2 inhibitors may influence the decision to transplant in a number of ways. The amelioration of clinical symptoms with JAK inhibitor therapy may delay consideration for transplant resulting in more advanced disease at the time of transplant. Most experts still agree that for patients where treatment intent is curative, transplant referral should be early on, irrespective of clinical response to JAK inhibitor therapy, as these drugs have not been shown definitively to reverse histologic abnormalities or reduce the risk of leukemic transformation.

On the other hand, by improving constitutional symptoms and splenomegaly, JAK inhibitors might turn out to be very useful in the pretransplant setting resulting in improved performance status. Reduction in splenomegaly may favor more rapid engraftment and down-regulation of inflammatory cytokines may lower the rates of rejection and/or acute GVHD.

Two prospective clinical trials are ongoing looking at ruxolitinib in the the pretransplant setting. In early reports from both these trials, ruxolitinib reduced spleen size and constitutional symptoms in the majority of patients before allogeneic stem cell transplantation.[78,79] There was no evidence that discontinuation of ruxolitinib at start of conditioning induced a rebound phenomenon.

The timing of JAK2 inhibitor therapy requires consideration due to possible negative impact on hematologic recovery post-transplant as these drugs are known to cause anemia and thrombocytopenia. A cohort of 14 patients treated with Ruxolitinib (median exposure 6.5 mos) and subsequently transplanted was, respectively, evaluated and showed a 93% engraftment rate.[80] Moreover, there is a reported cytokine storm with explosive splenomegaly in some cases upon withdrawal of these drugs.[81] Optimal timing will likely be in the pretransplant setting as the failure of these drugs to reduce *JAK2 V617F* allele burden makes them unlikely to eradicate MRD.

CONCLUSION

The decision to opt for an ASCT for patients with MF is currently based on multiple considerations: prognosis at the time of transplant, selection of conditioning regimen, type of donor, risk factors associated with transplant outcome, role for splenectomy, and the possible utilization of new agents prior to or following HSCT.

At present:

- Comparisons of myeloablative and RIC are retrospective and spread over many decades. However, RIC-HSCT has been shown to be safe and effective in patients of any age
- While patients with intermediate-2 and high-risk disease or adverse cytogenetics or transfusion dependence should unequivocally proceed to transplant, there is controversy about transplanting low-risk patients. Low-risk patients should be monitored closely for any sign of progression as they can enjoy an 80% survival if transplanted early in the disease course
- Utilizing disease-specific mutations, close monitoring of residual disease has become feasible and the outcome of post-transplant strategies has consequently improved. Strategies of using JAK1/2 inhibitor therapy in combination with transplantation is being explored in the context of a clinical trial (NCT01790295).

REFERENCES

1. Mesa RA, Hanson CA, Rajkumar SV, et al. Evaluation and clinical correlations of bone marrow angiogenesis in myelofibrosis with myeloid metaplasia. *Blood.* 2000;96(10):3374-80.
2. Cervantes F, Dupriez B, Pereira A, et al. New prognostic scoring system for primary myelofibrosis based on a study of the International Working Group for Myelofibrosis Research and Treatment. *Blood.* 2009;113(3):2895-901.
3. Barosi G, Viarengo G, Pecci A, et al. Diagnostic and clinical relevance of the number of circulating CD34(+) cells in myelofibrosis with myeloid metaplasia. *Blood.* 2001;98(12): 3249-55.

4. Xu M, Bruno E, Chao J, et al. The constitutive mobilization of bone marrow-repopulating cells into the peripheral blood in idiopathic myelofibrosis. *Blood.* 2005;105(4):1699-705.
5. Anderson JE, Tefferi A, Craig F, et al. Myeloablation and autologous peripheral blood stem cell rescue results in hematologic and clinical responses in patients with myeloid metaplasia with myelofibrosis. *Blood.* 2001;98(3):586-93.
6. Thiele J, Kvasnicka HM, Dietrich H, et al. Dynamics of bone marrow changes in patients with chronic idiopathic myelofibrosis following allogeneic stem cell transplantation. *Histol Histopathol.* 2005;20(3):879-89.
7. Chunduri S, Gaitonde S, Ciurea SO, et al. Pulmonary extramedullary hematopoiesis in patients with myelofibrosis undergoing allogeneic stem cell transplantation. *Haematologica.* 2008;93(10):1593-5.
8. Guardiola P, Anderson JE, Bandini G, et al. Allogeneic stem cell transplantation for agnogenic myeloid metaplasia: a European Group for Blood and Marrow Transplantation, Societe Francaise de Greffe de Moelle, Gruppo Italiano per il Trapianto del Midollo Osseo, and Fred Hutchinson Cancer Research Center Collaborative Study. *Blood.* 1999;93:2831-8.
9. Byrne JL, Beshti H, Clark D, et al. Induction of remission after donor leucocyte infusion for the treatment of relapsed chronic idiopathic myelofibrosis following allogeneic transplantation: evidence for a 'graft vs. myelofibrosis' effect. *Br J Haematol.* 2000;108:430-3.
10. Ni H, Barosi G, Rondelli D, et al. Studies of the site and distribution of CD34+ cells in idiopathic myelofibrosis. *Am J Clin Pathol.* 2005;123(6):833-9.
11. Kroger N, Holler E, Kobbe G, et al. Allogeneic stem cell transplantation after reduced-intensity conditioning in patients with myelofibrosis: a prospective, multicenter study of the Chronic Leukemia Working Party of the European Group for Blood and Marrow Transplantation. *Blood.* 2009;114:5264-70.
12. Lussana F, Rambaldi A, Finazzi MC, et al. Allogeneic hematopoietic stem cell transplantation in patients with polycythemia or essential thrombocythemia transformed to myelofibrosis or acute myeloid leukemia: report from the MPN subcommittee of the Chronic Malignancies Working Party of the European Group for Blood and Marrow Transplantation. *Haematologica.* 2014 Feb 7.
13. Daly A, Song K, Nevill T, et al. Stem cell transplantation for myelofibrosis: a report from two Canadian centers. *Bone Marrow Transplant.* 2003;32(1):35-40.
14. Ditschkowski M, Beelen DW, Trenschel R, et al. Outcome of allogeneic stem cell transplantation in patients with myelofibrosis. *Bone Marrow Transplant.* 2004;34(9):807-13.
15. Deeg HJ, Gooley TA, Flowers ME, et al. Allogeneic hematopoietic stem cell transplantation for myelofibrosis. *Blood.* 2003;102(12):3912-8.
16. Kerbauy DM, Gooley TA, Sale GE, et al. Hematopoietic cell transplantation as curative therapy for idiopathic myelofibrosis, advanced polycythemia vera, and essential thrombocythemia. *Biol Blood Marrow Transplant.* 2007;13(3):355-65.
17. Devine SM, Hoffman R, Verma A, et al. Allogeneic blood cell transplantation following reduced-intensity conditioning is effective therapy for older patients with myelofibrosis with myeloid metaplasia. *Blood.* 2002;99(6):2255-8.
18. Hessling J, Kroger N, Werner M, et al. Dose-reduced conditioning regimen followed by allogeneic stem cell transplantation in patients with myelofibrosis with myeloid metaplasia. *Br J Haematol.* 2002;119:769-72.
19. Snyder DS, Palmer J, Stein AS, et al. Allogeneic hematopoietic cell transplantation following reduced intensity conditioning for treatment of myelofibrosis. *Biol Blood Marrow Transplant.* 2006;12(11):1161-8.
20. Rondelli D, Barosi G, Bacigalupo A, et al. Allogeneic hematopoietic stem-cell transplantation with reduced-intensity conditioning in intermediate- or high-risk patients with myelofibrosis with myeloid metaplasia. *Blood.* 2005;105(10):4115-9.
21. Abelsson J, Merup M, Birgegard G, et al. The outcome of allo-HSCT for 92 patients with myelofibrosis in the Nordic countries. *Bone Marrow Transplant.* 2012;47(3):380-6.

22. Merup M, Lazarevic V, Nahi H, et al. Different outcome of allogeneic transplantation in myelofibrosis using conventional or reduced-intensity conditioning regimens. *Br J Haematol.* 2006;135(3):367-73.
23. Gupta V, Kröger N, Aschan J, et al. A retrospective comparison of conventional intensity conditioning and reduced-intensity conditioning for allogeneic hematopoietic cell transplantation in myelofibrosis. *Bone Marrow Transplant.* 2009;44(5):317-20.
24. Patriarca F, Bacigalupo A, Sperotto A, et al. Allogeneic hematopoietic stem cell transplantation in myelofibrosis: the 20-year experience of the Gruppo Italiano Trapianto di Midollo Osseo (GITMO). *Haematologica.* 2008;93(10):1514-22.
25. Lissandre S, Bay JO, Cahn JY, et al. Retrospective study of allogeneic haematopoietic stem-cell transplantation for myelofibrosis. *Bone Marrow Transplant.* 2011;46(4):557-61.
26. Kröger N, Zabelina T, Schieder H, et al. Pilot study of reduced-intensity conditioning followed by allogeneic stem cell transplantation from related and unrelated donors in patients with myelofibrosis. *Br J Haematol.* 2005;128(5):690-7.
27. Rondelli D, Goldberg JD, Marchioli R, et al. Results of Phase II Clinical Trial MPD-RC 101: allogeneic hematopoietic stem cell transplantation conditioned with fludarabine/melphalan in patients with myelofibrosis. *Biol Blood Marrow Transplant* 2012;18(2):S216.
28. Ballen KK, Shrestha S, Sobocinski KA, et al. Outcome of transplantation for myelofibrosis. *Biol Blood Marrow Transplant.* 2010;16(3):358-67.
29. Robin M, Tabrizi R, Mohty M, et al. Allogeneic haematopoietic stem cell transplantation for myelofibrosis: a report of the Societe Francaise de Greffe de Moelle et de Therapie Cellulaire (SFGM-TC). *Br J Haematol.* 2011;152(3):331-9.
30. Li Z, Gooley T, Applebaum FR, et al. Splenectomy and hemopoietic stem cell transplantation for myelofibrosis. *Blood.* 2001;97(7):2180-1.
31. Ciurea SO, Sadegi B, Wilbur A, et al. Effects of extensive splenomegaly in patients with myelofibrosis undergoing a reduced intensity allogeneic stem cell transplantation. *Br J Haematol.* 2008;141(1):80-3.
32. Mesa RA, Nagorney DS, Schwager S, et al. Palliative goals, patient selection, and perioperative platelet management: outcomes and lessons from 3 decades of splenectomy for myelofibrosis with myeloid metaplasia at the Mayo Clinic. *Cancer.* 2006;107(2):361-70.
33. Bacigalupo A, Soraru M, Dominietto A, et al. Allogeneic hemopoietic SCT for patients with primary myelofibrosis: a predictive transplant score based on transfusion requirement, spleen size and donor type. *Bone Marrow Transplant.* 2010;45(3):458-63.
34. Scott BL, Gooley TA, Sorror ML, et al. The Dynamic International Prognostic Scoring System for myelofibrosis predicts outcomes after hematopoietic cell transplantation. *Blood.* 2012;119(11):2657-64.
35. Stewart WA, Pearce R, Kirkland KE, et al. The role of allogeneic SCT in primary myelofibrosis: a British Society for Blood and Marrow Transplantation study. *Bone Marrow Transplant.* 2010;45(11):1587-93.
36. Michallet M, Corront B, Bosson JL, et al. Role of splenectomy in incidence and severity of acute graft-versus-host disease: a multicenter study of 157 patients. *Bone Marrow Transplant.* 1991;8(1):13-7.
37. Barosi G, Ambrosetti A, Centra A, et al. Splenectomy and risk of blast transformation in myelofibrosis with myeloid metaplasia. Italian Cooperative Study Group on Myeloid with Myeloid Metaplasia. *Blood.* 1998;91(10):3630-6.
38. Robin M, Espérou H, de Latour RP, et al. Splenectomy after allogeneic haematopoietic stem cell transplantation in patients with primary myelofibrosis. *Br J Haematol.* 2010;150(6):721-4.
39. Dupriez B, Morel P, Demory JL, et al. Prognostic factors in agnogenic myeloid metaplasia: a report on 195 cases with a new scoring system. *Blood.* 1996;88(3):1013-8.
40. Passamonti F, Cervantes F, Vannucchi AM, et al. A dynamic prognostic model to predict survival in primary myelofibrosis: a study by the IWG-MRT (International Working Group for Myeloproliferative Neoplasms Research and Treatment). *Blood.* 2010;115:1703-8.
41. Gangat N, Caramazza D, Vaidya R, et al. DIPSS plus: a refined Dynamic International Prognostic Scoring System for primary myelofibrosis that incorporates prognostic information from karyotype, platelet count, and transfusion status. *J Clin Oncol.* 2011;29:392-7.

42. Gooley TA, Chien JW, Pergam SA, et al. Reduced mortality after allogeneic hematopoietic-cell transplantation. *N Engl J Med.* 2010;363(22):2091-101.
43. Horan JT, Logan BR, Agovi-Johnson MA, et al. Reducing the risk for transplantation-related mortality after allogeneic hematopoietic cell transplantation: how much progress has been made? J *Clin Oncol.* 2011;29:805-13.
44. Sorror ML, Maris MB, Storb R, et al. Hematopoietic cell transplantation (HCT)-specific comorbidity index: a new tool for risk assessment before allogeneic HCT. *Blood.* 2005;106(8):2912-9.
45. Guardiola P, Anderson JE, Gluckman E. Myelofibrosis with myeloid metaplasia. *N Engl J Med.* 2000;343(9):659-60.
46. Nivison-Smith I, Dodds AJ, Butler J, et al. Allogeneic hematopoietic cell transplantation for chronic myelofibrosis in Australia and New Zealand: older recipients receiving myeloablative conditioning at increased mortality risk. *Biol Blood Marrow Transplant.* 2012;18:302-8.
47. Samuelson S, Sandmaier BM, Heslop HE, et al. Allogeneic haematopoietic cell transplantation for myelofibrosis in 30 patients 60-78 years of age. *Br J Haematol.* 2011;153(1):76-82.
48. Alchalby H, Badbaran A, Zabelina T, et al. Impact of JAK2V617F mutation status, allele burden, and clearance after allogeneic stem cell transplantation for myelofibrosis. *Blood.* 2010;116(18):3572-81.
49. Alchalby H, Yunus DR, Zabelina T, et al. Risk models predicting survival after reduced-intensity transplantation for myelofibrosis. *Br J Haematol.* 2012;157(1):75-85.
50. Klampfl T, Gisslinger H, Harutyunyan AS, et al. Somatic mutations of calreticulin in myeloproliferative neoplasms. *N Engl J Med.* 2013;369(25):2379-90.
51. Panagiota V, Thol F, Markus B, et al. Prognostic effect of calreticulin mutations in patients with myelofibrosis after allogeneic hematopoietic stem cell transplantation. *Leukemia.* 2014 Feb 7.
52. Ditschkowski M, Elmaagacli AH, Trenschel R, et al. Dynamic International Prognostic Scoring System scores, pre-transplant therapy and chronic graft-versus-host disease determine outcome after allogeneic hematopoietic stem cell transplantation for myelofibrosis. *Haematologica.* 2012;97:1574-81.
53. Tefferi A, Pardanani A, Gangat N, et al. Leukemia risk models in primary myelofibrosis: an International Working Group study. *Leukemia.* 2012;26(6):1439-41.
54. Ciurea SO, de Lima M, Giralt S, et al. Allogeneic stem cell transplantation for myelofibrosis with leukemic transformation. *Biol Blood Marrow Transplant.* 2010;16(4):555-9.
55. Ho GT, Parker A, MacKenzie JF, et al. Abnormal liver function tests following bone marrow transplantation: aetiology and role of liver biopsy. *Eur J Gastroenterol Hepatol.* 2004;1692):157-62.
56. Sakai M, Strasser SI, Shulman HM, et al. Severe hepatocellular injury after hematopoietic cell transplant: incidence, etiology and outcome. *Bone Marrow Transplant.* 2009;44(7):441-7.
57. Wong KM, Atenafu EG, Kim D, et al. Incidence and risk factors for early hepatotoxicity and its impact on survival in patients with myelofibrosis undergoing allogeneic hematopoietic cell transplantation. *Biol Blood Marrow Transplant.* 2012;18(10):1589-99.
58. Mahindra A, Bolwell B, Sobecks R, et al. Elevated pretransplant ferritin is associated with a lower incidence of chronic graft-versus-host disease and inferior survival after myeloablative allogeneic haematopoietic stem cell transplantation. *Br J Haematol.* 2009;146:310-6.
59. Mahindra A, Sobecks R, Rybicki L, et al: Elevated pretransplant serum ferritin is associated with inferior survival following nonmyeloablative allogeneic transplantation. *Bone Marrow Transplant.* 44:767-8, 2009
60. Armand P, Sainvil MM, Kim HT, et al. Pre-transplantation iron chelation in patients with MDS or acute leukemia and iron overload undergoing myeloablative allo-SCT. *Bone Marrow Transplant.* 2013;48(1):146-7.
61. Snyder DS, Palmer J, Gaal K, et al. Improved outcomes using tacrolimus/sirolimus for graft-versus-host disease prophylaxis with a reduced-intensity conditioning regimen for allogeneic

hematopoietic cell transplant as treatment of myelofibrosis. *Biol Blood Marrow Transplant.* 2010;16:281-6.

62. Park HB, Oh K, Garmaa N, et al. CP-690550, a Janus kinase inhibitor, suppresses CD4+ T-cell-mediated acute graft-versus-host disease by inhibiting the interferon-γ pathway. *Transplantation.* 2010;90(8):825-35.
63. Verstovsek S, Kantarjian H, Mesa RA, et al. Safety and efficacy of INCB018424, a JAK1 and JAK2 inhibitor, in myelofibrosis. *N Engl J Med.* 2010;363:1117-27.
64. Steckel NK, Koldehoff M, Ditschkowski M, et al. Use of the activating gene mutation of the tyrosine kinase (VAL617Phe) JAK2 as a minimal residual disease marker in patients with myelofibrosis and myeloid metaplasia after allogeneic stem cell transplantation. *Transplantation.* 2007;83:1518-20.
65. Kröger N, Badbaran A, Holler E, et al. Monitoring of the JAK2-V617F mutation by highly sensitive quantitative real-time PCR after allogeneic stem cell transplantation in patients with myelofibrosis. *Blood.* 2007;109(3):1316-21.
66. Tefferi A, Lasho TL, Huang J, et al. Low JAK2V617F allele burden in primary myelofibrosis, compared to either a higher allele burden or unmutated status, is associated with inferior overall and leukemia-free survival. *Leukemia.* 2008;22(4):756-61.
67. Lange T, Edelmann A, Siebolts U, et al. JAK2 p.V617F allele burden in myeloproliferative neoplasms one month after allogeneic stem cell transplantation significantly predicts outcome and risk of relapse. *Haematologica.* 2013.
68. Alchalby H, Badbaran A, Bock O, et al. Screening and monitoring of MPL W515L mutation with real-time PCR in patients with myelofibrosis undergoing allogeneic-SCT. *Bone Marrow Transplant.* 2010;45(9):1404-7.
69. Rumi E, Passamonti F, Arcaini L, et al. Molecular remission after allo-SCT in a patient with post-essential thrombocythemia myelofibrosis carrying the MPL (W515A) mutation. *Bone Marrow Transplant.* 2010;45(4):798-800.
70. Dazzi F, Szydlo RM, Cross NC, et al. Durability of responses following donor lymphocyte infusions for patients who relapse after allogeneic stem cell transplantation for chronic myeloid leukemia. *Blood.* 2000;96(8):2712-6.
71. Cervantes F, Rovira M, Urbano-Ispizua A, et al. Complete remission of idiopathic myelofibrosis following donor lymphocyte infusion after failure of allogeneic transplantation: demonstration of a graft-versus-myelofibrosis effect. *Bone Marrow Transplant.* 2000;26:697-9.
72. Kröger N, Alchalby H, Klyuchnikov E, et al. JAK2-V617F-triggered preemptive and salvage adoptive immunotherapy with donor-lymphocyte infusion in patients with myelofibrosis after allogeneic stem cell transplantation. *Blood.* 2009;113(8):1866-8.
73. Neave EL, Schwarb H, Shlebak A, et al. Lymphodepletion chemotherapy followed by donor leukocytes for post-transplantation relapse of myelofibrosis after previous donor leukocyte infusion failure. *Eur J Haematol.* 2013;90(1):76-8.
74. Gattinoni L, Finkelstein SE, Klebanoff CA, et al. Removal of homeostatic cytokine sinks by lymphodepletion enhances the efficacy of adoptively transferred tumor-specific CD8+ T cells. *J Exp Med.* 2005;202(7):907-12.
75. Antony PA, Piccirillo CA, Akpinarli A, et al. CD8+ T cell immunity against a tumor/ self-antigen is augmented by CD4+ T helper cells and hindered by naturally occurring T regulatory cells. *J Immunol.* 2005;174(5):2591-601.
76. Klebanoff CA, Khong HT, Antony PA, et al. Sinks, suppressors and antigen presenters: how lymphodepletion enhances T cell-mediated tumor immunotherapy. *Trends Immunol.* 2005;26(2):111-7.
77. Klyuchnikov E, Holler E, Bornhäuser M, et al. Donor lymphocyte infusions and second transplantation as salvage treatment for relapsed myelofibrosis after reduced-intensity allografting. *Br J Haematol.* 2012;159(2):172-81.
78. Kroger N, Alchalby H, Ditschkowski M, et al. Ruxolitinib as pretreatment before allogeneic stem cell transplantation for myelofibrosis. *ASH.* 2013. Abstract 392.

79. Robin M, Francois S. Huynh A, et al. Ruxolitinib before allogeneic hematopoietic stem cell transplantation (HSCT) in patients with myelofibrosis: a preliminary descriptive report of the JAK ALLO study, a phase ii trial sponsored by Goelams-FIM in collaboration with the SFGMTC. *ASH.* 2013. Abstract 306.
80. Jaekel N, Behre G, Behning A, et al. Allogeneic hematopoietic cell transplantation for myelofibrosis in patients pretreated with the JAK1 and JAK2 inhibitor ruxolitinib. *Bone Marrow Transplant.* 2014;49(2):179-84.
81. Tefferi A, Litzow MR, Pardanani A. Long-term outcome of treatment with ruxolitinib in myelofibrosis. *N Engl J Med.* 2011;365(15):1455-7.

CHAPTER 8 Novel Therapies in the Classical BCR-ABL Negative Myeloproliferative Neoplasms

Brady L Stein

INTRODUCTION AND BACKGROUND

Essential thrombocytosis (ET), polycythemia vera (PV), and myelofibrosis (MF), including primary, post-ET, and post-PV are clonal hematopoietic stem cell disorders which share an overproduction of mature blood elements, tendencies toward thrombotic or hemorrhagic events, varying degrees of extramedullary hematopoiesis, a transformation to MF (in ET and PV), and transformation to acute leukemia. The discovery of the acquired hematopoietic stem cell mutation Janus kinase 2 (JAK2) V617F (a change of valine to phenylalanine at the 617 position) in these three diseases substantiated the claim made by Dameshek of their shared pathogenesis.[1-5] Further, recognition of the JAK2 V617F mutation in ET, PV, and MF has ushered in a new era of scientific discovery in these diseases. Assessment of mutational status has resulted in a molecular classification and revision of diagnostic criteria, as well as an improvement in the understanding of disease pathogenesis. The recent discovery of calreticulin gene mutations in ET and MF only add to our enhanced understanding and diagnostic capabilities.[6,7]

Perhaps most important has been the rapid development of targeted therapy for the classical breakpoint cluster region-Abelson murine leukemia virus (BCR-ABL) negative myeloproliferative neoplasms (MPN); only 2 years after the JAK V617F discovery, small molecule JAK-inhibitors were in development, with the hope that targeted therapy in the MPN would parallel the success with tyrosine kinase inhibitor therapy in chronic myeloid leukemia (CML). At present, the major treatment strategies in ET and PV include management of myeloproliferation and vascular disease risk reduction with conventional agents, and the role of JAK-inhibition in these disorders is still being defined (Figure 8-1). Because MF has the most unfavorable prognosis, it has been the primary focus for study of JAK inhibitors and other novel therapies. The majority of MF patients, either at diagnosis or through the course of the disease, have symptoms related to cytopenias (particularly anemia), constitutional and systemic symptoms, and symptoms related to splenomegaly. Stem cell transplantation is considered in those with high-risk disease and can favorably alter its natural history, but is often not an option due to the presence of advanced age, competing comorbidities,

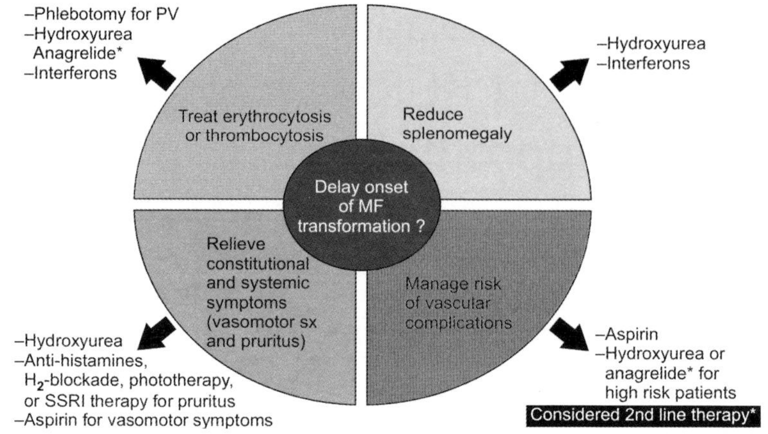

PV, polycythemia vera; MF, myelofibrosis; SSRI, selective serotonin reuptake inhibitor
*Barbui T, Barosi G, Birgegard G, et al. Philadelphia-negative classical myeloproliferative neoplasms: critical concepts and management recommendations from European LeukemiaNet. *J Clin Oncol.* 2011:29(6):761-70.

Figure 8-1 Current essential thrombocytosis (ET) and polycythemia vera (PV) management. The current therapy of ET and PV aims primarily to reduce the risk of vascular complications. Aspirin is an important component of vascular risk reduction, along with phlebotomy for PV patients. High-risk patients, who are age over 60 years, or with prior thrombosis, require cytoreduction, typically with hydroxyurea, anagrelide, or interferon therapy. Hydroxyurea and interferon may reduce the spleen size as well. Pruritus and vasomotor symptoms can compromise quality of life, and are treated with various agents as shown above. No therapy has been shown to reliably delay the risk of myelofibrosis transformation.

or the lack of a suitable donor. Therefore, most patients have been treated with conventional agents to palliate constitutional symptoms (hydroxyurea), treat anemia [androgens, erythropoietin stimulating agents (ESA) or immunomodulatory drugs (IMIDs)], or reduce splenomegaly [hydroxyurea, 2-chlorodeoxyadenosine (2-CDA)] (Figure 8-2). Unfortunately, the efficacy of conventional agents to treat these MF-related complications is usually modest and/or lacking in durability.

Accordingly, the introduction of novel therapies, particularly the JAK-inhibitors, was initially met with great enthusiasm. Ruxolitinib was the first in class of these JAK-inhibitors, and given its ability to relieve constitutional and systemic symptoms, and reduce the spleen size, has been approved for use. However, this agent has not led to complete remission, as can be case with tyrosine kinase inhibitors in CML. In fact, myelosuppression is an important adverse effect, as is the potential for early relapse of constitutional symptoms and splenomegaly with discontinuation of the medication. Nonetheless, ruxolitinib adds to the limited therapeutic options for MF patients, especially because it relieves constitutional symptoms and decreases splenomegaly (Figure 8-2).

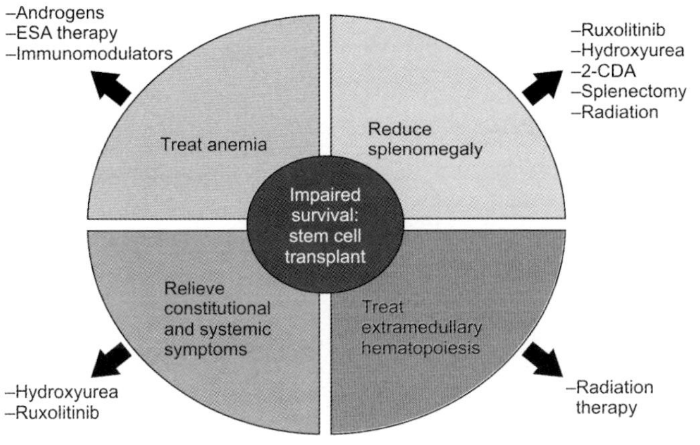

ESA, erythropoietin stimulating agents; 2-CDA, 2-chlorodeoxyademosine.

Figure 8-2 Current myelofibrosis management. While stem cell transplant provides a curative option for the treatment of myelofibrosis (MF), advanced age, competing comorbidities, and lack of donor availability are limiting factors. A risk-adapted approach would suggest that this procedure should be considered in patients with intermediate 2 or high-risk disease. For the majority of MF patients, palliation of symptoms with conventional approaches becomes the major focus. Conventional agents for the treatment of anemia include androgens, such as danazol, ESA, and immunomodulatory drugs, such as thalidomide and lenalidomide. Ruxolitinib relieves constitutional and systemic symptoms for a significant proportion of MF patients, likely replacing hydroxyurea as a first line treatment in this regard. Ruxolitinib is also effective at reducing splenomegaly, and also likely to replace hydroxyrurea as the first-line approach. Cladribine, or 2-chlorodeoxy-adenosive provides a more aggressive approach to the treatment of splenomegaly; if medical therapy fails, splenectomy is a consideration, though it carries considerable morbidity and mortality. Consequences of extramedullary hematopoiesis (non-hepatosplenic) are best treated with radiation therapy.

A number of other JAK-inhibitors are in clinical development, and some have unique features which might improve the course for MPN patients. However, in contrast to BCR-ABL in CML, JAK2 V617F or JAK/signal transducers and activators of transcription (STAT) activation is not the only lesion or pathway responsible for MPN; in fact, the classical MPN, especially MF, exhibit substantial clinical and molecular heterogeneity.[8,9] Therefore, JAK-inhibitor therapy is unlikely to address the full extent of clonal (and clinical) disease in the MPN, and there have been intense investigation of other acquired genetic and molecular abnormalities that might contribute to MPN disease pathogenesis, as outlined in chapter 2. These studies provide a rationale for novel treatment approaches that aim to improve upon the conventional approach to MPN/MF treatment (Figures 8-3 and 8-4), and in this chapter, the experience with IMIDs, interferons, epigenetic therapies, and mammalian target of rapamycin (mTOR) inhibition will be reviewed, along other novel strategies addressing unique aspects of disease pathogenesis.

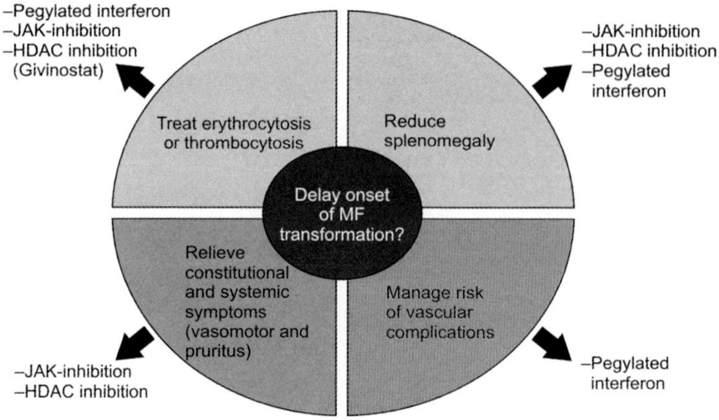

JAK, Janus kinase; HDAC, histone deaceftylase; MF, myelofibrosis.

Figure 8-3: Novel esssential thrombocytosis (ET) and polycythemia vera (PV) management. Note: Promising treatments for ET and PV include pegylated interferon, based on high rates of hematologic responses, along with molecular responses in a proportion of both newly and heavily pre-treated patients. For PV, histone deacetylase inhibitors and Janus kinase (JAK)-inhibitors have not only been shown control blood counts, but also relieve constitutional symptoms and reduce the spleen size. Pegylated interferon may reduce thrombosis rates, but this has not yet been proven. It is not known yet if JAK-inhibitors or pegylated interferon will delay the onset of myelofibrosis.

JANUS KINASE-INHIBITORS (TABLE 8-1)

Ruxolitinib

Ruxolitinib was the first oral, potent, and selective JAK1/JAK2 inhibitor to enter the clinic and is approved for use for intermediate and high-risk primary myelofibrosis (PMF), post-ETMF (essential thrombocytosis myelofibrosis), and post-PVMF (polycythemia vera myelofibrosis), as discussed in chapter 6. This approval was based on phase 3 studies demonstrating a significant reduction in spleen size, as detected by magnetic resonance imaging (MRI); ruxolitinib versus placebo: 41.9% versus 0.7%; ruxolitinib versus best available therapy: 28% versus 0%.[10,11] There was an improvement of 50% or more in the total symptom score (night sweats, itching, abdominal discomfort, pain under the ribs on the left side, early satiety, and muscle or bone pain) at 24 weeks in 45.9% of patients who received ruxolitinib as compared with 5.3% of patients who received placebo ($p < 0.001$).[10] Interestingly, both abdominal and non-abdominal symptoms improved even when spleen shrinkage was modest (<35% spleen volume by MRI). As compared to placebo, patients treated with ruxolitinib had improvements in fatigue and global health status, and compared to best-available therapy, they had improved health related quality-of-life and role functioning, along with considerable improvement in MF-associated symptoms, including appetite loss, dyspnea, fatigue, insomnia, and pain.[11] Finally, a survival benefit was reported in comparison to placebo and conventional therapy.[10,24]

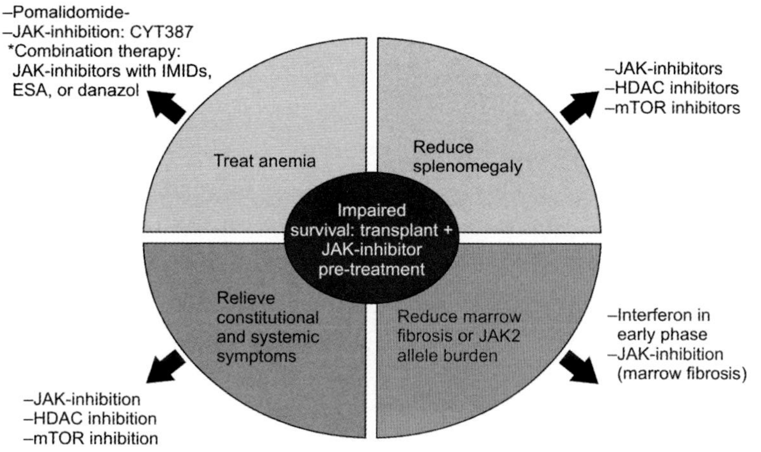

JAK, Janus kinase; IMIDs, immunomodulatory drugs; ESA, erythropoietin stimulating agents; HDAC, histone-deacetylase; mToR, mammation target of rapamycin.

Figure 8-4 Novel myelofibrosis management. Promising treatments for myelofibrosis (MF) are shown here, with the hope that these agents, either alone or in combination favorably alter the natural history for MF patients. To improve constitutional symptoms and splenomegaly, potentially improving the functional status before transplant, a study is planned to use ruxolitinib in the pretransplant period. For anemia, pomalidomide is promising in those patients that are JAK2 V617F negative, without splenomegaly or increased blasts. Of the Janus kinase (JAK)-inhibitors, CYT387 may uniquely ameliorate anemia. Trials combining JAK-inhibitors with immunomodulatory (IMIDs) agents, erythropoietin stimulating agents, and danazol are planned, hoping to counteract the myelosuppression attributed to JAK-inhibitors. Along with JAK-inhibitors, histone deacetylase inhibitors and mammalian target of rapamycin inhibitors have shown promise with regard to constitutional symptom relief, in addition to spleen size reduction. Interferons early in the course of MF and certain JAK-inhibitors (SA302503 and LY278544) may reduce the allele burden and marrow fibrosis.

Because myelosuppression was a limiting toxicity in trials that led to its approval, lower doses of ruxolitinib are being evaluated to determine whether it can be used safely in patients with baseline thrombocytopenia (clinical trials identifier: NCT01348490), and to lessen the rate of the initial decline in hemoglobin (clinical trials identifier: NCT01445769). Ruxolitinib is also in phase 3 trials for use in PV, based on prior results from the phase 2 study of 39 and 34 advanced ET and PV patients that were refractory or intolerant to hydroxyurea.[13] Complete hematologic responses, defined by normalization of blood counts and splenomegaly, were observed in 59% of patients with PV. By each individual parameter, 97% of patients had control of the hematocrit without phlebotomy, 59% had a 50% reduction in spleen size, and normalization of the white blood cell (WBC) and platelet count occurred in 63% and 69%, respectively. Symptom improvements were noted as well, especially those with pruritus, in whom 24 of 26 had complete resolution. JAK2

Table 8-1 Janus kinase-inhibitors in the Myeloproliferative Neoplasms

	Ruxolitinib	*Lestaurtinib (CEP-701)*	*Fedratinib (SAR302503)*	*Momelotinib (CYT387)*	*Pacritinib (SB1518)*	*LY2784544*
Selectivity	JAK1/JAK2	JAK2/FLT3	JAK2/FLT3	JAK1/JAK2	JAK2/FLT3	JAK2
Phase	3[10,11]	2[14] 1/2[15]	1/2[17]	1/2[19,20]	2[21,22]	1[23]
Improvement in splenomegaly	Phase 3: 35% reduction by imaging in 41.9%[10] 35% reduction by imaging in 28%[11]	Phase 2:[14] CI in 18% Phase 1/2:[15] Median decrease of 6.4 cm	CI in 47%	CI in 45%	57–88% with 25% reduction in volume by MRI	13 of 17 (76%) with >35% reduction by imaging
Alleviation of constitutional symptoms	45.9% improved total symptom score[10]	Phase 2: Not reported Phase 1/2: Not reported	Early satiety* Fatigue* NS* Cough* Pruritus*	Improvement in: pruritus NS Bone pain	Symptom improvement in 40–65%	Symptom reduction in 59%
Decrease in JAK2 V617F allele burden	Phase 1-2:[12] 13% after 12 cycles	Phase 2: No significant change Phase 1/2: Median decrease of 8.6%	16 of 20 patients with median 61% decrease	Not reported	Not reported	Not reported
Adverse effects	Myelosuppression	Myelosuppression Gastrointestinal	Myelosuppression Gastrointestinal	First dose effect** Thrombocytopenia	Gastrointestinal	Possible tumor lysis
Unique effects	Phase 1-2:[12] Reduction in level of proinflammatory cytokines Survival benefit noted	Phase 2: CI in anemia in 14%	Program discontinued due to reports of encephalopathy	Anemia response rate: 50%; 58% in transfusion-dependent patients	Tolerated in those with baseline cytopenias, despite JAK2 inhibition	Three of five patients experienced improvement in bone marrow fibrosis after five cycles
Trials in ET and PV patients	Complete hematological response in 59% PV and 49% ET[13]	Reduction in spleen size in 15/18, allele burden in 3/15 and phlebotomy in 3/5[16]	Clinical development halted			one PV patient included with complete resolution of splenomegaly

JAK, Janus kinase; CI, clinical improvement; NS, night sweats; PV, polycythemia vera; ET, essential thrombocytosis
*Percent complete resolution.
**Transient lightheadedness, hypotension.

V617F allele burden reduction was modest, with 42% of PV patients experiencing a 20% decrease.[13] However, myelosuppression was observed in this population, with grade 3 thrombocytopenia in 3% of patients and grade 2 anemia in 12%. This study suggests that JAK-inhibition in PV may be useful for the control of myeloproliferation and systemic symptoms, and a randomized phase 3 trial comparing ruxolitinib to best supportive care will further determine its net effect in PV patients (Figure 8-4). Although efficacy and tolerability were observed in those with ET, phase 3 trials are not planned for patients with ET.

Lestaurtinib (CEP-701)

Lestaurtinib (CEP-701) is an oral, potent inhibitor of JAK2 and fms-like kinase (FLT3), and has been evaluated in phase 2 in MF, and high-risk ET and PV patients. In the phase 2 study of MF patients,[14] 22 JAK2 V617F-positive, intermediate/high-risk patients were given 80 mg of lestaurtinib twice daily, and six responded, using the definitions of the International Working Group for Myelofibrosis Research and Treatment (IWG-MRT) criteria for clinical improvement. Of these six responders, three had a reduction in spleen size, two became transfusion independent, and one improved with regard to both spleen size and cytopenias. No significant changes in bone marrow fibrosis or JAK2 V617F allele burden were reported, and myelosuppression was the most common adverse effect (grade 3/4 anemia or thrombocytopenia: 14% and 23%, respectively). Gastrointestinal side effects, such as diarrhea, nausea, and vomiting were quite common.[14] Results from a second phase 1/2 study evaluating higher doses and encapsulated CEP-701 demonstrated a reduction in spleen size and JAK2 V617F allele burden, but gastrointestinal side effects have also been common with this preparation.[15]

Lestaurtinib was the first JAK-inhibitor evaluated in high-risk ET (n = 12) and PV (n = 27) patients.[16] The primary end-point, a reduction in the JAK2 V617F allele burden (>15% decline), was observed in 3 of 15 patients. A decrease in spleen size occurred in 15 of 18 patients, and pruritus was relieved in all 5 with this symptom. After 6 months of treatment, three of five experienced a reduction in phlebotomy requirements. Gastrointestinal toxicity was common and five patients experienced thrombotic events; furthermore, leukocytosis and thrombocytosis often worsened while patients remained on the drug.[16]

Fedratinib (SAR302503, Formerly TG101348)

SAR302503 is a potent, oral, selective JAK2-inhibitor that has completed phase 3 clinical testing. A phase 1/2 multi-center trial was conducted in 59 patients with intermediate or high-risk PMF, post-ETMF, and post-PVMF.[17] Most of the patients had PMF (75%), and were JAK2 V617F-positive (86%); 36% were red cell transfusion-dependent. In addition, patients with thrombocytopenia (but not $<50\times10^9$/L) were also included. In the dose-escalation phase, the limiting toxicity was hyperamylasemia; 43 patients continued onto the extension phase. After 12 cycles, a reduction in spleen size was seen in 47% of patients (overall cohort), and 56% and 88% of patients with baseline leukocytosis or thrombocytosis had normalization of these blood counts. Most participants had improvements in early satiety, fatigue, night sweats, cough, and pruritus, but in contrast to ruxolitinib, there were no significant changes in interleukin 6 (IL)-6, IL-2, IL-8, or tumor necrosis factor-alpha (TNF-α) levels, possibly due to selective inhibition of JAK2 compared to JAK1. Responses occurred in some patients who were JAK2 V617F negative. After six cycles, 16 of 20 patients with a baseline JAK2 V617F allele burden of more than 20% had a median 61% decrease in this measure.[17] Significant allele burden reduction is unique to this investigational agent, but its ultimate effect on outcomes is still unknown.

Not surprisingly, selective inhibition of JAK2 with SAR302503 resulted in myelosuppression: anemia (grade 3 or 4) emerged in 35% of patients who were not transfusion dependent at baseline, and grade 3 or 4 thrombocytopenia and neutropenia was observed in 24% and 10% of patients, respectively. Non-hematologic toxicities were often gastrointestinal in nature, including nausea, diarrhea, and vomiting, and were severe in 3.4, 10.2, and 3.4% of patients, respectively; 10.2% of patients had grade 3 or 4 increases in lipase.[17] Despite promising results, the report of Wernicke's encephalopathy has led to discontinuation of the fedratinib program.

Momelotinib (CYT387)

CYT387 is a potent JAK1/JAK2 inhibitor, and interim results for 163 intermediate/high-risk MF patients from six centers in the phase 1/2 study have been reported.[19] The study drug was given orally once daily at 150 or 300 mg, or twice daily at 150 mg, for a median of 6.6 months, with responses reported in accordance with IWG-MRT criteria. Most patients were JAK2 V617F positive (67%), and had PMF (64%). Treatment-related anemia has been rare (<1%); rather, anemia responses have been observed. Among 42 (33 transfusion-dependent) patients that could be evaluated for an anemia response, the overall response rate was 50% (58% in transfusion-dependent patients); responses have been reportedly durable.[19,20] Interestingly, responses were independent of JAK2 V617F status, karyotype, or blast count and the mechanism for this anemia response is unknown. Similar to other JAK-inhibitors, spleen size reduction observed was 45%, and a majority of patients have experienced resolution of pruritus, night sweats, and bone pain.[20] The most common toxicities were thrombocytopenia (16% with grade 3/4) hyperlipasemia (3% with grade 3/4) and transient (first dose) lightheadedness, and hypotension. Despite these adverse effects, 85% of participants have remained on study.[19,20] This agent will be studied in phase 3 in comparison to ruxolitinib with a hope of confirming anemia responses seen in early phases (NCT01969838).

Pacritinib (SB1518)

SB1518 is a selective inhibitor of JAK2 and FLT3. In phase 1 studies, a spleen response was observed in 41% of patients, including 24% with a 50% reduction.[25] The subsequent phase 2 study evaluated this agent in 33 patients with MF.[21] The primary objective was to examine spleen-volume reduction in those patients with splenomegaly more than or equal to 5 cm below the costal margin. Seventeen (57%) patients had a 25% reduction in spleen volume by MRI, which correlated with a 50% or more reduction by physical exam. Symptom improvement was also reported in 40–65% of patients treated for 6 months. Gastrointestinal side effects were common (nausea, vomiting, and abdominal pain), but were typically grade 1 or 2 in severity, except diarrhea (grade 3: 6%). There was no grade 3 or 4 neutropenia or thrombocytopenia, even in those with low platelet counts at enrollment.[21] Updated results from this study, which included 15 patients with baseline thrombocytopenia ($<100\times10^9$/L), demonstrated spleen size reductions in 30 patients (88%); of these, 15 had more than 50% reduction, and 6 had complete resolution of splenomegaly.[22] Two patients met criteria for an improvement in hemoglobin. There were 17 discontinuations due to adverse effects (8 patients), which were commonly gastrointestinal, disease progression (5 patients), and lack of efficacy (2 patients).[22] This agent will be studied in phase 3 compared to best available therapy, including in patients with baseline thrombocytopenia (NCT02055781 and NCT01773187).

LY2784544

LY2784544 is a selective JAK2 inhibitor, studied in patients with JAK2 V617F-positive MF, PV, and ET; phase 1 results from 19 patients (1 with PV, 18 with MF) have been reported.[23] Of 17 patients that could be evaluated, 13 experienced an at least 35% reduction in spleen length, including one PV patient with a 100% reduction. Symptom improvement occurred in the majority (59%) of patients, and importantly, three of five patients demonstrated a reduction in bone marrow fibrosis after five cycles of therapy. There were 4 discontinuations either for adverse events, disease progression, and investigator or patient decision. Drug-related adverse events included an increase in creatinine (transient), uric acid (grade 4), and potassium, sometimes characteristic of the tumor lysis syndrome (1 episode with laboratory evidence and 3 episodes with clinical evidence); diarrhea, nausea, and anemia were also reported, and were grade 1 or 2 in severity.[23]

Other Janus kinase-inhibitors

XL019, a selective JAK2 inhibitor, showed initial promise with regard to reduction in splenomegaly and leukocytosis, along with stabilization of hemoglobin, decrease in blast count, and relief from constitutional symptoms.[26] While hematologic toxicity was not observed, peripheral neuropathy occurred frequently leading to a discontinuation of the development of this agent. AZD-1480, NS-018, and BMS911543 are JAK2 inhibitors currently being tested in early phases.

NOVEL APPROACHES TO MYELOPROLIFERATIVE NEOPLASMS TREATMENT

Novel approaches to MPN treatment include immunomodulation, interferon therapy, epigenetic therapy, and mTOR inhibition (Table 8-2).

Immunomodulatory Drugs

The IMIDs exhibit anti-angiogenic and anti-inflammatory (mainly against TNF-α) activities, supporting their investigation in the treatment of MF. The first drug of

Table 8-2 Selected Novel Therapeutic Options for the Myeloproliferative Neoplasm

Agent	*Rationale*	*Promising results*
Immunomodulatory drugs		
Pomalidomide[27-30]	Immunomodulation Anti-angiogenesis and anti-inflammatory properties	Anemia responses (53%) in JAK2 V617F positive MF patients without splenomegaly or circulating blasts.[30] However, phase 3 testing may suggest similar efficacy when compared to placebo
Interferons		
Recombinant and pegylated interferon[31-36]	Suppression of hematopoietic and fibroblast progenitors	95% with complete hematologic response and 24% with complete molecular response in PV[31] CR or PR in 44% or MF patients[35] Improvement in marrow fibrosis and megakaryocyte atypia in minority of early MF patients[36]
Histone deacetylase inhibitors		
Panobinostat[37] Givinostat[38] Pracinostat[39]	Epigenetic regulation	Improvements in symptoms and splenomegaly in MF[37] Givinostat promising in PV, given overall response rate of 50%
Hypomethylating agents 5-azacytidine[40-42] Decitabine	Epigenetic regulation	Appear more encouraging in accelerated MPN (post-MPN AML or MDS), where the overall response rate was 52%[42]
Mammalian target of rapamycin inhibition		
Everolimus[43]	PI3K/AKT/mTOR pathway activation in MPN	Improvements in symptoms and splenomegaly

MF, myelofibrosis; PV, polycythemia vera; CR, complete response; PR, partial response; MPN, myeloproliferative neoplasm; AML, acute myeloid leukemia; MDS, myelodysplastic syndromes; mTOR, mammalian target of rapamycin this class to be used in MF, thalidomide, showed modest responses for anemia and thrombocytopenia that persisted for 2 years; in contrast, the alleviation of splenomegaly was not durable.[44,45] These studies observed that low dose thalidomide (50 mg daily) with prednisone (for 3 months) was better tolerated than single agent thalidomide. Thalidomide has also been used in combination with other agents, such as prednisone/cyclophosphamide [thalidomide prednisone cyclophosphamide (TPC)] and prednisone/etanercept [thalidomide prednisone etanercept (TPE)]. A pooled, long-term follow-up of the trials evaluating these combinations reported results in 50 intermediate 2 or high-risk patients.[46] From this pooled analysis, the tolerability and efficacy was best with low dose thalidomide (50 mg daily) combined with prednisone (tapering over 3 months) compared to this combination with cyclophosphamide or etanercept. Using IWG-MRT criteria, there was 1 partial response, 14 with clinical improvement, and 24 with stable disease. Typically, clinical improvement was seen in anemia (n = 11), rather than splenomegaly (n = 4), and the median response duration was 8.5 months. In this analysis, toxicity was primarily related to myelosuppression, with grade 3 anemia, neutropenia, and thrombocytopenia seen in three, three, and four patients respectively.[46] Adverse effects due to thalidomide can also include leukocytosis and thrombocytosis, along with constipation, sedation and neuropathy, limiting its long term use.

Lenalidomide, a second-generation IMID, was subsequently evaluated in MF. In a prospective phase 2 trial, 10 mg daily was given with prednisone (3 months) to 48 patients. However, only 19% and 10% experienced IWG-MRT defined improvement in anemia or splenomegaly, respectively.[47] There was no reduction in marrow fibrosis or angiogenesis. Lenalidomide was most useful in MF patients with deletions of 5q, akin to the experience in myelodysplastic syndromes (MDS) patients. Similarly, the IWG-MRT criteria were used to assess the efficacy of thalidomide and lenalidomide in three trials from a single center; lenalidomide was more effective (34–38% response rates) compared to thalidomide (16%).[48] In particular, lenalidomide with prednisone was the most durable (34 months) of these regimens, and best tolerated. Myelosuppression is the most common adverse effect of lenalidomide.

Pomalidomide is a potent IMID, and is currently under investigation in MF. The efficacy of this agent was initially demonstrated in a randomized, double-blind, multi-center study of 84 MF patients with anemia.[27] The four treatment arms included pomalidomide (2 mg/ daily) with placebo; pomalidomide (2 mg/daily) with prednisone; pomalidomide (0.5 mg/ daily) with prednisone; and prednisone plus placebo. For those completing at least three cycles, the responses rates were 38%, 23%, 40%, and 25%, respectively. Grade 3 or 4 toxicities included neutropenia (8%) and thrombocytopenia (11%), pneumonia and sepsis (11%), and venous thrombosis (4%). A subsequent dose-escalation study in 19 patients suggested that higher doses (3 mg/ daily) led to more myelosuppression, without increased efficacy.[28] Thereafter, the effects of low dose pomalidomide (0.5 mg/ daily) alone were evaluated in 58 MF patients with anemia.[29] Ten patients (17%) had an anemia response, which was significantly influenced by JAK2 V617F positivity (no JAK2 negative patient responded), the absence of splenomegaly, and the presence of drug-induced basophilia. An improvement in thrombocytopenia was also noted in 14 of 24 patients (58%) with a platelet count of less than 100×10^9/L. Grade 3 or 4 neutropenia or thrombocytopenia was infrequent (0 and 2%, respectively). A report of the long-term follow-up of 94 MF patients participating in pomalidomide trials revealed an overall anemia response of 27%; this number increased to 53% in JAK2 V617F positive patients without significant splenomegaly (<10 cm) and/or less than 5% circulating blasts.[30] The median response duration was 16 months, and 91% had discontinued therapy by 2 years; 4/30 (13%) patients treated for more than 1 year developed grade 1 neuropathy. Pomalidomide is currently being investigated in a phase 3, multi-center, double-blinded study compared to placebo (clinical trials identifier: NCT01178281). Preliminarily, and unfortunately, anemia responses reflecting rate or duration of transfusion independence to pomalidomide appeared similar to that of placebo.[49]

Interferons

Interferons suppress hematopoietic progenitors as well as bone marrow fibroblast progenitors, and inhibit platelet-derived growth factor (implicated in marrow fibrosis).[50] The most promising results have been demonstrated with pegylated interferon-α in ET and PV patients, justifying a potential up-front role for their use (Figure 8-4). In 40 newly treated patients with PV, 95% experienced complete hematologic remissions, judged by normalization of blood counts and spleen size; 90% of patients experienced a reduction in the JAK2 V617F allele burden, including 7 patients of 29 with complete molecular remissions.[31] Long-term follow-up suggests that these responses are durable, even in the minority of patients that have discontinued therapy.[32] A single center phase 2 study has reported significant hematologic and molecular responses in a cohort of pretreated ET and PV patients, confirmed by a retrospective analysis of clinical experiences with this agent in ET, PV, and MF patients.[33,34]

The experience with interferon in MF has been less encouraging.[51] However, a recent French multicenter retrospective study of 18 MF patients demonstrated complete (n = 6) or major (n = 2) responses in 44% of patients. Responses occurred in those with leukocytosis [5 of 9 with complete responses (CR)] and thrombocytosis (10 of 11 with CR), as well as in patients with anemia. Transfusion dependency was eliminated in two of three patients, and hemoglobin levels became normal in four of five. Changes in spleen size were less impressive, with only two responses; however, only two patients discontinued therapy.[35] Also intriguing was a prospective study of 17 early MF patients (low or intermediate-1 in risk), treated with recombinant or pegylated interferon.[36] In this report, 14 of 17 (82%) patients experienced clinical benefit or stability, including 2 CR, and 7 partial responses (PR). Nine of fifteen experienced complete splenomegaly responses, and 4 of 15 (2 CR) had improvement in marrow fibrosis and megakaryocyte atypia. Toxicity was frequent, but typically mild, and included systemic toxicity in 9 patients, 11 with hematologic toxicity, and 10 with metabolic toxicity.[36] Together, these studies suggest a potential benefit when interferon is given early in the natural history of MF.

Epigenetic Therapies

The association between epigenetic deregulation of transcription and disease pathogenesis in the MPN has been elucidated, as discussed in chapter 2. Somatic mutations of TET2, DNMT3A, EZH2, ASXL1, and IDH1/2, which contribute to epigenetic regulation, have been identified particularly in those with MF, providing a rationale for investigation of such epigenetic therapies as the histone-deacetylase inhibitors (HDACi) and hypomethylating agents.[52,53]

Histone Deacetylase Inhibitors

Panobinostat (LBH589) has been studied in phase 1 and 2 for MF patients. Preliminary results from the phase 1 study of 18 patients (intermediate and high-risk) suggested relief from systemic symptoms in all and reduction in splenomegaly in most (10 of 11 evaluable had a 30% reduction in size).[37] Five patients entered an extension phase, with a reported mean reduction in splenomegaly of 83% at 6 months; additionally, two patients had significant improvement in anemia, and one achieved a near CR, with resolution of splenomegaly, elimination of leukoerythroblastosis on the blood smear, a 4 g/dL improvement in hemoglobin, along with improvements in marrow histology (less megakaryocyte atypia and reduction of fibrosis). Thrombocytopenia was the dose-limiting toxicity. This study has proceeded with phase 2 enrollment[37] and the initial results have been published.[54]

In another phase 2 study, evaluating a higher dosing regimen, a correlative arm supported panobinostat's anti-MPN effects, including decreases in the JAK2 V617F allele burden, phosphorylated-STAT3, STAT5, and AKT; reductions in heat-shock protein 90 (HSP90) and histone deacetylase 6 (HDAC6) inhibition were also observed.[55] Clinical responses were less encouraging, however, in this study.

Givinostat, another oral HDAC inhibitor, was evaluated in the MPN. A phase 2, multi-center pilot study included patients with ET (n = 1), PV (n = 12), and MF (n = 16), and demonstrated tolerability, though gastrointestinal disturbance was common (62%), along with anemia (21%) and thrombocytopenia (10%), which were typically grade 1 or 2 in severity.[38] In ET/PV patients, the overall response rate was 7 of 12 (1 complete, 6 partial; 58%); 6 of 8 had improvement in splenomegaly (including 5 with complete resolution), and the majority had complete control of pruritus. The outcome in MF patients was less encouraging, with 3 of 16 (19%) achieving a major response; one patient had resolution of anemia and reduction in spleen size, while two others had reduction in splenomegaly and systemic symptoms.[38] Because this study suggested some efficacy in PV, a follow-up multicenter phase 2 study was initiated, givinostat was given in combination with hydroxyurea to 44 PV patients who were resistant to hydroxyurea alone. The combination was well-tolerated, with only grade 2 toxicities, including thrombocytopenia, leucopenia, and diarrhea; the complete and partial response rate was near 50%, and most had complete relief of pruritus. Therefore, the use of this HDAC-inhibitor is promising in PV (Figure 8-4).

Pracinostat, an oral, highly selective HDAC 1/2 inhibitor was studied in 22 MF patients with intermediate-1, intermediate 2, or high-risk disease, of whom 82% were JAK2 V617F positive.[39] Six patients (27%) experienced a reduction in spleen size (3 cm median reduction), but the response did not meet criteria for clinical improvement; five patients with hepatomegaly experienced a median 3 cm decrease in size. Anemia improved in two patients by IWG criteria, but only an insignificant reduction in the JAK2 V617F allele burden was noted. The most common adverse effect was fatigue (primarily grade 1), occurring in 20 (91%) of patients. Hematological toxicity included grade 3-4 neutropenia and thrombocytopenia in 13 and 21%, respectively. Twenty-one patients came off study, primarily due to lack of response or disease progression.[39] In summary, the effects were modest as a single agent, but the potential combination with JAK-inhibitors and HDAC inhibitor will be explored.

Hypomethylating Agents

Given the encouraging results in patients with MDS, and the awareness of epigenetic deregulation in MF, the hypomethylating agents have been investigated as potential therapeutic agents. Although 5-azacytidine (7 day schedule) induced global hypomethylation in a phase 2 study of 34 previously treated or intermediate/high-risk patients, clinical responses to were less impressive, and only noted in eight (24%) patients (one partial remission and seven with clinical improvement).[40] The median duration of response was 4 months (range 2–8.5), and myelosuppression was the most significant adverse event, with grade 3-4 neutropenia in 10 (29%) patients. In a second study of ten patients with MF, a 5 day regimen of 5-azacytidine was tested, but no patient achieved a clinical improvement, and eight of ten discontinued therapy primarily due to toxicity or disease progression.[41] Decitabine, another hypomethylating agent, was evaluated in 21 MF patients. Seven of nineteen evaluable patients, responded (37%).[18] The response was complete in one patient, and partial in two, with the rest experiencing hematologic improvement. Toxicity was considerable, with grade 3-4 neutropenia and thrombocytopenia in 95% and 52%, respectively.

While the efficacy of hypomethylating agents has been disappointing in MF, the results appear to be more encouraging in those whose MPN has accelerated. In a study of 54 patients with post-MPN acute myeloid leukemia (AML) (n = 26) or MDS (n = 28), the overall response rate was 52%, including 24% CR, with a median duration of 9 months.[42] These responses were more likely in those with MDS than AML, and those with antecedent ET rather than PV (71% vs. 33%); also, 39% of patients reverted back to their chronic phase MPN (thrombocytosis or erythrocytosis), sometimes requiring reinitiation of hydroxyurea or interferon. The median overall survival of the entire group was only 11 months, suggesting that some form of consolidation therapy would also be required.

Mammailiam Target of Rapamycin Inhibition

Based upon activation of the PI3K/Akt/mTOR pathway in MPN cells, and *in vitro* inhibition of proliferation of MPN and primary cell lines, everolimus (an mTOR inhibitor) has been studied in 39 MF patients in a multicenter phase 1/2 program.[56] Among 30 evaluable patients, response rates were highest with regard to splenomegaly (44% with response; 2 CR, 11 PR) and symptom reduction (69% and 80% for resolution of systemic symptoms and pruritus, respectively). As with JAK-inhibition, spleen responses occurred early (within 1 month), but progression was noted when the drug was discontinued. Hematologic responses rates were 15% for leukocytosis, and 25% each for anemia (five partial responses) and thrombocytosis. When applying IWG-MRT criteria, six patients clinically improved (spleen responses in five, improvement in hemoglobin in one), and one patient achieved a partial remission; the remaining 23 patients had stable disease. Grade 2/3 anemia occurred in 27% of patients, while grade 2 neutropenia and thrombocytopenia occurred in 7 and 3% of patients; among non-hematologic toxicity, grade 1/2 stomatitis occurred in 70% of patients.[56] Significant changes in the JAK2 V617F allele burden did not occur, nor were there meaningful changes in levels of proinflammatory cytokines. Interestingly, there was synergistic inhibition of the growth of MPN cells with the combination of PI3K/mTOR inhibitors and JAK1/2 inhibitors, suggesting a possible future therapeutic strategy.[43]

TARGETING OTHER MECHANISMS OF DISEASE PATHOGENESIS IN MYELOFIBROSIS

Results from other early phase studies exploring novel mechanisms, such as inhibition of anti-apoptotic proteins, proteasomes, VEGF, and farnesyltransferase have only resulted in modest activity at best. However, there are a number of novel, promising strategies that are being investigated in MF. These include anti-fibrotic agents, such as PRM-151, also studied in pulmonary fibrosis, GC1008; NCT01291784), an antibody against transforming growth factor β, and a monoclonal antibody against lysyl oxidase, (GS-6624). Imetelstat, a telomerase inhibitor, has shown promise in a small study of MF patients.[57] Finally, other novel strategies that will be tested in the clinic include inhibitors of the sonic hedgehog pathway and heat shock protein 90.

CONCLUSION

The discovery that JAK/STAT activation contributes significantly to disease pathogenesis in the MPN has led to a new era of enthusiasm and discovery, manifest by the clinical development and approval of the first specific MPN therapy, the JAK-inhibitors. While the initial excitement about these agents have been tempered by recognition that JAK2 V617F represents only one component of lesions driving the heterogeneity of the MPN, these agents consistently alleviate constitutional symptoms and reduce spleen size and offer an important palliative option for MF patients. Clinical studies indicate individual JAK-inhibitors have additional unique effects: ruxolitinib results in a significant reduction in the level of proinflammatory cytokines; momeltonib (CYT387) may ameliorate anemia; pacritinib (SB1518) may result in efficacy without myelosuppression; and in a small number of patients, LY2784544 resulted in improvements in marrow fibrosis.

As clinical development advances, the therapeutic potential of these agents might be realized, not as single agents but when administered in combination with other novel agents, given the biologic and molecular complexity of the MF and the other classical MPN (Figure 8-4). Promising future strategies include the use of JAK-inhibitors to reduce splenomegaly and constitutional symptoms prior to transplantation;[58] JAK-inhibitors in combination with other conventional or novel agents used to treat anemia (androgens, ESA, IMIDs), counteracting the myelosuppression associated with wild-type JAK2 inhibition; and in combination with interferons, epigenetic therapies, or mTOR inhibitors, to address other relevant contributors to disease pathogenesis in MF and the MPN.[59] Hopefully, these rational combinations add to the therapeutic landscape, and positively alter the natural history of the MPN.

REFERENCES

1. Dameshek W. Some speculations on the myeloproliferative syndromes. *Blood.* 1951;6(4): 372-5.
2. Baxter EJ, Scott LM, Campbell PJ, et al. Acquired mutation of the tyrosine kinase JAK2 in human myeloproliferative disorders. *Lancet.* 2005;365(9464):1054-61.
3. James C, Ugo V, Le Couedic JP, et al. A unique clonal JAK2 mutation leading to constitutive signalling causes polycythaemia vera. *Nature.* 2005;434(7037):1144-8.
4. Kralovics R, Passamonti F, Buser AS, et al. A gain-of-function mutation of JAK2 in myeloproliferative disorders. *N Engl J Med.* 2005;352(17):1779-90.
5. Levine RL, Wadleigh M, Cools J, et al. Activating mutation in the tyrosine kinase JAK2 in polycythemia vera, essential thrombocythemia, and myeloid metaplasia with myelofibrosis. *Cancer Cell.* 2005;7(4):387-97.

6. Klampfl T, Gisslinger H, Harutyunvan AS, et al. Somatic mutations of calreticulin in myeloproliferative neoplasms. *New Eng J Med.* 2013;369()25:2379-90.
7. Nangalia J, Massie CE, Baxter EJ et al. Somatic CALR mutations in myeloproliferative neoplasms with nonmutated JAK2. *New Eng J Med.* 2013;369(25):2397-405
8. Tefferi A. Novel mutations and their functional and clinical relevance in myeloproliferative neoplasms: JAK2, MPL, TET2, ASXL1, CBL, IDH and IKZF1. *Leukemia.* 2010;24(6):1128-38.
9. Stein BL, Moliterno AR. Primary myelofibrosis and the myeloproliferative neoplasms: the role of individual variation. *JAMA.* 2010;303(24):2513-8.
10. Verstovsek S, Mesa RA, Gotlib J, et al. A double-blind, placebo-controlled trial of ruxolitinib for myelofibrosis. *N Engl J Med.* 2012;366(9):799-807.
11. Harrison C, Kiladjian JJ, Al-Ali HK, et al. JAK inhibition with ruxolitinib versus best available therapy for myelofibrosis. *N Eng J Med.* 2012;366(9):787-98.
12. Verstovsek S, Kantarjian H, Mesa RA, et al. Safety and efficacy of INCB018424, a JAK1 and JAK2 inhibitor, in myelofibrosis. *N Engl J Med.* 2010;363(12):1117-27.
13. Verstovsek S, Passamonti F, Rambaldi A, et al. Durable Responses with the JAK1/ JAK2 Inhibitor, INCB018424, In Patients with Polycythemia Vera (PV) and Essential Thrombocythemia (ET) Refractory or Intolerant to Hydroxyurea (HU). *ASH Annual Meeting Abstracts.* 2010.
14. Santos FP, Kantarjian HM, Jain N, et al. Phase 2 study of CEP-701, an orally available JAK2 inhibitor, in patients with primary or post-polycythemia vera/essential thrombocythemia myelofibrosis. *Blood.* 2010;115(6):1131-6.
15. Hexner E, Goldberg JD, Prchal JT, et al. A Multicenter, Open Label Phase I/II Study of CEP701 (Lestaurtinib) in Adults with Myelofibrosis; a Report On Phase I: A Study of the Myeloproliferative Disorders Research Consortium (MPD-RC). *ASH Annual Meeting Abstracts.* 2009.
16. Moliterno AR, Hexner E, Roboz GJ, et al. An Open-Label Study of CEP-701 in Patients with JAK2 V617F-Positive PV and ET: Update of 39 Enrolled Patients. *ASH Annual Meeting Abstracts.* 2009.
17. Pardanani A, Gotlib JR, Jamieson C, et al. Safety and efficacy of TG101348, a selective JAK2 inhibitor, in myelofibrosis. *J Clin Oncol.* 2011;29(7):789-96.
18. Odenike OM, Godwin JE, Van Besien K, et al. Phase II Trial of Low Dose, Subcutaneous Decitabine in Myelofibrosis. *ASH Annual Meeting Abstracts.* 2008;112(11):2809.
19. Pardanani A, Gotlib J, Gupta V, Roberts AW, Wadleigh M, Sirhan S, et al. An Expanded Multicenter Phase I/II Study of CYT387, a JAK- 1/2 Inhibitor for the Treatment of Myelofibrosis. *ASH Annual Meeting Abstracts.* 2011 November 18, 2011.
20. Pardanani AC, D George, G Lasho, et al. Safety and efficacy of CYT387, a JAK-1/2 inhibitor, for the treatment of myelofibrosis. *Clin Oncol.* 2011;29(Suppl; abstract 6514).
21. Deeg HJO, O Scott, BL Estrov, et al. Phase II study of SB1518, an orally available novel JAK2 inhibitor, in patients with myelofibrosis. *J Clin Oncol.* 2011;29(Suppl; abstract 6515).
22. Komrokji RS, Wadleigh M, Seymour JF, et al. Results of a Phase 2 Study of Pacritinib (SB1518), a Novel Oral JAK2 Inhibitor, In Patients with Primary, Post-Polycythemia Vera, and Post-Essential Thrombocythemia Myelofibrosis. *ASH Annual Meeting Abstracts.* 2011.
23. Verstovsek S, Mesa RA, Rhoades SK, et al. Phase I Study of the JAK2 V617F Inhibitor, LY2784544, in Patients with Myelofibrosis (MF), Polycythemia Vera (PV), and Essential Thrombocythemia (ET). *ASH Annual Meeting Abstracts.* 2011.
24. Cervantes F, Vannucchi AM, Kiladjian JJ, et al. Three year efficacy, safety, and survival finding from COMFORT-II, a phase 3 study comparing ruxolitinib with best available therapy for myelofibrosis. Blood. 2013;122(25):4047-53.
25. Verstovsek S, Odenike O, Scott B, et al. Phase I Dose-Escalation Trial of SB1518, a Novel JAK2/ FLT3 Inhibitor, in Acute and Chronic Myeloid Diseases, Including Primary or Post-Essential Thrombocythemia/ Polycythemia Vera Myelofibrosis. *ASH Annual Meeting Abstracts.* 2009.
26. Shah NP, Olszynski P, Sokol L, et al. A Phase I Study of XL019, a Selective JAK2 Inhibitor, in Patients with Primary Myelofibrosis, Post-Polycythemia Vera, or Post-Essential Thrombocythemia Myelofibrosis. *ASH Annual Meeting Abstracts.* 2008.

27. Tefferi A, Verstovsek S, Barosi G, et al. Pomalidomide is active in the treatment of anemia associated with myelofibrosis. *J Clin Oncol.* 2009;27(27):4563-9.
28. Mesa RA, Pardanani AD, Hussein K, et al. Phase1/-2 study of Pomalidomide in myelofibrosis. *Am J Hematol.* 2010;85(2):129-30.
29. Begna KH, Mesa RA, Pardanani A, et al. A phase-2 trial of low-dose pomalidomide in myelofibrosis. *Leukemia.* 2011;25(2):301-4.
30. Begna KH, Pardanani A, Mesa R, et al. Long-term outcome of pomalidomide therapy in myelofibrosis. *Am J Hematol.* 2012;87(1):66-8.
31. Kiladjian JJ, Cassinat B, Chevret S, et al. Pegylated interferon-alfa-2a induces complete hematologic and molecular responses with low toxicity in polycythemia vera. *Blood.* 2008;112(8):3065-72.
32. Turlure P, Cambier N, Roussel M, et al. Complete Hematological, Molecular and Histological Remissions without Cytoreductive Treatment Lasting After Pegylated-Interferon {alpha}-2a (peg-IFN{alpha}-2a) Therapy in Polycythemia Vera (PV): Long Term Results of a Phase 2 Trial. *ASH Annual Meeting Abstracts.* 2011.
33. Quintas-Cardama A, Kantarjian H, Manshouri T, et al. Pegylated interferon alfa-2a yields high rates of hematologic and molecular response in patients with advanced essential thrombocythemia and polycythemia vera. *J Clin Oncol.* 2009;27(32):5418-24.
34. Gowin K, Thapaliya P, Samuelsson J, et al. Experience with pegylated Interferon alpha-2a in advanced myeloproliferative neoplasms in an international cohort of 118 patients. *Haematologica.* 2012;97(10)1570-3.
35. Ianotto JC, Kiladjian JJ, Demory JL, et al. PEG-IFN-alpha-2a therapy in patients with myelofibrosis: a study of the French Groupe d'Etudes des Myelofibroses (GEM) and France Intergroupe des syndromes Myeloproliferatifs (FIM). *Br J Haematol.* 2009;146(2):223-5.
36. Silver RT, Vandris K, Goldman JJ. Recombinant interferon-alpha may retard progression of early primary myelofibrosis: a preliminary report. *Blood.* 2011;117(24):6669-72.
37. Mascarenhas J, Mercado A, Rodriguez A, et al. Prolonged Low Dose Therapy with a Pan-Deacetylase Inhibtor, Panobinostat (LBH589), in Patients with Myelofibrosis. *ASH Annual Meeting Abstracts.* 2011;118(21):794-.
38. Rambaldi A, Dellacasa CM, Finazzi G, et al. A pilot study of the Histone-Deacetylase inhibitor Givinostat in patients with JAK2V617F positive chronic myeloproliferative neoplasms. *Br J Haematol.* 2010;150(4):446-55.
39. Quintas-Cardama A, Kantarjian H, Estrov Z, et al. Therapy with the histone deacetylase inhibitor pracinostat for patients with myelofibrosis. *Leuk Res.* 2012;36(9):1124-7.
40. Quintas-Cardama A, Tong W, Kantarjian H, et al. A phase II study of 5-azacitidine for patients with primary and post-essential thrombocythemia/polycythemia vera myelofibrosis. *Leukemia.* 2008;22(5):965-70.
41. Mesa RA, Verstovsek S, Rivera C, et al. 5-Azacitidine has limited therapeutic activity in myelofibrosis. *Leukemia.* 2009;23(1):180-2.
42. Thepot S, Itzykson R, Seegers V, et al. Treatment of progression of Philadelphia-negative myeloproliferative neoplasms to myelodysplastic syndrome or acute myeloid leukemia by azacitidine: a report on 54 cases on the behalf of the Groupe Francophone des Myelodysplasies (GFM). *Blood.* 2010;116(19):3735-42.
43. Vannucchi AM, Bogani C, Bartalucci N, et al. Inhibitors of PI3K/Akt and/or mTOR Inhibit the Growth of Cells of Myeloproliferative Neoplasms and Synergize with JAK2 Inhibitor and Interferon. *ASH Annual Meeting Abstracts.* 2011.
44. Mesa RA, Elliott MA, Schroeder G, et al. Durable responses to thalidomide-based drug therapy for myelofibrosis with myeloid metaplasia. *Mayo Clin Proc.* 2004;79(7):883-9.
45. Mesa RA, Steensma DP, Pardanani A, et al. A phase 2 trial of combination low-dose thalidomide and prednisone for the treatment of myelofibrosis with myeloid metaplasia. *Blood.* 2003;101(7):2534-41.
46. Thapaliya P, Tefferi A, Pardanani A, et al. International working group for myelofibrosis research and treatment response assessment and long-term follow-up of 50 myelofibrosis patients treated with thalidomide-prednisone based regimens. *Am J Hematol.* 2011;86(1):96-8.

47. Mesa RA, Yao X, Cripe LD, et al. Lenalidomide and prednisone for myelofibrosis: Eastern Cooperative Oncology Group (ECOG) phase 2 trial E4903. *Blood.* 2010;116(22):4436-8.
48. Jabbour E, Thomas D, Kantarjian H, Zhou L, Pierce S, Cortes J, et al. Comparison of thalidomide and lenalidomide as therapy for myelofibrosis. Blood. 2011;118(4):899-902.
49. Tefferi A, Passamanti F, Tiziano Barbui T, et al. Phase 3 study of pomalidomide in myelopraliferative neoplasms (NPN)-associated myelofibrosis with RBC-transfusion-dependence. *Blood* 2013;122(21):394.
50. Kiladjian JJ, Chomienne C, Fenaux P. Interferon-alpha therapy in bcr-abl-negative myeloproliferative neoplasms. *Leukemia.* 2008;22(11):1990-8.
51. Kiladjian JJ, Mesa RA, Hoffman R. The renaissance of interferon therapy for the treatment of myeloid malignancies. *Blood.* 2011;117(18):4706-15.
52. Vannucchi AM, Biamonte F. Epigenetics and mutations in chronic myeloproliferative neoplasms. *Haematologica.* 2011;96(10):1398-402.
53. Abdel-Wahab O, Pardanani A, Bernard OA, et al. Unraveling the genetic underpinnings of myeloproliferative neoplasms and understanding their effect on disease course and response to therapy: Proceedings from the 6th international post-ASH symposium. *Am J Hematol.* 2012;87(5):562-8.
54. Mascarenhas J, Lu M, Li T, et al. A phase I study of panobinostat (LBH589) in patients with primary myelofibrosis (PMF) and post-polycythemia vera/essential thrombocythaemia myelofibrosis (post-PV/ET MF). *Br J Haematol.* 2013;120(7:1367-79.)
55. DeAngelo DJ, Tefferi A, Fiskus W, et al. A Phase II Trial of Panobinostat, an Orally Available Deacetylase Inhibitor (DACi), in Patients with Primary Myelofibrosis (PMF), Post Essential Thrombocythemia (ET), and Post Polycythemia Vera (PV) Myelofibrosis. *ASH Annual Meeting Abstracts.* 2010;116(21):630-.
56. Guglielmelli P, Barosi G, Rambaldi A, et al. Safety and efficacy of everolimus, a mTOR inhibitor, as single agent in a phase 1/2 study in patients with myelofibrosis. *Blood.* 2011;118(8):2069-76.
57. Tefferi A, Begna K, Laborde RR, et al. Imetelstat, a telomerase inhibitor, induces morphologic and molecular remissions in myelofibrosis and reversal of bone marrow fibrosis. *Blood.* 2013;122(21):662.
58. Gupta V, Hari P, Hoffman R. Allogeneic hematopoietic cell transplantation for myelofibrosis in the era of JAK inhibitors. *Blood.* 2012;120(7):1367-79.
59. Harrison C, Verstovsek S, McMullin MF, et al. Janus kinase inhibition and its effect upon the therapeutic landscape for myelofibrosis: from palliation to cure? *Br J Haematol.* 2012; 157(4):426-37.

CHAPTER

9 Hypereosinophilic Syndromes

Sonia L Ali, Casey O'Connell

HISTORY OF HYPEREOSINOPHILIC DISORDERS

Peripheral blood eosinophilia can accompany a variety of disorders, ranging from infectious to rheumatologic to neoplastic. While the presence of eosinophilia complicating a treatable etiology, such as parasitic infection is reversible and usually not associated with long-term damage, eosinophilia with evidence of otherwise unexplained organ dysfunction has puzzled clinicians for almost a century. A number of eponymous syndromes were coined to name eosinophilic infiltrates confined to a single organ. In 1932, Löeffler described a syndrome consisting of pulmonary infiltrates in the setting of peripheral blood eosinophilia.[1] Patients with this syndrome experienced a nonfatal and relatively short course of disease. Harkavy later described 16 patients with similar pulmonary findings, but these patients also demonstrated electrocardiographic abnormalities along with manifestations of damage in various other organs.[2] Four patients succumbed to pericarditis and autopsy revealed dense eosinophilic infiltration of the pericardium. Later, Churg and Strauss described histological findings of granulomatous nodules and eosinophilic infiltrates among patients with peripheral blood eosinophilia and vasculitis, the syndrome now a well-known connective tissue disease.[3]

In 1968, Hardy and Anderson used the term "hypereosinophilic syndrome (HES)" to describe patients in whom persistent, unexplained eosinophilia could not be attributed to any known cause.[4] Diagnostic criteria were proposed by Chusid et al. in 1975 and consisted of: greater than 6 months of elevated eosinophils greater than $1.5 \times 10^9/L$; lack of evidence of parasitic, allergic, or other etiologies for eosinophilia; and signs and symptoms of organ involvement. The first major molecular breakthrough in the understanding of hypereosinophilia came in 2003, only after the clinical observation that some patients had significant and durable responses to the tyrosine kinase inhibitor imatinib. Cools and colleagues demonstrated a novel fusion of the Fip1-like 1 (FIP1L1) gene to the platelet-derived growth factor receptor-alpha (PDGFRA) gene resulting from an interstitial deletion on chromosome 4q.[5] The resulting tyrosine kinase is constitutively active and is inhibited by imatinib at significantly lower concentrations than are required to inhibit the previously described breakpoint cluster region (BCR)-Abelson leukemia virus (ABL) fusion protein in chronic myeloid leukemia (CML).

As a result of these findings, the most recent iteration of the World Health Organization's (WHO) classification of hematopoietic disorders has subclassified those cases of hypereosinophilia with characteristic molecular abnormalities, distinguishing them from idiopathic cases and from chronic eosinophilic leukemia not otherwise specified (CEL-NOS).[6]

EPIDEMIOLOGY

Unfortunately, accurate epidemiologic information regarding the incidence and prevalence of HES is hampered by delay in diagnosis, lack of International Classification of Diseases, Ninth Revision (ICD-9) codes distinguishing the various subtypes of HES, and coders' or clinicians' improper coding for the diagnosis. A crude age-adjusted incidence rate of 0.036 per 100,000 person-years was calculated based on Surveillance, Epidemiology and End Results Program (SEER) 17 data for the period 2001-2005 in the United States.[7] Of the 131 incident cases recorded, 78 were male and 53 female (1.47 male: female ratio). Median age at diagnosis was 52.5 years, with the peak incidence occurring between 65 years and 74 years of age. Prior reports suggested an earlier average age at presentation with more of a male predominance in gender distribution. The fused FIP1L1-PDGFRA abnormality is present in 10–20% of all cases of hypereosinophilia, with much higher prevalence in males.[5]

EOSINOPHIL DEVELOPMENT

Eosinophil maturation begins in the bone marrow, where clusters of differentiation (CD)34$^+$ progenitor cells develop into an initial precursor common to both the eosinophil and basophil.[8] The action of at least three classes of transcription factors [GATA-1, PU.1, CCAAT/enhancing binding protein (C/EBP) members] drives lineage specification.[9,10] Murine studies have shown that deletion of the GATA-binding site in the GATA-1 promoter and deficiency of C/EBP-α both disrupt the development of eosinophils.[11,12] Additionally, eosinophil development is influenced by levels of circulating cytokines [granulocyte colony-stimulating factor (G-CSF), granulocyte-macrophage colony-stimulating factor (GM-CSF), interleukin (IL)-3, IL-5];[13] however, IL-5 appears to be the only eosinophil-specific cytokine.[14] Full bone marrow maturation takes approximately 2–6 days to complete,[15] at which point the newly-formed eosinophils are released into the peripheral blood circulation where they have a half-life of 8–18 hours.[14] IL-5 appears to greatly influence this release,[16,17] as murine models of IL-5 overexpression develop profound eosinophilia.[18,19] Eosinophils then migrate to mucosal-associated tissues (nasal mucosa,[20] lungs,[21] gastrointestinal mucosa,[22] uterus,[23] and skin[24]) and lymphocyte-associated tissue (lymph nodes,[22] thymus,[25] and spleen[22]).

EOSINOPHIL TRAFFICKING

The process of eosinophil migration from the vasculature into tissues is guided by chemoattractants and can be divided into four steps: (1) tethering, (2) rolling, (3) adhesion, and (4) transmigration (Figure 9-1).[26,27] Tethering involves interactions between eosinophil and endothelial selectins (specialized transmembrane carbohydrate-binding proteins) as well as integrins (membrane heterodimeric proteins).[28,29] Of the three types of selectins (E-, L- and P-selectin), eosinophils utilize L-and P-selectin during their interaction with the endothelium.[28,30-33] The eosinophil L-selectins interact with endothelial CD34, GlyCAM-1, and mucosal addressin cell-adhesion molecule-1 (MAdCAM-1), and the endothelial P-selectins interact with eosinophil P-selectin glycoprotein ligand 1 (PSGL-1).[28] P-selectins are preformed and stored in the endothelial transmembrane; their expression

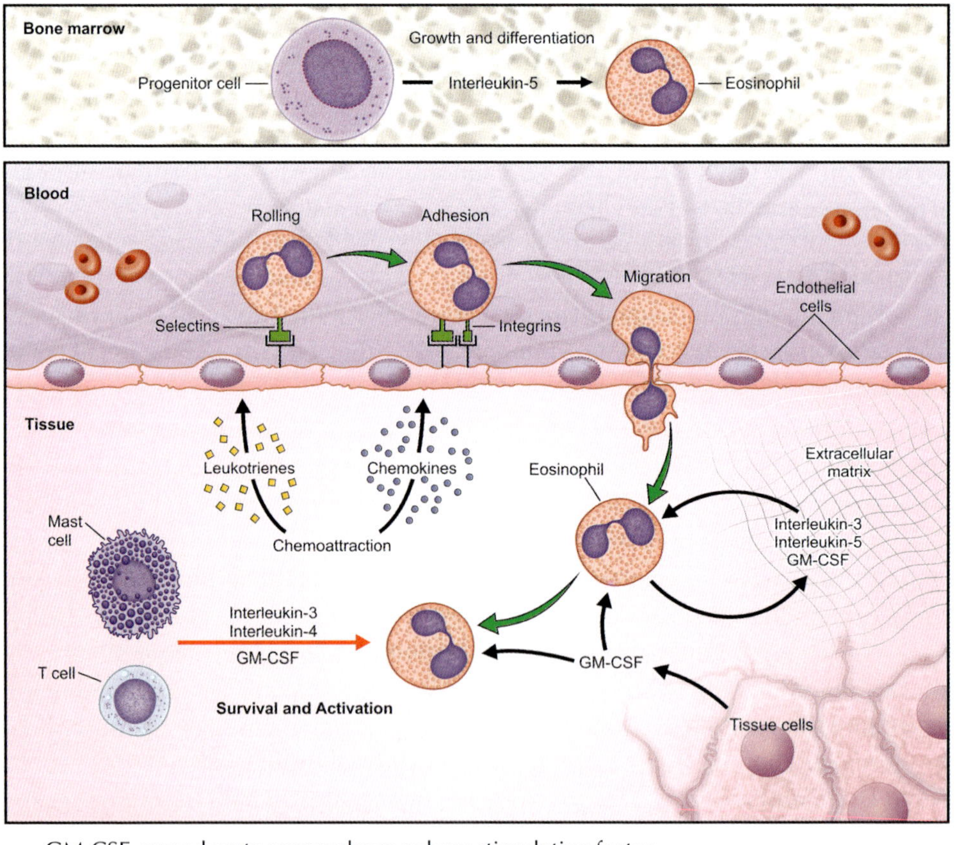

GM-CSF, granulocyte-macrophage colony stimulating factor.

Figure 9-1 Process of eosinophil migration from the vasculature into tissues (guided by chemoattractants).

on the surface is governed by thrombin, histamine, hydrogen peroxide, and C5a.[28] Integrins are utilized in both tethering and rolling.[28] During tethering, the eosinophil integrin very late antigen 4 (VLA-4) interacts with its endothelial counter-receptor, vascular cell-adhesion molecule-1 (VCAM-1) (CD106).[31,34] Expression of both endothelial P-selectin and VCAM-1 is induced by IL-4 or IL-13.[35-38] Following tethering, eosinophils roll along the endothelial surface until stimulated by a chemoattractant,[27] which results in firm attachment.

In order for adhesion to occur, the endothelium must first be primed.[28] Priming occurs following stimulation by various agents including lipopolysaccharide (LPS), tumor necrosis factor-alpha (TNF-α), interferons (IFNs), interleukin-1 beta (IL-1β), IL-4, and IL-13. Priming causes surface expression of adhesion molecules, such as additional P-selectins, intercellular-adhesion molecule-1 (ICAM-1) (CD54), ICAM-2 (CD102), and VCAM-1. These adhesion molecules interact with eosinophil integrins and result in the arrest of rolling.

The next step in eosinophil trafficking is transmigration. In addition to priming caused by the agents previously mentioned, C3a and C5a cause generation of nitric oxide from eosinophils.[39] Nitric oxide, combined with histamine and leukotriene C4 (LTC4) from other cells, causes an increase in vascular permeability, which likely results in increased transmigration of eosinophils.[28] In order for this to occur, the eosinophil must attach itself on the leading edge, and break its adhesive interactions on the tail end.[27] Termed "diapedesis", this process is incompletely understood; however, *in vitro* studies have found that C5a causes endothelial cell retraction, leading to gaps which facilitate diapedesis.[28,40] Having penetrated the endothelial layer, the eosinophil must now traverse the basement membrane. This process requires proteolysis. The eosinophil, equipped with granules containing metalloprotease-9, is able to degrade many of the components of the subendothelial extracellular matrix (ECM).[41-43]

EOSINOPHIL STRUCTURE AND FUNCTION

The membrane-bound granules contained within eosinophils are its most prominent feature. There are three main granules: (1) primary granules, (2) small granules, and (3) specific or secondary granules.[24] Primary granules are formed early in the development and contain Charcot-Leyden crystal protein.[14] Small granules serve as sites for hydrolytic enzymes. Secondary granules contain four basic proteins: (1) the major basic protein (MBP), (2) eosinophil cationic protein (ECP), (3) eosinophil peroxidase (EPO), and (4) eosinophil protein X (EPX)/eosinophil-derived neurotoxin (EDN).[44] The release of these proteins is governed by vesicotubular structures.[45] Secondary granules contain a crystalloid core, the major component of which is MBP.[14]

In addition to the main granules, eosinophils also contain lipid bodies, which are non-membrane-bound lipid-rich organelles containing the principal eosinophil eicosanoiden-forming enzymes, whose function is not fully understood.[26]

The contents of these granules are released in one of four different mechanisms: (1) classical exocytosis, (2) compound exocytosis, (3) piecemeal degranulation, and (4) necrosis (cytolysis).[27] The mode of degranulation utilized appears to be based upon the type of disease encountered; for example, in allergic disease, piecemeal and necrosis are most commonly observed, whereas compound exocytosis is typical of parasitic and fungal disease.[27] With the exception of necrosis, all other methods of degranulation seem to require specific intracellular membrane-associated proteins, including soluble NSF attachment proteins (SNAP) receptors. The ability of eosinophil granules to selectively extrude their contents allows them to function as a secretory "organelles".[45]

In addition to granules, eosinophils are structurally notable for their bilobed nucleus, highly condensed chromatin, and an array of cell-surface molecules.[14] Included in the cell-surface molecules are immunoglobulin (Ig) receptors for IgG and IgA, complement receptors, cytokine receptors, chemokines, adhesion molecules, leukotriene receptors, prostaglandin receptors, platelet-activating factor-receptor, toll-like receptors, and several inhibitory receptors.

Functionally, eosinophils have immunomodulatory capabilities.[46] The majority of eosinophil effector functions are secondary to the cationic proteins contained within its secondary granules. MBP has been shown in vitro to have toxic activity against parasites, including helminthes and schistosomula.[47] In addition, MBP has antibacterial properties[48] and has been shown to be cytotoxic to airways.[49] The toxicity of MBP is thought to be secondary to increased membrane permeability resulting from surface charge interactions.[13,14] Both ECP and EDN are ribonuclease (RNAse); however, ECP is 100 times less potent than EDN.[26,50,51] ECP has also been shown to be toxic to helminthes, function as a bactericidal agent, and also promote mast cell degranulation.[48,51] Though it does function as an RNAse, its main toxicity is thought to be secondary to pore formation in target membranes.[52] EDN has been implicated in antiviral activity against respiratory syncytial virus in a manner directly dependent on its RNAse activity.[53] Eosinophil peroxidase, through catalyzing the peroxidative oxidation of halides and pseudohalides, is associated with bactericidal killing.[54-56]

In addition to the effects of the cationic proteins, eosinophils are capable of producing a number of cytokines and chemokines including transforming growth factor-beta (TGF-β), IL-3, IL-4, IL-5, IL-8, IL-10, IL-12, IL-13, IL-16, IL-18, TNF-α, CCL5 [chemokine (C-C motif) ligand 5], and CCL11 (C-C motif chemokine 11).[14] Many of these cytokines are inducers of immune responses in inflammatory diseases.[13] Interestingly, the cytokines of eosinophils, in contrast to those of T cells (which generate much larger quantities of cytokines), are preformed and stored in secretory vesicles.[57] This allows for their immediate release.

Finally, eosinophils have recently been shown to act as true professional antigen-presenting cells (APCs).[58] Eosinophils have been found to travel to lymph nodes following antigen challenge[59] and major histocompatibility complex (MHC) class II expression has been observed in eosinophils from allergic and parasitic inflammation.[60-62]

CLASSIFICATION OF EOSINOPHILIA

Eosinophilia is defined as mild when the peripheral blood eosinophil count ranges from 0.5×10^9/L to 1.5×10^9/L and it is considered marked when counts exceed 1.5×10^9/L.[63] When marked eosinophilia is present on two separate examinations distanced by at least a 1 month time-period and tissue hypereosinophilia is present, the term "hypereosinophilia" is appropriate.[64] The term HES is utilized if the criteria for hypereosinophilia have been met and there is evidence of organ damage secondary to tissue hypereosinophilia. HES can be categorized into three main groups: (1) secondary eosinophilia, (2) clonal eosinophilia, and (3) idiopathic eosinophilia (Figure 9-2). The diagnosis of idiopathic eosinophilia is made only after all other causes are ruled out.

Secondary eosinophilia can be divided into two separate subgroups: those with infectious etiologies and those with noninfectious etiologies, including neoplastic conditions with reactive hypereosinophilia.[64,65] Worldwide, parasites are the most

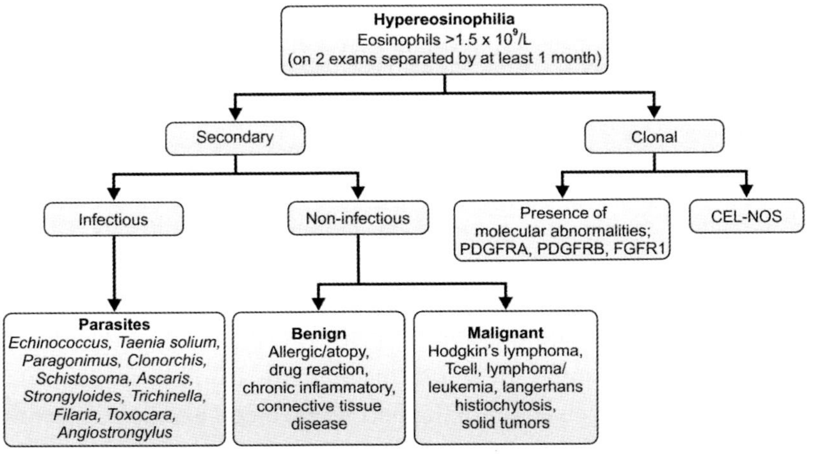

PDGFRA, platelet-derived growth factor receptor-alpha; PDGFRB, platelet-derived growth factor receptor-beta; FGFR1, fibroblast growth factor receptor-1; CEL-NOS, chronic eosinophilic leukemia not otherwise specified.

Figure 9-2 Classification of hypereosinophilic syndrome into secondary eosinophilia, clonal eosinophilia, and idiopathic eosinophilia.

common cause of secondary eosinophilia; however, a variety of noninfectious etiologies must also be considered. Drug reactions (allergic or toxic), allergic reactions, atopic diseases, chronic graft-versus-host disease, chronic inflammatory disorders, autoimmune diseases, and lymphoid variant of HES (L-HES) are included in the differential diagnoses for noninfectious secondary eosinophilia, with allergic diseases causing the majority of cases in developed countries. L-HES is a subset of HES in which the chronic reactive hypereosinophilia is secondary to IL-5 overproduction by T cells.[66] Due to the generation of eosinopoietic cytokines, Hodgkin's disease, B- or T-cell lymphoma/leukemia, Langerhans cell histiocytosis and solid tumors can also result in reactive eosinophilia. These are differentiated from hypereosinophilia caused by clonal expansion, which is the result of a somatic mutation within and eosinophil precursor.[64,65]

Clonal eosinophilia refers to any eosinophilia in which there exists an underlying clonal myeloid or stem cell disorder, and as such, is diagnosed after review of bone marrow histology, cytogenetics, and molecular genetics.[66,67] Molecular studies have established an association between eosinophilia and fusion genes involving platelet-derived growth factor receptor-alpha (PDGFRA), platelet-derived growth factor receptor-beta (PDGFRB), fibroblast growth factor receptor-1 (FGFR1), and other tyrosine kinases.[66] These findings resulted a distinct classification within the WHO scheme of myeloid neoplasms: "myeloid and lymphoid neoplasms with eosinophilia and abnormalities of PDGFRA, PDGFRB, or FGFR1"[68] (Chapter 1). The fusion tyrosine kinase FIP1L1-PDGFRA was first reported in 2003[5] and was the first description of a gain-of-function fusion protein resulting from deletion of genetic material.[5] This fusion protein is thought to result in eosinophilia by modification of both expression and activity of lineage-specific transcription factors (C/EBP-α, GATA-1, and GATA-2) through Ras/MEK and p38MAPK (mitogen-activated protein kinase) cascades.[69] Identification of PDGFR mutations is of therapeutic importance given the responsiveness of these mutations to therapy with imatinib.[70,71]

Also included within the domain of clonal eosinophilia is CEL-NOS, a subclassification of the WHO major category "myeloproliferative neoplasms".[68] This is defined as a condition in which eosinophilia is present (eosinophilia count $>1.5 \times 10^9$/L); there is no abnormality of PDGFRA, PDGFRB, or FGFR1; there is no Philadelphia chromosome, BCR-ABL fusion gene, or other myeloproliferative neoplasm; and the blast cell count in the peripheral blood and bone marrow is less than 20% [thus excluding acute myeloid leukemia (AML)].

Finally, the diagnosis of idiopathic hypereosinophilic syndrome (IHES) is considered only after a full investigation has been performed to rule out causes for secondary and clonal hypereosinophilia.[64] According to the most recent WHO criteria, IHES requires the presence of hypereosinophilia for at least 6 months with concurrent tissue damage.[66] The preferred terminology for persistent hypereosinophilia of duration greater than 6 months without evidence of tissue damage and absence of criteria for secondary or clonal hypereosinophilia is "idiopathic hypereosinophilia".

TREATMENT INDICATIONS AND OPTIONS FOR HYPEREOSINOPHILIA

When considering treatment for hypereosinophilia, the clinician must first identify and treat secondary causes requiring specific treatment not directed at eosinophilia.[72] Once secondary causes have been ruled out, identification of organ involvement is of utmost importance, because, if present, empiric high-dose corticosteroid should be administered to induce rapid decline in eosinophil counts in an effort to prevent progression of organ damage.[63,72] Therefore, a workup consisting of serum troponins, serum creatinine kinase, echocardiogram, and electrocardiography (EKG) to evaluate for cardiac involvement; serum liver enzymes, serum lipase, and abdominal computed tomography (CT) to evaluate for gastrointestinal involvement; and serum creatinine and urinalysis to evaluate for kidney and urinary tract involvement should be performed in all patients to assess for the presence of HES.[73] Furthermore, if the patient shows signs of neurological, skin, and/or vascular involvement, a workup consisting of neuroimaging, skin biopsy, and angiography, respectively, should also be obtained.

If no end-organ damage is initially identified, treatment is guided by the type of HES variant present. For asymptomatic patients with idiopathic eosinophilia, there is no data to support initiation of therapy and these patients should be periodically monitored for signs of organ involvement.[63,64,73] Serum troponin levels, electrocardiogram, echocardiogram, and pulmonary function tests can be performed every 6 months and therapy should be initiated if organ involvement is suggested.[64,74]

However, if the clinician is concerned about worsening signs and symptoms, the initiation of steroid treatment should not be delayed by investigational studies.[72] An approach to the treatment of HES is outlined in figure 9-3. Dosing options for corticosteroids include intravenous (IV) methylprednisolone 1 mg/kg/day or oral prednisone 1 mg/kg/day for 1–2 weeks then tapered over the following 2–3 months, once symptoms are controlled and eosinophil counts drop below 1.5×10^9/L.[63,71,72] A multicenter retrospective analysis found that maintenance doses of prednisone ranged from 10 mg to 40 mg, with complete or partial responses obtained in 85% of patients after 1 month.[75] This study also investigated the results of patients with high serum levels of thymus- and activation-regulated chemokine (TARC). Because TARC is expressed on T cells following stimulation with IL-4,[76] and patients with L-HES have been shown to have higher levels of TARC, it has been proposed as a surrogate

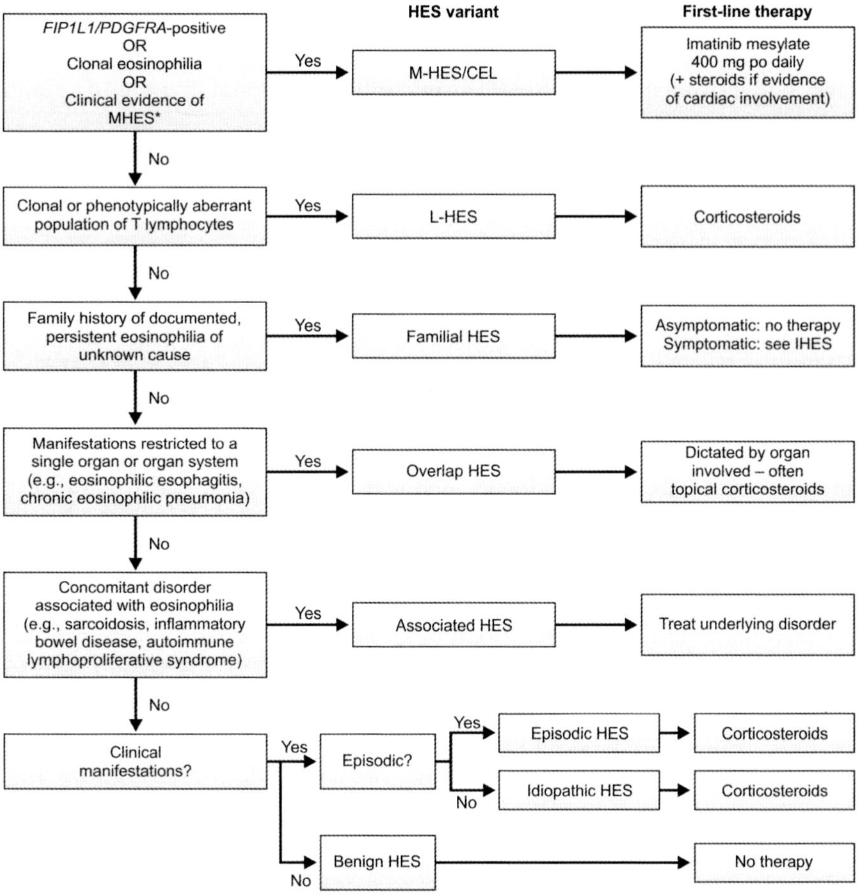

FIP1L1, Fip1-like 1; PDGFRA, platelet-derived growth factor receptor-alpha; HES, hypereosinophilic syndrome; M-HES, myeloproliferative variant of hypereosinophilic syndrome; CEL, chronic eosinophilic leukemia; L-HES, lymphoid variant of hypereosinophilic syndrome; IHES, idiopathic hypereosinophilic syndrome.

*Four or more of the following: dysplastic eosinophils, serum B12 greater than 737.8 pM (1,000 pg/mL), serum tryptase greater than 12 ng/mL, anemia and/or thrombocytopenia, splenomegaly, bone marrow cellularity greater than 80%, myelofibrosis, spindle-shaped mast cell greater than 25%.

Figure 9-3 Treatment-based approach to the patient with presumed hypereosinophilic syndrome.

marker of disease activity in these patients.[77] Compared to corticosteroid non-responders, patients showing response to corticosteroids has higher levels of serum TARC. Additionally, significantly elevated levels of serum TARC (>10,000 pg/mL) were only observed in the group of patients who responded to corticosteroids. This data suggests that corticosteroids may have greater benefit in patients with more severe disease. In patients with L-HES, corticosteroids remain first-line treatment for symptomatic patients.[66] Of note, high-dose steroids administered to a patient with occult strongyloides infection places them at risk for hyperinfection syndrome. For this reason, ivermectin (200 µg/kg on 2 consecutive days) should be administered with corticosteroids to any patient with a history of travel to endemic areas.[78]

Due to the side effects of long-term corticosteroid use, cytoreductive therapy with corticosteroid-sparing treatments, such as hydroxyurea and IFN-α are warranted in patients with return of symptoms or organ damage, or in patients requiring maintenance prednisone doses greater than 10 mg/day.[66,73,78] A retrospective analysis revealed that patients requiring therapy with either hydroxyurea or IFN-α, in addition to steroids, achieved response rates of 69% and 75%, respectively.[75] The median maximum dose of hydroxyurea in this study was 1 g/day. A single-center prospective study was able to achieve higher response rates with increased doses of hydroxyurea (2 g/day) combined with corticosteroids.[79] Unfortunately, the therapeutic effect of hydroxyurea may be delayed by at least 2 weeks, thus precluding its utility in the acute setting.

Interferon-α is an immunomodulatory agent that seems to work through a variety of mechanisms including reducing Th2-mediated IL-5 production, reducing the synthesis of GM-CSF, impairing release of eosinophil neurotoxin and cationic protein, as well as by indirectly inhibiting eosinophil differentiation.[80-82] It has been shown to be effective as monotherapy with long-term results,[74,83,84] and because of its effects on both eosinophils and T cells, it can potentially be used in all FIP1L1/PDGFRA-negative disease variants.[73,85] As such, it is the primary corticosteroid-sparing agent of choice for patients with L-HES.[66] In the previously described large retrospective analysis of therapies, 25% of the patients were treated with IFN-α.[75] The median maximum dose was 14 million units per week, with a range of 3–40 million units per week. Twenty-six percent of these patients were treated with IFN-α as monotherapy. Among these, 17% achieved complete response after 1 month of therapy, and 33% achieved a partial response. Unfortunately, 88% of these patients were forced to discontinue therapy, most commonly (50%) due to side effects. Despite the fact that resistance to IFN-α does not typically occur and doses can be tapered over time, its side-effect profile appears to be its most limiting factor. In a majority of patients, a flu-like syndrome occurs within 1–2 hours of administration, may last up to 24 hours, and may be dose-limiting; however, this may be avoided by initial slow uptitration of the dose.[73] Subacute and chronic side effects, if present, usually develop after 2–4 weeks and include, but are not limited to severe depression, suicidal ideation, fatigue, myalgia, induction of autoantibodies, or exacerbation of autoimmune disease (including autoimmune thyroiditis and psoriasis), myelosuppression, and transaminitis. Fortunately, the relatively recent introduction of pegylated-IFN-α has allowed for once weekly injections, which have been shown to be equally effective, with perhaps fewer side effects.[73,80]

Other agents have been used for the treatment of HES; however, the data supporting their use is scant. Vincristine alone or in combination with either 6-thioguanine or mercaptopurine was reported to induce responses in case reports.[86] 2-chlorodeoxyadenosine, alone or in combination with cytarabine, has been shown to have activity in HES.[87,88] Jabbour et al. treated nine patients with the combination and achieved complete remission in 55% of the patients, with a median disease-free survival of 26 months. Of the four subjects who did not achieve complete remission, three had progression of disease and one showed no change. Cyclosporine was used in 6/188 patients in the large retrospective study performed by Ogbogu.[75] One patient achieved complete response and two patients achieved partial response; unfortunately, 82% of the patients discontinued therapy secondary to medication intolerance. Another study evaluated the use of methotrexate and cyclophosphamide in patients with idiopathic eosinophilia and clonal T cells.[89] Of the patients studied, one received methotrexate and one received cyclophosphamide. Both patients achieved complete clinical remission within 3 months; however, their T cell clones remained present. In summary, these alternative treatment strategies cannot be uniformly recommended, as they have been used with varied success in a limited number of patients.

Myeloid and lymphoid neoplasms with eosinophilia and abnormalities of PDGFRA, PDGFRB, or FGFR1 have been shown to respond to imatinib,[70,71,90] and molecular remission in patients with FIP1L1/PDGFRA gene rearrangements has been achieved.[91] Because of this responsiveness, imatinib is used as the first-line treatment of choice in patients with these gene rearrangements, regardless of their clinical severity.[66,72,73] However, if cardiac involvement is present, concomitant corticosteroids should be administered as outlined above to prevent acute myocarditis.[63,78] The optimal dose of imatinib varies from patient to patient, and the range needed to achieve remission has been reported at 100–600 mg daily.[92] Imatinib therapy should be continued indefinitely[73] due to the observed molecular relapse with therapy withdrawal.[93] Additionally, secondary resistance to imatinib has been reported in patients with a T6741I mutation in the adenosine triphosphate (ATP)-binding domain of PDGFRA.[5] In these instances, other tyrosine kinase inhibitors, such as nilotinib and sorafenib have been shown to be of use.[94,95] Finally, the efficacy of imatinib seems to be limited to patients with abnormalities of PDGFRA, PDGFRB, or FGFR1 as patients without these gene rearrangements showed no long-term benefit.[90]

Initial studies utilizing mepolizumab, a monoclonal anti-IL-5 antibody, in the treatment of refractory HES provided promising results.[96,97] It was later shown to be effective as a corticosteroid-sparing agent in HES patients lacking PDGRFA/FIP1L1 gene rearrangements.[98] In this international, randomized, double-blind, placebo-controlled trial, 85 patients previously maintained on prednisone single-agent therapy with doses ranging from 20–60 mg daily were administered mepolizumab 750 mg IV every 4 weeks versus placebo while tapering down the corticosteroid dose. The study's primary endpoint of decreasing the daily prednisone requirement to less than 10 mg for at least 8 consecutive weeks was achieved in 84% of the treatment arm and 43% of the placebo group. Additionally, of the patients in the treatment arm, 95% were able to maintain absolute eosinophil counts of less than $0.6 \times 10^9/L$ for at least 8 consecutive weeks, and 56% were tapered completely off of prednisone. The time to treatment failure was significantly shorter in the placebo group, with 69% of the placebo group and 21% on the treatment group failing therapy. Finally, the results suggested increased responsiveness to mepolizumab in patients with more severe disease (patients requiring greater than 30 mg prednisone at the start of the trial). A subsequent study of mepolizumab on L-HES patients also showed similar results.[99] Utilizing the same inclusion and primary end-point criteria, patients with L-HES on the treatment arm compared with L-HES patients in the placebo group were significantly more likely to achieve the endpoint. However, compared to 100% of patients on the treatment arm without L-HES, only 71% of L-HES patients receiving mepolizumab were able to maintain an eosinophil count less than $0.6 \times 10^9/L$ for the duration of the trial, suggesting incomplete control. These studies are currently the only available to evaluate the safety of mepolizumab in HES and L-HES patients. In the study performed by Rothenberg et al., adverse events occurred in 16 of the 43 patients in the treatment arm. Serious adverse events included asthma, HES flare, pneumonia, renal failure, bronchitis, cardiac arrest, dehydration, hepatitis, pancreatitis, pyrexia, rhinitis resulting in hospitalization, and spinal compression fracture, though the investigators felt that none of these were related to the study drug. The one death occurring in the treatment arm was secondary to cardiac arrest; however, this patient had a cardiac history, and the death was thought to be secondary to implantable cardioverter-defibrillator (ICD) failure. Based on these studies, it appears as though mepolizumab is well-tolerated; however, further studies evaluating its safety are needed. As a result, its use is currently limited to a compassionate use trial for patients with life-threatening disease refractory to other therapies.[100]

Alemtuzumab, an anti-CD52 monoclonal antibody targets the surface CD52 glycoprotein on lymphocytes and eosinophils and has shown promising results in patients with HES refractory to other therapies.[101-103] The study performed by Verstovsek was enrolled 11 patients.[103] Initial administered doses of 5 mg IV were titrated up to 10 mg and 30 mg IV daily on days 2 and 3, respectively, in the absence of grade 3 or 4 toxicity. If tolerated, the dose was maintained and given three times per week for a total of 12 weeks. Thereafter, the dosage interval was decreased to once weekly. In the presence of a partial response, further doses were administered three times a week for an additional 4 weeks. Ninety-one percent of the study patients achieved complete hematologic response at 2 weeks. Of these responders, 70% relapsed; however, relapse occurred after discontinuation of the drug, suggesting the necessity of maintenance therapy. The most common adverse reaction in the study was secondary to complications of chronic immunosuppression; cytomegalovirus reactivation occurred in 18% and was effectively controlled with initiation of antiviral therapy.

The role of transplant among patients with HES is incompletely understood. Allogeneic stem cell transplant may be most effective among patients with L-HES and imatinib-resistant patients with PDGFRA-FIP1L1 associated disease who fail all other available treatments.[73,104,105] Its efficacy among other treatment-refractory patients with HES is not well described and may improve with alternative conditioning strategies.

REFERENCES

1. Loeffler W. Zur differential-Diagnose der Lundeninfiltrierundgen, uber fluchtige Succedean-Infiltrate (mit Eosinophilie). *Beitr Z Klin Tuberk.* 1932;79:368.
2. Harkavy J. Vascular allergy. *Clinics.* 1946;5(2):504-49.
3. Churg J, Strauss L. Allergic granulomatosis, allergic angiitis, and periarteritis nodosa. *Am J Pathol.* 1951;27(2):277-301.
4. Hardy WR, Anderson RE. The hypereosinophilic syndromes. *Ann Intern Med.* 1968; 68(6): 1220-9.
5. Cools J, DeAngelo DJ, Gotlib J, et al. A tyrosine kinase created by fusion of the PDGFRA and FIP1L1 genes as a therapeutic target of imatinib in idiopathic hypereosinophilic syndrome. *N Engl J Med.* 2003;348(13):1201-14.
6. Bain BJ, Gilliland DG, Horny HP, et al. Myeloid and lymphoid neoplasms with eosinophilia and abnormalities of PDGFRA, PDGFRB, or FGFR1. In: Swerdlow SH, Campo E, Harris NL, Jaffe ES, Pileri SA, Stein H, Theile J, Vardiman JW (Eds). WHO Classification of Tumours. Pathology and Genetics of Tumours of Haematopoietic and Lymphoid Tissues. Lyon, France: IARC Press; 2008. pp. 68-73.
7. Crane MM, Chang CM, Kobayashi MG, et al. Incidence of myeloproliferative hypereosinophilic syndrome in the United States and an estimate of all hypereosinophilic syndrome incidence. *J Allergy Clin Immunol.* 2010;126:179-80.
8. Boyce JA, Friend D, Matsumoto R, et al. Differentiation in vitro of hybrid eosinophil/ basophil granulocytes: autocrine function of an eosinophil developmental intermediate. *J Exp Med.* 1995;182(1):49-57.
9. Nerlov C, McNagny KM, Doderlein G, et al. Distinct C/EBP functions are required for eosinophil lineage commitment and maturation. *Genes Dev.* 1998;12(15):2413-23.
10. Nerlov C, Graf T. PU.1 induces myeloid lineage commitment in multipotent hematopoietic progenitors. *Genes Dev.* 1998;12(15):2403-12.
11. Hirasawa R, Shimizu R, Takahashi S, et al. Essential and instructive roles of GATA factors in eosinophil development. *J Exp Med.* 2002;195(11):1379-86.
12. Zhang DE, Zhang P, Wang ND, et al. Absence of granulocyte colony-stimulating factor signaling and neutrophil development in CCAAT enhancer binding protein alpha-deficient mice. *Proc Natl Acad Sci USA.* 1997;94(2):569-74.
13. Hogan SP, Rosenberg HF, Moqbel R, et al. Eosinophils: biological properties and role in health and disease. *Clin Exp Allergy.* 2008;38(5):709-50.
14. Stone KD, Prussin C, Metcalfe DD. IgE, mast cells, basophils, and eosinophils. *J Allergy Clin Immunol.* 2010;125(2 Suppl 2):S73-80.

15. Mazza JJ. Manual of Clinical Hematology, 3rd edition. Philadelphia, PA, USA: Lippincott Williams & Wilkins; 2001.
16. Kay AB, Klion AD. Anti-interleukin-5 therapy for asthma and hypereosinophilic syndrome. *Immunol Allergy Clin North Am.* 2004;24(4):645-66.
17. Menzies-Gow A, Flood-Page P, Sehmi R, et al. Anti-IL-5 (mepolizumab) therapy induces bone marrow eosinophil maturational arrest and decreases eosinophil progenitors in the bronchial mucosa of atopic asthmatics. *J Allergy Clin Immunol.* 2003;111(4):714-9.
18. Dent LA, Strath M, Mellor AL, et al. Eosinophilia in transgenic mice expressing interleukin 5. *J Exp Med.* 1990;172(5):1425-31.
19. Tominaga A, Takaki S, Koyama N, et al. Transgenic mice expressing a B cell growth and differentiation factor gene (interleukin 5) develop eosinophilia and autoantibody production. *J Exp Med.* 1991;173(2):429-37.
20. Amin K, Rinne J, Haahtela T, et al. Inflammatory cell and epithelial characteristics of perennial allergic and nonallergic rhinitis with a symptom history of 1 to 3 years' duration. *J Allergy Clin Immunol.* 2001;107(2):249-57.
21. Amin K, Ludviksdottir D, Janson C, et al. Inflammation and structural changes in the airways of patients with atopic and nonatopic asthma. BHR Group. *Am J Respir Crit Care Med.* 2000;162(6):2295-301.
22. Kato M, Kephart GM, Talley NJ, et al. Eosinophil infiltration and degranulation in normal human tissue. *Anat Rec.* 1998;252(3):418-25.
23. Press MF, King WJ. Distribution of peroxidase and granulocytes in the human uterus. *Lab Invest.* 1986;54(2):188-203.
24. Leiferman KM, Peters MS, Gleich GJ. The eosinophil and cutaneous edema. *J Am Acad Dermatol.* 1986;15(3):513-7.
25. Muller E. Localization of eosinophils in the thymus by the peroxidase reaction. *Histochemistry.* 1977;52(3):273-9.
26. Rothenberg ME. Mechanisms of disease: eosinophilia. *New Engl J Med.* 1998;338(22):1592-600.
27. Greer JP, Foerster J, Rodgers GM, Paraskevas F, Glader B, Arber DA, Means RT (Eds). Wintrobe's Clinical Hematology, 12th edition. Philadelphia, PA, USA: Lippincott Williams & Wilkins; 2008.
28. DiScipio RG, Schraufstatter IU. The role of the complement anaphylatoxins in the recruitment of eosinophils. *Int Immunopharmacol.* 2007;7(14):1909-23.
29. Wickham TJ. Adhesion molecules: integrins. In: Crystal RG, West JB, Barnes PJ, Weibel ER, editors. The Lung: Scientific Foundations, 2nd subedition. Philadelphia, PA, USA: Lippincott Williams & Wilkins; 1997. pp. 201-14.
30. Kitayama J, Fuhlbrigge RC, Puri KD, et al. P-selectin, L-selectin, and alpha 4 integrin have distinct roles in eosinophil tethering and arrest on vascular endothelial cells under physiological flow conditions. *J Immunol.* 1997;159(8):3929-39.
31. Alon R, Kassner PD, Carr MW, et al. The integrin VLA-4 supports tethering and rolling in flow on VCAM-1. *J Cell Biol.* 1995;128(6):1243-53.
32. Patel KD, McEver RP. Comparison of tethering and rolling of eosinophils and neutrophils through selectins and P-selectin glycoprotein ligand-1. *J Immunol.* 1997;159(9):4555-65.
33. Knol EF, Tackey F, Tedder TF, et al. Comparison of human eosinophil and neutrophil adhesion to endothelial cells under nonstatic conditions. Role of L-selectin. *J Immunol.* 1994;153(5):2161-7.
34. Elices MJ, Osborn L, Takada Y, et al. VCAM-1 on activated endothelium interacts with the leukocyte integrin VLA-4 at a site distinct from the VLA-4/fibronectin binding site. *Cell.* 1990;60(4):577-84.
35. Woltmann G, McNulty CA, Dewson G, et al. Interleukin-13 induces PSGL-1/P-selectin dependent adhesion of eosinophils, but not neutrophils, to human umbilical vein endothelial cells under flow. *Blood.* 2000;95(1):3146-52.

36. Sano H, Nakagawa N, Nakajima H, et al. Role of vascular cell adhesion molecule-1 and platelet-activating factor in selective eosinophil migration across vascular endothelial cells. *Int Arch Allergy Immunol.* 1995;107(4):533-40.
37. Schleimer RP, Sterbinsky SA, Kaiser J, et al. IL-4 induces adherence of human eosinophils and basophils but not neutrophils to endothelium: association with expression of VCAM-1. *J Immunol.* 1992;148(4):1086-92.
38. Bochner BS, Klunk DA, Sterbinsky SA, et al. IL-13 selectively induces vascular cell adhesion molecule-1 expression in human endothelial cells. *J Immunol.* 1995;154(2):799-803.
39. MacPherson JC, Comhair SA, Erzurum SC, et al. Eosinophils are a major source of nitric oxide-derived oxidants in severe asthma: characterization of pathways available to eosinophils for generating reactive nitrogen species. *J Immunol.* 2001;166(9):5763-72.
40. Schraufstatter IU, Trieu K, Sikora L, et al. Complement C3a and C5a induce different signal transduction cascades in endothelial cells. J Immunol. 2002;169(4):2102-10.
41. Denis M. Human monocytes/macrophages: NO or no NO. *J Leukoc Biol.* 1994;55(5):682-4.
42. Okada S, Kita H, George TJ, et al. Migration of eosinophils through basement membrane components in vitro: role of matrix metalloproteinase-9. *Am J Respir Cell Mol Biol.* 1997;17(4):519-28.
43. Fujisawa T, Kato Y, Terada A, et al. Matrix metalloproteinase-9 in peripheral blood eosinophils. *Int Arch Allergy Immunol.* 1999;120(Suppl 1):65-9.
44. Bystrom J, Amin K, Bishop-Bailey D. Analysing the eosinophil cationic protein--a clue to the function of the eosinophil granulocyte. *Respir Res.* 2011;12:10.
45. Neves JS, Weller PF. Functional extracellular eosinophil granules: novel implications in eosinophil immunobiology. *Curr Opin Immunol.* 2009;21(6):694-9.
46. Akuthota P, Xenakis JJ, Weller PF. Eosinophils: offenders or general bystanders in allergic airway disease and pulmonary immunity? *J Innate Immun.* 2011;3(2):113-9.
47. Butterworth AE. Cell-mediated damage to helminths. *Adv Parasitol.* 1984;23:143-235.
48. Lehrer RI, Szklarek D, Barton A, et al. Antibacterial properties of eosinophil major basic protein and eosinophil cationic protein. *J Immunol.* 1989;142(12):4428-34.
49. Hisamatsu K, Ganbo T, Nakazawa T, et al. Cytotoxicity of human eosinophil granule major basic protein to human nasal sinus mucosa in vitro. *J Allergy Clin Immunol.* 1990;86(1):52-63.
50. Slifman NR, Loegering DA, McKean DJ, et al. Ribonuclease activity associated with human eosinophil-derived neurotoxin and eosinophil cationic protein. *J Immunol.* 1986;137(9):2913-7.
51. Gleich GJ, Loegering DA, Bell MP, et al. Biochemical and functional similarities between human eosinophil-derived neurotoxin and eosinophil cationic protein: homology with ribonuclease. *Proc Natl Acad Sci USA.* 1986;83(10):3146-50.
52. Young JD, Peterson CG, Venge P, et al. Mechanism of membrane damage mediated by human eosinophil cationic protein. *Nature.* 1986;321(6070):613-6.
53. Rosenberg HF, Domachowske JB. Eosinophils, eosinophil ribonucleases, and their role in host defense against respiratory virus pathogens. *J Leukoc Biol.* 2001;70(5):691-8.
54. Weiss SJ, Test ST, Eckmann CM, et al. Brominating oxidants generated by human eosinophils. *Science.* 1986;234(4773):200-3.
55. Mayeno AN, Curran AJ, Roberts RL, et al. Eosinophils preferentially use bromide to generate halogenating agents. *J Biol Chem.* 1989;264(10):5660-8.
56. Thomas EL, Bozeman PM, Jefferson MM, et al. Oxidation of bromide by the human leukocyte enzymes myeloperoxidase and eosinophil peroxidase. Formation of bromamines. *J Biol Chem.* 1995;270:2906-13.
57. Lacy P, Moqbel R. Eosinophil cytokines. *Chem Immunol.* 2000;76:134-55.
58. Akuthota P, Wang H, Weller PF. Eosinophils as antigen-presenting cells in allergic upper airway disease. *Curr Opin Allergy Clin Immunol.* 2010;10:14-9.
59. Shi HZ, Humbles A, Gerard C, et al. Lymph node trafficking and antigen presentation by endobronchial eosinophils. *J Clin Invest.* 2000;105:945-53.

60. Sedgwick JB, Calhoun WJ, Vrtis RF, et al. Comparison of airway and blood eosinophil function after in vivo antigen challenge. *J Immunol.* 1992;149:3710-8.
61. Hansel TT, Braunstein JB, Walker C, et al. Sputum eosinophils from asthmatics express ICAM-1 and HLA-DR. *Clin Exp Immunol.* 1991;86:271-7.
62. Mawhorter SD, Pearlman E, Kazura JW, et al. Class II major histocompatibility complex molecule expression on murine eosinophils activated in vivo by Brugia malayi. *Infect Immun.* 1993;61:5410-2.
63. Tefferi A, Gotlib J, Pardanani A. Hypereosinophilic syndrome and clonal eosinophilia: point-of-care diagnostic algorithm and treatment update. *Mayo Clin Proc.* 2010;85:158-64.
64. Valent P, Klion AD, Horny HP, et al. Contemporary consensus proposal on criteria and classification of eosinophilic disorders and related syndromes. *J Allergy Clin Immunol.* 2012;130(3):607-12.
65. Valent P, Gleich G, Reiter A, et al. Pathogenesis and classification of eosinophil disorders: a review of recent developments in the field. *Expert Rev. Hematology.* 2012;5(2):157-76.
66. Gotlib J. World Health Organization-defined eosinophilic disorders: 2011 update on diagnosis, risk stratification, and management. *Am J Hematol.* 2011;86:677-88.
67. Pardanani A, Tefferi A. Primary eosinophilic disorders: a concise review. *Curr Hematol Malig Rep.* 2008;3(1):37-43.
68. Tefferi A, Thiele J, Vardiman JW. The 2008 World Health Organization classification system for myeloproliferative neoplasms. *Cancer.* 2009;115:3842-7.
69. Fukushima K, Matsumura I, Ezoe S, et al. FIP1L1-PDGFRalpha imposes eosinophil lineage commitment on hematopoietic stem/progenitor cells. *J Biol Chem.* 2009;284:7719-32.
70. Pardanani A, Brockman SR, Paternoster SF, et al. FIP1L1-PDGFRA fusion: prevalence and clinicopathologic correlates in 89 consecutive patients with moderate to severe eosinophilia. *Blood.* 2004;104(10):3038-45.
71. Apperley JF, Gardembas M, Melo JV, et al. Response to imatinib mesylate in patients with chronic myeloproliferative diseases with rearrangements of the platelet-derived growth factor receptor beta. *N Engl J Med.* 2002;347:481-7.
72. Klion AD. How I treat hypereosinophilic syndromes. *Blood.* 2009;114:3736-41.
73. Cogan E, Roufosse F. Clinical management of the hypereosinophilic syndromes. *Expert Rev Hematology.* 2012;5(3):275-90.
74. Ogbogu PU, Bochner BS, Butterfield JH, et al. Hypereosinophilic syndrome: a multicenter, retrospective analysis of clinical characteristics and response to therapy. *J Allergy Clin Immunol.* 2009;124(6):1319.
75. Yoon TY, Ahn GB, Chang SH. Complete remission of hypereosinophilic syndrome after interferon-alpha therapy: Report of a case and literature review. *J Dermatol.* 2000;27:110-5.
76. Wirnsberger G, Hebenstreit D, Posselt G, et al. IL-4 induces expression of TARC/CCL17 via two STAT6 binding sites. *Eur J Immunol.* 2006;36(7):1882-91.
77. De Lavareille A, Roufosse F, Schmid-Grendelmeier P, et al. High serum thymus and activation-regulated chemokine levels in the lymphocytic variant of the hypereosinophilic syndrome. *J Allergy Clin Immunol.* 2002;110(3):476-9.
78. Roufosse F, Weller PF. Practical approach to the patient with hypereosinophilia. *J Allergy Clin Immunol.* 2010;126:39-44.
79. Schöffski P, Ganser A, Pascheberg U, et al. Complete haematological and cytogenetic response to interferon alpha-2a of a myeloproliferative disorder with eosinophilia associated with a unique t(4;7) aberration. *Ann Hematol.* 2000;79(2):95-8.
80. Butterfield JH. Interferon treatment for hypereosinophilic syndromes and systemic mastocytosis. *Acta Haematol.* 2005;114(1):26-40.
81. Zella D, Romerio F, Curreli S, et al. IFN-α2b reduces IL-2 production and IL-2 receptor function in primary CD4+ T cells. *J Immunol.* 2000;164:2296-302.
82. Schandene L, Del Prete GF, Cogan E, et al. Recombinant interferon-alpha selectively inhibits the production of interleukin-5 by human CD4+ T cells. *J Clin Invest.* 1996;97:309-15.

83. Ceretelli S, Capochiani E, Petrini M. Interferon-alpha in the idiopathic hypereosinophilic syndrome: consideration of five cases. *Ann Hematol.* 1998;77:161-4.
84. Butterfield JH, Gleich GJ. Response of six patients idiopathic hypereosinophilic syndrome to interferon alfa. *J Allergy Clin Immunol.* 1994;94(6):1318-25.
85. Butterfield JH. Treatment of hypereosinophilic syndromes with prednisone, hydroxyurea, and interferon. *Immunol Allergy Clin North Am.* 2007;27(3):493-518.
86. Sakamoto K, Erdreich-Epstein A, deClerck Y, et al. Prolonged clinical response to vincristine treatment in two patients with idiopathic hypereosinophilic syndrome. *Am J Pediatr Hematol Oncol.* 1992;14:348-51.
87. Jabbour E, Verstovsek S, Giles F, et al. 2-Chlorodeoxyadenosine and cytarabine combination therapy for idiopathic hypereosinophilic syndrome. *Cancer.* 2005;104(3):541-6.
88. Ueno NT, Zhao S, Robertson LE, et al. 2-Chlorodeoxyadenosine therapy for idiopathic hypereosinophilic syndrome. *Leukemia.* 1997;11:1386-90.
89. Vaklavas C, Tefferi A, Butterfield J, et al. 'Idiopathic' eosinophilia with an Occult T-cell clone: prevalence and clinical course. *Leuk Res.* 2007;31(5):691-4.
90. Baccarani M, Cilloni D, Rondoni M, et al. The efficacy of imatinib mesylate in patients with FIP1 L1-PDGFRalpha-positive hypereosinophilic syndrome. Results of a multicenter prospective study. *Haematologica.* 2007;92(9):1173.
91. Klion AD, Robyn J, Akin C, et al. Molecular remission and reversal of myelofibrosis in response to imatinib mesylate treatment in patients with the myeloproliferative variant of hypereosinophilic syndrome. *Blood.* 2004;103(2):473-8.
92. Musto P, Falcone A, Sanpaolo G, et al. Heterogeneity of response to imatinib-mesylate (glivec) in patients with hypereosinophilic syndrome: implications for dosing and pathogenesis. *Leuk Lymphoma.* 2004;45:1219-22.
93. Klion AD, Robyn J, Maric I, et al. Relapse following discontinuation of imatinib mesylate therapy for FIP1L1/PDGFRA-positive chronic eosinophilic leukemia: implications for optimal dosing. *Blood.* 2007;110:3552-6.
94. Lierman E, Folens C, Stover EH, et al. Sorafenib is a potent inhibitor of FIP1L1-PDGFRalpha and the imatinib-resistant FIP1L1-PDGFRalpha T674I mutant. *Blood.* 2006;108:1374-6.
95. Stover EH, Chen J, Lee BH, et al. The small molecule tyrosine kinase inhibitor AMN107 inhibits TEL-PDGFRbeta and FIP1 L1-PDGF Ralpha in vitro and in vivo. *Blood.* 2005; 106(9):3206-13.
96. Koury MJ, Newman JH, Murray JJ. Reversal of hypereosinophilic syndrome and lymphomatoid papulosis with mepolizumab and imatinib. *Am J Med.* 2003;115:587-9.
97. Garrett JK, Jameson SC, Thomson B, et al. Anti-interleukin-5 (mepolizumab) therapy for hypereosinophilic syndromes. *J Allergy Clin Immunol.* 2004;113:115-9.
98. Rothenberg ME, Klion AD, Roufosse FE, et al. Treatment of patients with the hypereosinophilic syndrome with mepolizumab. *N Engl J Med.* 2008;358:1215-28.
99. Roufosse F, de Lavareille A, Schandené L, et al. Mepolizumab as a corticosteroid-sparing agent in lymphocytic variant hypereosinophilic syndrome. *J Allergy Clin Immunol.* 2010; 126:828-35.
100. Mepolizumab: 240563, anti-IL-5 monoclonal antibody-GlaxoSmithKline, anti-interleukin-5 monoclonal antibody - GlaxoSmithKline, SB 240563. *Drugs R D.* 2008;9(2):125-30.
101. Pitini V, Teti D, Arrigo C, et al. Alemtuzumab therapy for refractory idiopathic hypereosinophilic syndrome with abnormal T cells: a case report. *Br J Haematol.* 2004;127(5):477.
102. Sefcick A, Sowter D, DasGupta E, et al. Alemtuzumab therapy for refractory idiopathic hypereosinophilic syndrome. *Br J Haematol.* 2004;124(4):558-9.
103. Verstovsek S, Tefferi A, Kantarjian H, et al. Alemtuzumab therapy for hypereosinophilic syndrome and chronic eosinophilic leukemia. *Clin Cancer Res.* 2009;15(1):368-73.
104. Esteva-Lorenzo FJ, Meehan KR, Spitzer TR, et al. Allogeneic bone marrow transplantation in a patient with hypereosinophilic syndrome. *Am J Hematol.* 1996;51:164-5.
105. Halaburda K, Prejzner W, Szatkowski D, et al. Allogeneic bone marrow transplantation for hypereosinophilic syndrome: long-term follow-up with eradication of FIP1L1-PDGFRA fusion transcript. *Bone Marrow Transplant.* 2006;38:319-20.

CHAPTER

10 Mast Cell Diseases/Systemic Mastocytosis

Mahboobeh Mahdavinia, Anne M Ditto

INTRODUCTION

Mast cells (MCs) play a major role in the pathogenesis of a variety of diseases, with a dominant role in allergic conditions such as asthma, atopic dermatitis, urticaria, and anaphylaxis. MCs are tissue dependent cells, found throughout the body in tissues, such as the skin, gastrointestinal (GI) tract, mucosal surfaces of the upper and lower airway, and bone marrow. When activated, either spontaneously or after various stimuli, MCs release multiple mediators, resulting in a variety of symptoms depending on the organ(s) affected. Systemic mastocytosis (SM) is a rare neoplastic disease involving both MCs and their marrow-derived myelomastocytic progenitor cells. Various clinical and biological features characterize this heterogeneous disease. The symptoms of SM tend to be generalized, due to the systemic release of biologic mediators, and include generalized pruritus, flushing, diarrhea, asthma, anaphylaxis including cardiovascular collapse, and even neuropsychiatric symptoms. Furthermore, pathologic infiltration and clustering of MCs in tissues can cause tissue specific presentations, such as urticaria pigmentosa (UP), bone marrow invasion, hepatosplenomegaly, osteosclerosis, as well as GI and cardiopulmonary manifestations.[1,2] The symptoms of mastocytosis might be confused with multiple other immunologic, allergic, rheumatologic, or endocrine diseases, and it is of utmost importance to think of possible underlying malignant MC disease in patients who experience any of the above symptoms like unexplained anaphylaxis, vascular instability, flushing, or diarrhea.[3] In this chapter, we aim to provide a summary of mastocytosis, its classification, diagnostic criteria, clinical and laboratory characteristics, and the available treatment options.

CLASSIFICATION

The classification of tumors of the hematopoietic and lymphoid tissues was published and revised last in 2008 by the World Health Organization (WHO) in collaboration with the Society for Hematopathology and the European Association of Hematopathology.[4] The WHO classification of mastocytosis, which is a part of this publication, is widely accepted and used to categorize mastocytosis into three major groups as detailed in box 10.1.[4,5]

Box 10-1 World Health Organization Classification of Mastocytosis[4]

- Cutaneous mastocytosis
- Systemic mastocytosis
  - Indolent systemic mastocytosis, includes smoldering systemic mastocytosis and isolated bone marrow mastocytosis
  - Systemic mastocytosis with associated hematologic non-mast cell clonal disease
  - Aggressive systemic mastocytosis
  - Mast cell leukemia
- Extracutaneous mast cell neoplasms

The first category is cutaneous mastocytosis (CM) which is a benign disease seen most commonly in the pediatric population. In CM, MC infiltration is confined to the skin and in most cases, regresses spontaneously. Therefore, no workup for systemic involvement is needed unless symptoms direct otherwise. However, adults with CM need to be monitored for systemic involvement. All adult patients and also all patients with unexplained organomegaly or evidence of other organ involvement, such as cytopenia need further work up. A bone marrow biopsy is strongly recommended in these cases to rule out SM.[6]

The second category is SM, which is seen mostly in adults and is further divided into four subtypes.[5] The first subtype is indolent systemic mastocytosis (ISM), which is the most common form of SM, and mainly involves the skin and bone marrow. The second subtype is SM with an associated non-mast cell, clonal, hematological disease (SM-AHNMD), with the most common associated hematological diseases being chronic myelomonocytic leukemia (CMML)[7] and hypereosinophilic syndrome (HES) carrying the fip1-like-1 platelet-derived growth factor receptor a (*FIPL1/PDGFRA*) hybrid gene.[8,9] The third subtype of SM is aggressive systemic mastocytosis (ASM). This subtype is characterized by multiple organ function impairment due to MC infiltration. These patients have markedly increased tryptase levels and present clinically with cytopenia, hepatosplenomegaly, pathologic fractures due to osteolysis, and severe GI symptoms, such as abdominal pain, vomiting, diarrhea, and malabsorption. The fourth subtype is mast cell leukemia (MCL), the least common variant of human leukemia and the most aggressive form of SM. MCL presents with rapidly progressive impairment in involved organs and a dense infiltration of the bone marrow of MCs with blast-like morphology, comprising almost 20% of the bone marrow as seen on aspiration.[3] Smoldering systemic mastocytosis (SSM) is considered an intermediate between ISM and ASM.[10] Patients with SSM tend to have a higher MC burden and organomegaly, but do not exhibit significant functional impairment.

The other category of mastocytosis is a localized extracutaneous MC neoplasm and is extremely rare. It either presents in a malignant form termed MC sarcoma, or as a benign tumor, termed an extracutaneous mastocytoma.

DIAGNOSTIC CRITERIA

The diagnosis of mastocytosis is made using widely accepted international criteria[5] that are based on histologic and molecular manifestations of mastocytosis, and include one major criterion and four minor criteria as detailed in box 10.2. To confirm the diagnosis of SM, one major and one minor criterion, or a minimum of three minor criteria need to be fulfilled.

CM is diagnosed based on the presence of mast cell infiltrates in a skin biopsy. For a diagnosis of SM, extracutaneous organs need to be involved.

The major criterion for SM is the histologic presence of compact focal MCs infiltrating more than one site in a tissue, termed a multifocal pattern. The main tissue in which SM is diagnosed is the bone marrow, but the presence of dense mast cell infiltrates in extramedullary tissues like the spleen, lymph nodes, or mucosa can also be indicative of the disease.[3] Of note, in most cases of intestinal or splenic mastocytosis, there is also bone marrow involvement but a more meticulous study of the bone marrow may be needed to reveal this.

Minor criteria include typical cytological characteristics of MCs and molecular markers including *Kit* D816V mutation, co-expression of Kit (CD117) with CD2, and/or CD25 as well as a serum total tryptase level of more than 20 ng/mL.[5]

Clinical manifestations of mastocytosis are called B and C findings, and are used to distinguish the different forms of SM. B findings refer to organomegaly including hepatosplenomegaly and/or lymphadenopathy. C findings are manifestations indicative of organ dysfunction caused by widespread mast cell infiltration, such as cytopenia due to diffuse infiltration of bone marrow in ASM or ascites secondary to severe liver infiltration. These findings are listed in box 10.3.

Box 10-2 International Criteria to Diagnose Mastocytosis[5]

Cutaneous mastocytosis: Typical skin lesions, typical clinical signs and positive histology

Systemic mast cell disease "Systematic mastocytosis criteria"

- Major criterion:
  - Multifocal dense mast cell infiltrates detected in bone marrow sections and/or other extracutaneous organ(s) by tryptase immunohistochemistry or other stain (Kit)
- Minor criteria:
  - In mast cell infiltrates detected in sections of bone marrow or other cutaneous organs, more than 25% of mast cells are spindle-shaped or in bone marrow spears, atypical mast cells comprise more than 25% of all mast cells
  - Detection of Kit point mutation at codon 816 in bone marrow, blood, or extracutaneous organ(s)
  - Mast cells in bone marrow coexpress CD117 and either CD2, CD25, or both as detected by flow cytometry
  - Serum total tryptase concentration persistently more than 20 ng/mL (invalid in case of an associated clonal hematological non-mast cell lineage disease)

Box 10-3 B and C Findings in Systemic Mastocytosis[71]

B findings: Indication of high mast cell burden and expansion of the genetic defect into various myeloid lineages

- Infiltration of mast cells in bone marrow more than 30% as seen on (>30% histology) and serum total tryptase levels less than 200 ng/mL
- Hypercellular bone marrow with loss of fat cells, discrete signs of dysmyelopoiesis without substantial cytopenias, or World Health Organization criteria for myelodysplastic syndrome or myeloproliferative disorder
- Organomegaly defined as palpable hepatomegaly, splenomegaly, or lymphadenopathy (>2 cm on computed tomography or ultrasound) without impaired organ function

C findings: Indication of impaired organ function because of mast cell infiltration (confirmed by biopsy in most patients)

- Cytopenia(s): Absolute neutrophil count less than 1.0×10^3/L, hemoglobin <10 g/dL, or platelets $<100 \times 10^5$/L
- Hepatomegaly with ascites and impaired liver function
- Palpable splenomegaly with hypersplenism
- Malabsorption with hypoalbuminemia and weight loss
- Skeletal lesions large-osteolyses or/and severe osteoporosis causing pathologic fractures
- Life-threatening organomegaly in other organ systems that is definitively caused by an infiltration of the tissue by mast cells.

CLINICAL MANIFESTATIONS

Patients with mastocytosis most commonly present with skin lesions, hepatosplenomegaly, GI symptoms, or symptoms from recurrent generalized mast cell degranulation, such as flushing, diarrhea, and anaphylaxis. We will focus on some of the more important clinical manifestations of mastocytosis.

Cutaneous Manifestations

The pathognomonic skin lesion, UP, is one of the major physical examination findings suggestive of mastocytosis. The rash consists of telangiectasic and hyperpigmented papules, and plaques measuring up to a few centimeters, and tends to involve mostly the trunk and extremities, sparing the sun-exposed areas, such as the face and hands.[6] A burning or itching sensation can be induced by stroking these skin lesions with resultant urtication of the lesion (Darier sign). Apart from CM, which is primarily a pediatric disease presenting with only UP, almost all adult patients with UP have evidence of systemic disease, with pathologic mast cell infiltration of the bone marrow and/or other organs. UP is seen in majority of SM cases but may be absent in the more advanced and aggressive categories of SM.

Mast Cell Mediator Release Associated Symptoms

As previously mentioned, systemic unloading of mast cell mediators can cause a variety of symptoms including episodic flushing, lightheadedness, syncope or near syncope, tachycardia, GI cramping, nausea, vomiting, and diarrhea. In SM, these episodes are usually recurrent and self-limited, lasting from a few minutes to several hours. Interestingly, recurrent angioedema and urticaria are not very common in any form of mastocytosis,[11,12] however, anaphylaxis can occur and SM should always be in the differential of idiopathic anaphylaxis (IA).[13,14]

Gastrointestinal Symptoms

Any part of the GI tract from the esophagus to the rectum can be involved in mastocytosis. GI manifestations of SM include abdominal pain, nausea, vomiting, diarrhea, and malabsorption. Abdominal pain is the most common GI symptom, reported in up to 50% of patients.[15,16] Diarrhea and nausea/vomiting occur in 30–40% of the cases and have a significant effect on a patient's quality of life.[11,15] In some studies, 25% of patients with mastocytosis were found to have peptic ulcer disease and GI bleeding was reported in up to 10% of patients.[17] Gastric lesions associated with mucosal and submucosal mast cell infiltrates have been reported in several studies.[15-17]

Bone Mineralization Abnormalities

Pathological changes in bones can be seen in all types of mastocytosis. The abnormalities of bone mineralization can cause persistent bone pain, bone sclerosis, osteoporosis, and pathological fractures. Skeletal lesions are found in 70–75% of SM cases, and are seen mostly at the ends of the long bones and the axial skeleton.[18] At times, pathological fractures or the incidental finding of sclerosis and osteoporosis on imaging are the initial presenting signs leading to the diagnosis.[19]

Hepatobiliary Manifestations

Hepatomegaly is an important finding in mastocytosis and is considered a B finding. A recent study reported hepatomegaly or morphological hepatic alterations in 34% of patients. In this study, 75% of patients had abnormally high cholesterol levels. Furthermore, elevations of liver transaminases and bilirubin were found in 36% and 40% of these patients, respectively.[20]

Neurologic and Psychiatric Symptoms

Neuropsychiatric symptoms have been reported in many patients with mastocytosis and are often significantly disabling.[21] A recent large retrospective cohort study of patients with mastocytosis showed that 35% of patients suffered from headache,[22] which was reported in as many as 69% of patients in other studies.[21] Syncope, another clinically significant symptom, has been reported in 5% of patients in one study with unexplained syncope preceding the formal diagnosis of mastocytosis in several cases.[22] Multiple neuropsychiatric symptoms including depression, anxiety, and memory loss have been reported in patients with mastocytosis.[23,24] Depression has been reported in as many as 50–70% of patients and memory loss in up to 66%.[22,23]

LABORATORY STUDIES

Tryptase Level

Elevated total serum tryptase is a well-established marker of SM. The tryptase level is in fact a marker of the total MC burden, and is on average about 5 ng/mL in healthy controls.[25] A level higher than 20 ng/mL is one of the minor criteria for the diagnosis of SM. The tryptase level is persistently elevated in most cases of SM as opposed to IA, where it is only elevated during an acute episode.[25,26]

Complete Blood Count

Although the complete blood count (CBC) is typically normal in the case of ISM, in ASM or AHNMD significant findings, such as cytopenia, leukocytosis, eosinophilia, basophilia, monocytosis, or circulating MCs are important clues to the diagnosis. Furthermore, in aggressive subtypes of SM it is common to see elevated lactate dehydrogenase (LDH) and liver enzymes, low albumin, and/or abnormal coagulation markers.[27,28]

Bone Marrow Biopsy

The bone marrow is the most frequently affected organ and thus is the preferred tissue for evaluation of SM. Typical lesions are multifocal mast cell collections of fifteen or more MCs, called multifocal dense mast cell infiltrations, and these are considered the major criterion in the diagnosis of mastocytosis. Sometimes, the MCs are scattered and no focal dense infiltration sites are found. In these cases, the diagnosis could be made based on morphologic features, such as spindle-shaped MCs, and the pathologist may need additional biopsy material.[3,29] In some subtypes of SM, such as in the leukemic variant, the normal marrow is replaced by MC infiltrates which have a diffuse and dense pattern.[29,30] These MCs may be extremely immature and hypogranulated, and therefore, hard to identify as MCs unless specifically stained for tryptase.[31]

Immunohistochemistry

Staining with antibodies against tryptase is a useful diagnostic tool to characterize and grade MC infiltration in lesions as all MCs express this marker regardless of their stage of maturation or tissue of localization.[31,32] For patients in whom the diagnostic criteria are not fulfilled based on histologic examination, additional disease-related markers, such as *Kit* mutation analysis and flow cytometry expression of CD25 or CD2 are suggested. Kit (CD117) is another marker that can be used to stain MCs as normal tissue MCs express considerable amounts of Kit (CD117) on their surface.[33] On the other hand, aberrant expression of CD25 and CD2 on MCs as detected by immunohistochemistry appears to be a reliable tool to detect abnormal MCs in SM.[34] Both these markers are absent in normal and reactive bone marrow MCs, and different studies have found aberrant expression of these markers on MCs in SM.[34] Both CD2 and CD25 can be detected by flow cytometry or immunohistochemistry.[34,35]

Other Tissue Biopsies

Splenomegaly with increased MCs in the splenic biopsy should lead to the suspicion of mastocytosis (SM) as the concentrations of MCs are normally very low in this organ.[36] In some organs, such as the GI tract, it is normal to see high concentrations of MCs; therefore, an increase of MC infiltrates is not always diagnostic of mastocytosis. However, regardless of the type of the tissue, the finding of a multifocal, dense, well-demarcated infiltrate of MCs is not normal in any tissue and thus, is the major diagnostic criterion for SM.

Molecular Studies

Kit Mutations

Kit (CD117) is a type III receptor tyrosine kinase, highly expressed by MCs and hematopoietic progenitor cells, and functionally necessary for normal MC development and hematopoiesis.[37] *Kit* D816V is a gain-of-function point mutation in the tyrosine kinase domain of Kit.[38] This mutation is found in the majority of cases of adult SM.[39] It results in ligand-independent activation of Kit signaling, causing uncontrolled proliferation of MCs and their resistance to apoptosis.[38,40] The *Kit* D816V mutation can be detected by polymerase chain reaction (PCR) techniques that are widely available and is now a target for newly developed therapies.

Fip1-like-1 Platelet-derived Growth Factor Receptor A Hybrid Gene

A subset of patients with SM present with blood or bone marrow eosinophilia. In these cases it is worthwhile to screen for *FIP1L1-PDGFRA* by either the fluorescence *in situ* hybridization or real time PCR method. The *FIP1L1-PDGFRA* oncogene results from a deletion in chromosome 4q12, leading to the constitutive activation of the *PDGFRA* kinase.[9,41] Checking for this mutation is important because of its therapeutic implications as these patients are responsive to the tyrosine kinase inhibitor imatinib.[42] Patients with MC hyperplasia who carry these gene rearrangements in *PDGFRA*/platelet-derived growth factor receptor-beta (*PDGFRB*) are classified as "myeloid or lymphoid neoplasms with eosinophilia and abnormalities of *PDGFRA, PDGFRB,* or *FGFR1*" per the WHO classification.[4]

DIFFERENTIAL DIAGNOSIS

The differential diagnosis for SM includes other diseases with increased MC burden such as mast cell hyperplasia, myelodysplastic mast cell syndrome, and acute myeloid leukemia (AML) with the expression of tryptase and/or the *Kit* mutation at codon 816. One must also consider diseases without MC proliferation but similar episodic symptoms of flushing, diarrhea or anaphylaxis, such as monoclonal mast cell activation syndrome (MMAS), mast cell activation syndrome (MCAS), IA, and carcinoid syndrome.

Mast cell hyperplasia is a condition with local or systemic increases in MCs, usually associated with an underlying process like malignancy or inflammation but without the typical mastocytosis skin lesions required to fulfill the criteria for the diagnosis of SM.[43] Myelodysplastic mast cell syndrome, which is also referred to as "mastocytic differentiation in myelogenous neoplasm other than mastocytosis," is characterized by an increase in very immature (blast-like) MCs in the bone marrow and/or peripheral blood with underlying myelodysplastic syndrome (MDS), myeloproliferative syndrome (MPS), or AML.[4] These patients also do not have the typical skin lesions of mastocytosis.

Tryptase staining or the 816 mutation in *Kit* can be seen in some AML patients. In this disease, maturation arrest in the bone marrow prevents differentiation of immature progenitors into MCs. They do not fulfill the necessary criteria for the diagnosis of mastocytosis but might have 2–3 of the minor criteria.[43]

Mast cell activation syndrome is characterized by episodes of hypotension, flushing, hives, abdominal pain, diarrhea, paresthesias, or cognitive dysfunction due to sudden unprovoked, synchronous mast cell mediator release in patients who have no evidence of mast cell proliferation.[44] The clonal markers of mast cell disease including the *Kit* mutation or aberrant CD25 expression (two of the minor criteria for SM) may be found in these patients thus categorizing them as MMAS,[45] but distinguishing them from SM based on the presence or absence of other WHO diagnostic criteria.[46,5] In these patients, histamine-induced symptoms usually respond to treatment with MC stabilizers and histamine receptor antagonists.[43]

Idiopathic anaphylaxis is another clinical entity that should be distinguished from SM. In patients with idiopathic anaphylaxis-generalized type (IA-G), the episodes may consist of angioedema, bronchospasm, urticaria, digestive symptoms, and cardiovascular collapse. These patients have no evidence of mast cell proliferation and the tryptase level is not chronically elevated, but is usually elevated during an acute event.[13,14] Unlike MMAS these patients have no clonal marker of mast cell disease.

Carcinoid syndrome is characterized by episodic symptoms of flushing, diarrhea, bronchospasm, and hemodynamic instability due to release of peptide mediators, such as serotonin and bradykinins produced by carcinoid tumors. Elevated urinary 5-hydroxyindoleacetic acid (5-HIAA) levels provide an indicator for this disease. Tryptase levels are normal in these patients.[47]

TREATMENT

The clinical outcome for patients with mastocytosis varies, depending on the severity of the disease. CM and ISM patients tend to remain in an indolent stage for many years, but those with ASM, SM-AHNMD, or MCL can have a progressive clinical course with life-threatening organ dysfunction. Therefore, treatment of SM needs to be decided on a patient by patient basis, based on the aggressiveness of the disease.

The prognosis of patients with ISM is usually favorable, with patients benefiting from anti-mediator drugs, such as anti-histamines, aspirin, and MC stabilizers, such as ketotifen and cromolyn sodium.[48-54] These drugs are used in a step-wise manner and individual drugs should be selected based on the symptoms and the organ(s) involved. Ketotifen is recommended for patients who have bone pain and/or flushing,[50,53] H2 blockers and proton-pump inhibitors for patients with gastric ulcers[50] and aspirin for patients with flushing and tachycardia.[54] Low-dose corticosteroids including budesonide respules taken orally have been effective in the treatment of abdominal pain crises, malabsorption and diarrhea.[15,55] Cytoreductive biologic agents, such as interferon alpha (IFN-α) are indicated in patients with severe osteoporosis or in patients who continue to have a poor quality of life despite symptom-directed therapy.[56,57] Cutaneous lesions may be treated with psoralen and ultraviolet A photo chemotherapy (PUVA) or local corticosteroids, but the response is transient in most cases.[58,59]

In contrast to ISM, ASM patients have a poor prognosis and quality of life. These patients need to be treated with cytoreductive therapy, such as IFN-a with or without corticosteroids,[60,61] cladribine (2-chlorodeoxyadenosine),[62] or imatinib.[63-65] However, not all patients with ASM respond to these treatments, and long-lasting remission is hard to achieve. Cladribine and IFN-α have been shown to be the most effective drugs.[66,67] Imatinib is an effective therapy in patients with mastocytosis and eosinophilia associated with *FIP1L1/PDGFRA* mutation and in patients with SM who carry *Kit* mutations outside of exon 17 but not in patients with the D816V mutation.[65] Hematopoietic stem cell transplantation has been tried in ASM and has resulted in only a transient remission.[68] Patients with SSM may also benefit from biologic cytoreductive therapy with IFN-α.[43]

There is no known curative therapy for MCL. These patients mostly present with rapid onset of disease and a high MC burden. They have been traditionally treated with a trial of experimental chemotherapy regimens similar to AML or bone marrow transplantation[43,48] but unfortunately there is not enough data on the response of MCL in these high-risk therapies.

In patients with SM-AHNMD, separate treatment plans for SM and AHNMD need to be established with the main focus on the associated hematologic disease.[48,69] The AHNMD component could be managed with the standard guidelines for the hematologic disease, the same as patients who do not have MC disease and they should also be treated with IFN-α (with or without corticosteroids) or cladribine depending on the severity of the disease and the MC burden. Splenectomy may be considered in patients with significant splenomegaly and hypersplenism.[70]

Several new biologic agents are currently under investigation for the treatment of SM, with most of these agents targeting the active *Kit* D816V mutant tyrosine kinase. As mentioned previously this mutation leads to constitutively active Kit receptor, which plays a central role in the pathogenesis of SM. These biologic markers are designed to inhibit the phosphorylation of Kit and its downstream targets Akt and STAT3. Some of these new drugs including midostaurin are being evaluated in clinical trials.[48,65,71-74]

REFERENCES

1. Valent P, Sperr WR, Schwartz LB, et al. Diagnosis and classification of mast cell proliferative disorders: delineation from immunologic diseases and non-mast cell hematopoietic neoplasms. *J Allergy Clin Immunol.* 2004;114(1):3-11.
2. Horny HP, Sotlar K, Valent P. Mastocytosis: state of the art. *Pathobiology.* 2007;74(2):121-32.
3. Horny HP,Valent P. Histopathological and immunohistochemical aspects of mastocytosis. *Int Arch Allergy Immunol.* 2002;127(2):115-7.
4. Swerdlow SH, Campo E, Harris NL, Jaffe ES, Pileri SA, Stein H, Thiele J, et al. WHO Classification of Tumours of Haematopoietic and Lymphoid Tissues, 4th edition. Lyon, USA: International Agency for Research on Cancer Press; 2008.
5. Valent P, Horny HP, Escribano L, et al. Diagnostic criteria and classification of mastocytosis: a consensus proposal. *Leuk Res.* 2001;25(7):603-25.
6. Wolff K, Komar M, Petzelbauer P. Clinical and histopathological aspects of cutaneous mastocytosis. *Leuk Res.* 2001;25(7):519-28.
7. Sperr WR, Horny HP, Lechner K, et al. Clinical and biologic diversity of leukemias occurring in patients with mastocytosis. *Leuk Lymphoma.* 2000;37(5-6):473-86.
8. Klion AD, Noel P, Akin C, et al. Elevated serum tryptase levels identify a subset of patients with a myeloproliferative variant of idiopathic hypereosinophilic syndrome associated with tissue fibrosis, poor prognosis, and imatinib responsiveness. *Blood.* 2003;101:4660-6.
9. Tefferi A, Lasho TL, Brockman SR, et al. FIP1L1-PDGFRA and c-kit D816V mutation- based clonality studies in systemic mast cell disease associated with eosinophilia. *Haematologica.* 2004;89(7):871-3.
10. Valent P, Spanblöchl E, Sperr WR, et al. Induction of differentiation of human mast cells from bone marrow and peripheral blood mononuclear cells by recombinant human stem cell factor/kit-ligand in long-term culture. *Blood.* 1992;80(9):2237-45.
11. Horan RF, Austen KF. Systemic mastocytosis, retrospective review of decade's of clinical experience at the Brigham and Women's Hospital. *J Invest Dermatol.* 1991;96(3 suppl):5S-13 S.
12. Travis WD, Li CY, Bergstralh EJ, et al. Systemic mast cell disease. Analysis of 58 cases and literature review. *Medicine (Baltimore).* 1988;67(6):345-68.
13. Greenberger PA. Idiopathic anaphylaxis. *Immunol Allergy Clin North Am.* 2007;27(2):273-93.
14. Ditto AM, Harris KE, Krasnick J, et al. Idiopathic anaphylaxis: a series of 335 cases. *Ann Allergy Asthma Immunol.* 1996;77(4):285-91.
15. Sokol H, Georgin-Lavialle S, Grandpeix-Guyodo C, et al. Gastrointestinal involvement and manifestations in systemic mastocytosis. *Inflamm Bowel Dis.* 2010;16(7):1247-53.
16. Jensen RT. Gastrointestinal abnormalities and involvement in systemic mastocytosis. *Hematol Oncol Clin North Am.* 2000;14(3):579-623.

17. Scolapio JS, Wolfe J 3rd, Malavet P, et al. Endoscopic findings in systemic mastocytosis. *Gastrointest Endosc.* 1996;44(5):608-10.
18. Delsignore JL, Dvoretsky PM, Hicks DG, et al. Mastocytosis presenting as a skeletal disorder. *Iowa Orthop J.* 1996;16:126-34.
19. Chines A, Pacifici R, Avioli LV, et al. Systemic mastocytosis presenting as osteoporosis: a clinical and histomorphometric study. *J Clin Endocrinol Metab.* 1991;72(1):140-4.
20. Alfter K, von Kügelgen I, Haenisch B, et al. New aspects of liver abnormalities as part of the systemic mast cell activation syndrome. *Liver Int.* 2009;29(2):181-6.
21. Hermine O, Lortholary O, Leventhal PS, et al. Case-control cohort study of patients' perceptions of disability in mastocytosis. *PLoS One.* 2008;3(5):e2266.
22. Smith JH, Butterfield JH, Pardanani A, et al. Neurologic symptoms and diagnosis in adults with mast cell disease. *Clin Neurol Neurosurg.* 2011;113(7):570-4.
23. Rogers MP, Bloomingdale K, Murawski BJ, et al. Mixed organic brain syndrome as a manifestation of systemic mastocytosis. *Psychosom Med.* 1986;48(6):437-47.
24. Soter NA, Austen KF, Wasserman SI. Oral disodium cromoglycate in the treatment of systemic mastocytosis. *N Engl J Med.* 1979;301(9):465-9.
25. Schwartz LB, Metcalfe DD, Miller JS, et al. Tryptase levels as an indicator of mast cell activation in systemic anaphylaxis and mastocytosis. *N Engl J Med.* 1987;316(26):1622-6.
26. Schwartz LB, Clinical utility of tryptase levels in systemic mastocytosis and associated hematologic disorders. *Leuk Res.* 2001;25(7):553-62.
27. Lawrence JB, Friedman BS, Travis WD, et al. Hematologic manifestation of systemic mast cell disease: a prospective study of laboratory and morphologic features and their relation to prognosis. *Am J Med.* 1991;91(6):612-24.
28. Horny HP, Ruck M, Wehrmann M, et al. Blood findings in generalized mastocytosis: evidence of frequent simultaneous occurrence of myeloproliferative disorders. *Br J Haematol.* 1990;76(2):186-93.
29. Lennert K, Parwaresch MR. Mast cells and mast cell neoplasia: a review. *Histopathology.* 1979;3(5):349-65.
30. Horny HP, Valent P. Diagnosis of mastocytosis: General histopathological aspects, morphological criteria, and immunohistochemical findings. *Leuk Res.* 2001;25(7):543-51.
31. Horny HP, Sillaber C, Menke D, et al. Diagnostic value of immunostaining for tryptase in patients with mastocytosis. *Am J Surg Pathol.* 1998;22(9):1132-40.
32. Hughes DM, Kurtin PJ, Hanson CA, et al. Identification of normal and neoplastic mast cells by immunohistochemical demonstration of tryptase in paraffin sections. *J Surg Pathol.* 1995;1:87-96.
33. Valent P, Ashman LK, Hinterberger W, et al. Mast cell typing: demonstration of a distinct hemopoietic cell type and evidence for immunophenotypic relationship to mononuclear phagocytes. *Blood.* 1989;73(7):1778-85.
34. Escribano L, Diaz-Agustin B, Bellas C, et al. Utility of flow cytometric analysis of mast cells in the diagnosis and classification of adult mastocytosis. *Leuk Res.* 2001;25(7):563-70.
35. Escribano L, Orfao A, Díaz-Agustin B, et al. Indolent systemic mast cell disease in adults: immunophenotypic characterization of bone marrow mast cells and its diagnostic implications. *Blood.* 1998;91(8):2731-6.
36. Horny HP, Ruck MT, Kaiserling E. Spleen findings in generalized mastocytosis. A clinicopathologic study. *Cancer.* 1992;70(2):459-68.
37. Miettinen M, Lasota J. KIT (CD117): A review on expression in normal and neoplastic tissues, and mutations and their clinicopathologic correlation. *Appl Immunohistochem Mol Morphol.* 2005;13(3):205-20.
38. Furitsu T, Tsujimura T, Tono T, et al. Identification of mutations in the coding sequence of the proto-oncogene c-kit in a human mast cell leukemia cell line causing ligand-independent activation of c-kit product. *J Clin Invest.* 1993;92(4):1736-44.

39. Buttner C, Henz BM, Welker P, et al. Identification of activating c-kit mutations in adult-, but not in childhood-onset indolent mastocytosis: A possible explanation for divergent clinical behavior. *J Invest Dermatol.* 1998;111(6):1227-31.
40. Valent P, Spanblöchl E, Sperr WR, et al. Induction of differentiation of human mast cells from bone marrow and peripheral blood mononuclear cells by recombinant human stem cell factor/kit-ligand in long-term culture. *Blood.* 1992;80(9):2237-45.
41. Robyn J, Lemery S, McCoy JP, et al: Multilineage involvement of the fusion gene in patients with FIP1L1/PDGFRA-positive hypereosinophilic syndrome. *Br J Haematol.* 2006; 132(3):286-92.
42. Pardanani A, Ketterling RP, Brockman SR, et al. CHIC2 deletion, a surrogate for FIP1L1-PDGFRA fusion, occurs in systemic mastocytosis associated with eosinophilia and predicts response to imatinib mesylate therapy. *Blood.* 2003;102(9):3093-6.
43. Valent P, Horny HP, Escribano L, et al. Diagnostic criteria and classification of mastocytosis: a consensus proposal. *Leuk Res.* 2001;25(7):603-25.
44. Valent P, Horny HP, Triggiani M, et al. Clinical and laboratory parameters of mast cell activation as basis for the formulation of diagnostic criteria. *Int Arch Allergy Immunol.* 2011;156(2):119-27.
45. Sonneck K, Florian S, Müllauer L, et al. Diagnostic and subdiagnostic accumulation of mast cells in the bone marrow of patients with anaphylaxis: Monoclonal mast cell activation syndrome. *Int Arch Allergy Immunol.* 2007;142(2):158-64.
46. Valent P, Akin C, Escribano L, et al. Standards and standardization in mastocytosis: consensus statement on diagnostics, treatment recommendations and response criteria. *Eur J Clin Invest.* 2007;37(6):435-53.
47. Bendelow J, Apps E, Jones LE, et al. Carcinoid syndrome. Eur J Surg Oncol. 2008;34(3):289-96.
48. Pardanani A. Systemic mastocytosis in adults: 2012 Update on diagnosis, risk stratification, and management. *Am J Hematol.* 2012;87(4):401-11.
49. Marone G, Spadaro G, Granata F, et al. Treatment of mastocytosis: pharmacologic basis and current concepts. *Leuk Res.* 2001;25(7):583-94.
50. Graves L 3rd, Stechschulte DJ, Morris DC, et al. Inhibition of mediator release in systemic mastocytosis is associated with reversal of bone changes. *J Bone Miner Res.* 1990;5(11):1113-9.
51. Horan RF, Scheffer AL, Austen KF. Cromolyn sodium in the management of systemic mastocytosis. *J Allergy Clin Immunol.* 1990;85(5):852-5.
52. Soter NA, Austen KF, Wasserman SI. Oral disodium cromoglycate in the treatment of systemic mastocytosis. *N Engl J Med.* 1979;301(9):465-9.
53. Póvoa P, Ducla-Soares J, Fernandes A, et al. A case of systemic mastocytosis; therapeutic efficacy of ketotifen. *J Intern Med.* 1991;229(5):475-7.
54. Roberts LJ 2nd, Sweetman BJ, Lewis RA, et al. Increased production of prostaglandin D2 in patients with systemic mastocytosis. *N Engl J Med.* 1980;303(24):1400-4.
55. Metcalfe DD. The treatment of mastocytosis: an overview. *J Invest Dermatol.* 1991;96(3 suppl):55S-56S.
56. Weide R, Ehlenz K, Lorenz W, et al. Successful treatment of osteoporosis in systemic mastocytosis with interferon alpha-2b. *Ann Hematol.* 1996;72(1):41-3.
57. Lehmann T, Beyeler C, Lämmle B, et al. Severe osteoporosis due to systemic mast cell disease: successful treatment with interferon alpha-2B. *Br J Rheumatol.* 1996;35(9):898-900.
58. Godt O, Proksch E, Streit V, et al. Short- and long-term effectiveness of oral and bath PUVA therapy in urticaria pigmentosa and systemic mastocytosis. *Dermatology.* 1997;195(1):35-9.
59. Vella-Briffa D, Eady RA, James MP, et al. Photochemotherapy (PUVA) in the treatment of urticaria pigmentosa. *Br J Dermatol.* 1983;109(1):67-75.
60. Kluin-Nelemans HC, Jansen JH, Breukelman H, et al. Response to interferon alpha-2b in a patient with systemic mastocytosis. *N Engl J Med.* 1992;326(9):619-23.
61. Butterfield JH. Response of severe systemic mastocytosis to interferon alpha. *Br J Dermatol.* 1998;138(3):489-95.

62. Kluin-Nelemans HC, Oldhoff JM, Van Doormaal JJ, et al. Cladribine therapy for systemic mastocytosis. *Blood.* 2003;102(13):4270-6.
63. Pardanani A, Elliott M, Reeder T, et al. Imatinib for systemic mast-cell disease. *Lancet.* 2003;362(9383):535-6.
64. Vega-Ruiz A, Cortes JE, Sever M, et al. Phase II study of imatinib mesylate as therapy for patients with systemic mastocytosis. *Leuk Res.* 2009;33(11):1481-4.
65. Ustun C, DeRemer DL, Akin C. Tyrosine kinase inhibitors in the treatment of systemic mastocytosis. *Leuk Res.* 2011;35(9):1143-52.
66. Pardanani A, Tefferi A. Systemic mastocytosis in adults: a review on prognosis and treatment based on 342 Mayo Clinic patients and current literature. *Curr Opin Hematol.* 2010;17(2):125-32.
67. Lim KH, Pardanani A, Butterfield JH, et al. Cytoreductive therapy in 108 adults with systemic mastocytosis: Outcome analysis and response prediction during treatment with interferon-alpha, hydroxyurea, imatinib mesylate or 2-chlorodeoxyadenosine. *Am J Hematol.* 2009;84:790-4.
68. Nakamura R, Chakrabarti S, Akin C, et al. A pilot study of nonmyeloablative allogeneic hematopoietic stem cell transplant for advanced systemic mastocytosis. *Bone Marrow Transplant.* 2006;37(4):353-8.
69. Parker RI. Hematologic aspects of mastocytosis. II. Management of hematologic disorders in association with systemic mast cell disease. *J Invest Dermatol.* 1991;96(3 suppl):53S-54S,60S-65S.
70. Friedman B, Darling G, Norton J, et al. Splenectomy in the management of systemic mast cell disease. *Surgery.* 1990;107(1):94-100.
71. Quintas-Cardama A, Aribi A, Cortes J, et al. Novel approaches in the treatment of systemic mastocytosis. *Cancer.* 2006;107(7):1429-39.
72. Gotlib J, Berube C, Growney JD, et al. Activity of the tyrosine kinase inhibitor PKC412 in a patient with mast cell leukemia with the D816V KIT mutation. *Blood.* 2005;106(8):2865-70.
73. Shah NP, Lee FY, Luo R, et al. Dasatinib (BMS-354825) inhibits KITD816V, an imatinib-resistant activating mutation that triggers neoplastic growth in the majority of patients with systemic mastocytosis. *Blood.* 2006;108(1):286-91.
74. Gleixner KV, Mayerhofer M, Aichberger KJ, et al. PKC412 inhibits in vitro growth of neoplastic human mast cells expressing the D816V-mutated variant of KIT: comparison with AMN107, imatinib, and cladribine (2CdA) and evaluation of cooperative drug effects. *Blood.* 2006;107(2):752-9.

Index

Page numbers followed by *f* refer to figure, *t* refer to table and *b* refer to box.

C

D

E

I

J

K

L

M

N

O

P

R

U

V

W

X